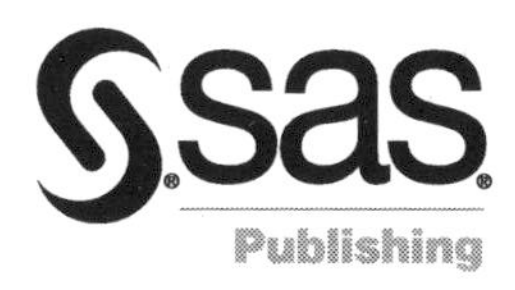

Analysis of Observational Health Care Data Using SAS®

Douglas E. Faries
Andrew C. Leon
Josep Maria Haro
Robert L. Obenchain

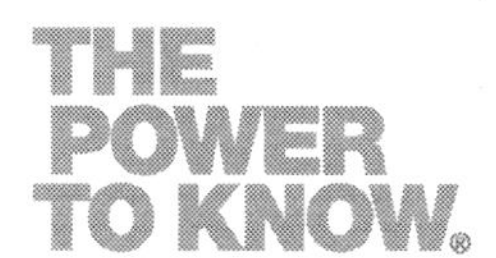

The correct bibliographic citation for this manual is as follows: Faries, Douglas, Andrew C. Leon, Josep Maria Haro, and Robert L. Obenchain. 2010. *Analysis of Observational Health Care Data Using SAS®*. Cary, NC: SAS Institute Inc.

Analysis of Observational Health Care Data Using SAS®

ISBN 978-1-60764-227-5

SAS Institute Inc., SAS Campus Drive, Cary, North Carolina 27513.

1st printing, February 2010

Contents

Part 6 Designing Observational Studies

Preface

Introduction

The use and importance of observational data—such as naturalistic real-world trials, patient registries, and health care claims database analyses—have grown in recent years. Observational research produces real-world data—information on how treatments or policies work in practice—that is critical to consumers interested in actual practice information. Such data are now commonly used by researchers and health care decision-makers to assess treatment strategies and make policy decisions. However, techniques and standards for statistical analysis are less well-developed for observational data compared with randomized clinical trials. Quality analyses of observational data are more challenging due to such issues as selection bias. Literature reviews of recent manuscripts from various types of observational data have criticized the lack of quality, consistency, and transparency of observational data reporting. Low-quality analyses and limited experience with such data by many decision-makers has led to a lack of optimal use and even mistrust of such work. Several research groups, recognizing these analytical and reporting issues, are starting to provide general guidance on improving the quality of such analyses. However, there is still a lack of practical detailed guidance on implementing such methodology.

Our goal for creating this book was to provide a resource that would make high-quality, thorough, transparent analysis of observational data easy to perform. Each chapter includes background information, data examples, SAS code, output, and references to allow for implementation of these methods in accordance with the highest quality manuscripts and guidelines that exist for these topics. As a result, this book should be beneficial to a wide variety of researchers who use observational data (from sources such as prospective and retrospective observational studies, patient registries, survey research, and claims [billing] databases) for analyses and decision-making. Given the breadth of observational research, potential users include statisticians, health outcomes researchers, epidemiologists, medical researchers, health care administrators, statistical programmers, analysts, economists, professors, and graduate students, among others.

Outline of the Book

The main objective of this book is to provide information allowing researchers to perform high-quality analyses of observational data, to present the data in a transparent manner, and to ensure accurate interpretation and appropriate decision-making based on the data. To achieve this, the book includes detailed sections on the general methodological issues of both cross-sectional and longitudinal bias adjustment, followed by shorter sections focused on claims database analyses, economic analyses, and design of observational research.

Chapter 1 provides an overview of the issues involved in analyzing observational data. From a statistical perspective, the most common challenge in observational data analysis is addressing the selection bias (confounding) resulting from a lack of randomization. When the groups of interest are not randomized, they are likely to differ on many key characteristics and might not be comparable. Thus, standard statistical methods will most likely produce associations, not causal inferences. This book includes a detailed section with six chapters covering the core issue of bias adjustment. This section includes the commonly used propensity scoring approaches (applied via regression, stratification, and matching), as well as alternatives of doubly robust estimation, instrumental variables, and newly developed approaches such as local control. In addition, a separate chapter discusses the practical issue of addressing missing covariate data.

Cross-Sectional Selection Bias Adjustment:

- Chapter 2, "Propensity Score Stratification and Regression"
- Chapter 3, "Propensity Score Matching for Estimating Treatment Effects"
- Chapter 4, "Doubly Robust Estimation of Treatment Effects"
- Chapter 5, "Propensity Scoring with Missing Values"
- Chapter 6, "Instrumental Variable Method for Addressing Selection Bias"
- Chapter 7, "Local Control Approach Using JMP"

The analysis of longitudinal naturalistic data includes these challenges along with the potential for patients to switch treatments, time-dependent confounding, and censored records. The next section of the book provides details on performing four different analysis methods designed for longitudinal naturalistic data:

- Chapter 8, "A Two-Stage Longitudinal Propensity Adjustment for Analysis of Observational Data"
- Chapter 9, "Analysis of Longitudinal Observational Data Using Marginal Structural Models"
- Chapter 10, "Structural Nested Models"
- Chapter 11, "Regression Models on Longitudinal Propensity Scores"

Claims database analyses have become a growing area of research because such billing databases provide immediate access to data from thousands of patients. Such databases are being used more frequently to assess questions such as resource utilization, patient outcomes, treatment costs, and safety information that can not be practically addressed in clinical trials. For instance, detecting rare events requires many more patients than are typically included in clinical trials. Also, issues such as drug combinations and patient subsets might be assessed in such data. This book includes a chapter providing general guidance on such analyses as well as a chapter demonstrating a safety analysis from a health care database:

- Chapter 12, "Good Research Practices for the Conduct of Observational Database Studies"
- Chapter 13, "Dose-Response Analyses Using Large Health Care Databases"

With rising medical costs becoming a major issue, another growing area of research with observational data is cost and cost-effectiveness analyses. Clinical trials are typically not the best source of data for assessing real-world costs that health care payers must cover—trials have strict entry criteria, restrictions on co-morbidities, polypharmacy, concomitant medications, required compliance, and mandatory visits and procedures. Thus, observational data are the preferred source for such information. However, proper analysis and presentation of cost data can be difficult, and a recent literature review has raised issues with the lack of consistency of methodology and the quality of reporting of cost analyses.[1]

- Chapter 14, "Cost and Cost-Effectiveness Analysis Using Propensity Score Bin Bootstrapping"
- Chapter 15, "Incremental Net Benefit"
- Chapter 16, "Cost and Cost-Effectiveness Analysis with Censored Data"

---

[1] See Doshi, J.A., H.A. Glick, and D. Polsky 2006. "Analyses of cost data in economic evaluations conducted alongside randomized controlled trials." *Value in Health* 9: 334–340.

While the majority of the material focuses on analytical methods for existing data, researchers often are faced with the challenge of designing observational studies. The last section includes guidance on sample size determination and dealing with broader issues such as measurement and sponsor bias:

- Chapter 17, "Addressing Measurement and Sponsor Biases in Observational Research"
- Chapter 18, "Sample Size Calculation for Observational Studies"

List of Contributors

Aristide Achy-Brou, Johns Hopkins University
Daniel Almirall, University of Michigan
Peter Austin, University of Toronto, Institute for Clinical Evaluative Sciences
Heejung Bang, Weill Medical College of Cornell University
John Brooks, University of Iowa
Maria Chiu, Institute for Clinical Evaluative Sciences
Cynthia Coffman, VA-Durham and Duke University
William Crown, i3 Innovus
Peter Davey, University of Dundee
Marie Davidian, North Carolina State University
Elizabeth DeLong, Duke University
Douglas E. Faries, Lilly USA
Constantine Frangakis, Johns Hopkins University
Michelle Funk, University of North Carolina
Hassan Ghomrawi, Weill Medical College of Cornell University
Ron Goeree, McMaster University
Michael Griswold, Johns Hopkins University
Josep Maria Haro, St. John of God, Barcelona
Don Hedeker, University of Chicago
Dave Hutchins, Advanced PCS Health Systems
Sin-Ho Jung, Duke University
Zbigniew Kadziola, Eli Lilly
Dennis T. Ko, Institute for Clinical Evaluative Sciences
Taiyeong Lee, SAS Institute
Andrew C. Leon, Weill Medical College of Cornell University
R. Scott Leslie, MedImpact Healthcare Systems
Chunshan Li, Weill Medical College of Cornell University
Xiang Ling, Amgen
Ilya Lipkovich, Eli Lilly
Bradley Martin, University of Arkansas Medical School
Brenda Motheral, Care Scientific
Susan A. Murphy, University of Michigan
Robert L. Obenchain, Risk Benefit Statistics
Xiaomei Peng, Lilly USA
Yongming Qu, Eli Lilly
Paul Stang, West Chester University
David Suarez, St. John of God, Barcelona
Jack V. Tu, Institute for Clinical Evaluative Sciences, University of Toronto
Honkun Wang, University of Virginia
Ouhong Wang, Amgen
Chris Weisen, University of North Carolina
Daniel Westreich, University of North Carolina
Andrew Willan, University of Toronto

Will S. Yancy Jr., Duke University
Hongwei Zhao, Texas A&M University

Author Pages

Each SAS Press author has an author page, which contains several features that relate to the author, including a biography; book descriptions for upcoming titles and other titles by the author; contact information; links to sample chapters, and example code and data; events and extras; and more.

You can access the author pages from http://support.sas.com/authors.

For an alphabetical listing of all books for which example code is available, see http://support.sas.com/bookcode. Select a title to display the book's example code.

If you are unable to access the code through the Web site, send e-mail to saspress@sas.com.

Acknowledgments

The authors would like to thank the reviewers who provided multiple quality suggestions to improve this text. In addition, the authors would like to thank Alex Dmitrienko, research advisor at Eli Lilly and Company, for his inspiration to start this work. Special thanks go to George McDaniel, acquisitions editor at SAS Press, for his guidance and hard work in helping us complete this project. Also, we would like to thank the entire SAS Press team who made this possible. These individuals include Kathy Restivo, copy editor; Mary Beth Steinbach, managing editor; Candy Farrell, technical publishing specialist; Patrice Cherry, cover designer; Jennifer Dilley, designer; and Stacey Hamilton and Shelly Goodin, marketing specialists.

Additional Resources

SAS offers a rich variety of resources to help build your SAS skills and explore and apply the full power of SAS software. Whether you are in a professional or academic setting, we have learning products that can help you maximize your investment in SAS.

Bookstore	http://support.sas.com/publishing/
Training	http://support.sas.com/training/
Certification	http://support.sas.com/certify/
Knowledge Base	http://support.sas.com/resources/
Support	http://support.sas.com/techsup/
Learning Center	http://support.sas.com/learn/
Community	http://support.sas.com/community/

Comments or Questions?

If you have comments or questions about this book, contact the authors through SAS as follows:

Mail:

SAS Institute Inc.
SAS Press
Attn: <Author's name>
SAS Campus Drive
Cary, NC 27513

E-mail: saspress@sas.com

Fax: (919) 677-4444

Please include the title of the book in your correspondence.

For a complete list of books available through SAS Press, visit http://support.sas.com/publishing.

SAS Publishing News: Receive up-to-date information about all new SAS publications via e-mail by subscribing to the SAS Publishing News monthly eNewsletter. Visit http://support.sas.com/subscribe.

Part 1

Introduction

Chapter 1

Introduction to Observational Studies

Heejung Bang

1.1 Observational vs. Experimental Studies

When a researcher designs and performs an experimental study, the assignment of exposure (or treatment)* is under the researcher's control and is done randomly. Random assignment uses chance to form treatment groups that are expected to be comparable. Studies without this feature are collectively referred to as *observational* or *non-experimental* studies. In research involving human subjects, experimental studies are typically called *randomized controlled trials* (RCTs).

Whereas subjects in RCTs are assigned to treatment or control in a randomized fashion, in observational studies the subjects assign themselves or are assigned to one of the groups in a non-random manner and the investigators just *observe* what happens. Observational studies are non-interventional; that is, the treatment and care of the patient are not influenced by the study but are conducted as in usual practice. Cochran (1965) defined an observational study as an empirical comparison of control and treated groups in which:

> The objective is to elucidate cause-and-effect relationships . . . [in which it] is not feasible to use controlled experimentation, in the sense of being able to impose the procedures or treatments whose effects it is desired to discover, or to assign subjects at random to different procedures.

The advantages and disadvantages of an observational study compared to an RCT have been well-documented (Concato et al., 2000; Benson and Hartz, 2002; Grimes and Schulz, 2002; Roy-Byrne et al., 2003; Rubin, 2007). The main strength of an RCT is that the average causal effects

* Throughout this chapter, we use the terms *exposure* and *treatment* interchangeably. Treatment can be viewed as a part of exposure, and the effectiveness of treatment is a common research question for both RCTs and observational studies.

can be estimated from a well-designed and well-conducted RCT using standard statistical analyses, where *well* means being sufficiently powered and eliminating or minimizing subject withdrawal, noncompliance, loss to follow-up, differential attrition, unblinding, compensated reactions, and other factors that can cause bias in RCTs (Little and Rubin, 2000; Bang and Davis, 2007; Park et al., 2008). Therefore, randomization itself is not a panacea. Due to randomization, it is hoped that the comparison groups are much alike (or approximately equal on average) in all aspects except for the treatments, where *all* includes both observed and unobserved characteristics. Hence, if there is a difference in the outcomes, it is likely *caused* by the treatment. Indeed, this property makes RCTs the best approach for evaluating the efficacy/effectiveness of treatment, placing it in the highest position within a widely accepted hierarchy of study designs (see Figure 1.1 in Section 1.3). In an RCT, researchers hope to reduce not only bias and any potential confounding but also variability (by having homogeneous samples), with a goal to maximize the treatment effect should one exist.

However, RCTs involve a high level of restrictions and regulations. They typically evaluate the efficacy of treatments in a narrow subset of individuals with the illness in question, and they have carefully planned treatment rules specified in the protocol (e.g., treatment allocation, dosing, compliance, visit structure, procedures, and concomitant treatments). Due to the strict inclusion/exclusion criteria, the generalizability of an RCT can be quite limited. Conversely, by excluding people with specific co-morbidities or concomitant medications, RCTs might fail to identify subjects who, in clinical practice, are found to be at increased risk for certain adverse events (Levi et al., 2008) or even rule out the enrollment of people who could benefit. Most importantly, it is impossible to conduct RCTs to answer many research questions due to infeasibility; permissibility; or ethical, financial, or other practical reasons. For example, researchers cannot randomize people to smoking or gender to study their effects on lung cancer. Can researchers design experimental studies to determine the effects of pollution or global warming on people? The answer is no. Indeed, randomization could be a fear factor to patients (Rimm and Bortin, 1978)!

The fact that observational studies do not use randomization presents analytical challenges. Due to the lack of randomization, the treatment and control groups tend to differ in many ways, because allocation is not under the control of the investigator. It is typically hard or impossible to determine exactly why and how they differ. As a result, standard statistical techniques applied to observational studies may yield biased estimates of true effects. In fact, strong additional assumptions and advanced methods are required to adjust for bias and confounding. In addition, when randomization is not used, an understanding of the scientific context of the study becomes much more important. (Sometimes, observational research is conducted without any plans to compare groups—such as studies to assess usual care treatment patterns, risk factors, and burden of illness.)

On the other hand, observational settings reflect less artificial and more naturalistic circumstances; people's lives and behaviors are not being modified by restrictive rules or specific recommendations, and the natural history of disease occurrence and progression can be better observed. As such, these studies may provide opportunities to evaluate the effectiveness of treatment in people who are more like those who are in need of treatment in the community. Also, observational data are helpful in examining the safety or unintended (particularly, rare or late) effects of treatment. If health care professionals were to wait for RCTs to be designed and conducted, relevant information would not be available for several years. Thus, health care providers and policy makers must act, at least in the near term, on the currently available findings, mostly from observational studies (Ware, 2003). In fact, the growing availability of large amounts of relatively inexpensive data in health care claims databases and electronic medical records, compared to prospective RCTs, will result in an increased use of observational data in medical decision-making.

Here, it is worthwhile to mention landmark observational studies that have changed our lives in various ways. Among others, let me introduce two studies: the Framingham Heart Study (FHS) and the Women's Health Initiative (WHI). In 1948, the FHS embarked on an ambitious project in health research, under the direction of the National Institutes of Health (NIH). At the time, little was known about the general causes of heart disease and stroke, but the death rates for cardiovascular disease had been increasing steadily since the beginning of the century and had become an American epidemic. Fifty years of data collected from this epidemiologic study identified major risk factors associated with cardiovascular disease, paved the way for researchers to undertake singular clinical trials based on Framingham findings, created a revolution in preventive medicine, and changed the way the medical community and general public view the genesis of disease (http://www.framinghamheartstudy.org/). In 1991, the NIH also established the WHI to address the most common causes of death, disability, and impaired quality of life in postmenopausal women, including cardiovascular disease, cancer, and osteoporosis. The WHI was a 15-year endeavor and one of the largest US prevention studies of its kind. The three major components of the WHI were:

1. an RCT of promising but unproven approaches to prevention
2. an observational study to identify predictors of disease
3. a community prevention study to investigate healthful behaviors

where the observational study provided information that complemented the findings obtained in the RCT (http://www.nhlbi.nih.gov/whi/).

1.2 Issues in Observational Studies

1.2.1 Association vs. Causation

To study whether an exposure causes an outcome, we first must understand the difference between *association* or *correlation* (meaning that one is found more commonly in the presence of the other) vs. *causation*. It is not infrequent for observational data to produce counterintuitive (i.e., contrary to what we expect or to the way that mechanisms are thought to work) or inconsistent findings concerning treatment-outcome relationships. Typical scenarios with nonrandomized treatment are provided here: Sicker people tend to take more medications at higher doses (selection by indication). As a result, high-dose medication takers may show poorer outcomes in a naive analysis. Similarly, some treatments, supplements, or diets are thought to be beneficial, even if this is not so. Why? It is possibly because persons who take these are different from those who do not in other ways (such as by being economically better off or doing additional things for their health). Another example is that people tend to have low expectations of inexpensive products (or services), so these products may provide higher satisfaction than expensive ones. One could naively conclude that the less expensive product results in greater satisfaction. In circumstances of this kind, it can be inappropriate to interpret a crude association as a causal relationship because such findings are likely simple associations. If RCTs were conducted for the same comparisons, it is possible to reach reversed results.

Why is *cause* considered so important? Rose (1985) points out that if causes can be removed, susceptibility ceases to matter. Neither associates nor correlates have this power. A treatment is said to have a true causal effect if the values that would have been observed under all possible assignments of treatments, including treatments that had not been given to experimental units (i.e., contrary to the fact or *counterfactual*), differ; see Rubin (1978), Maldonado and Greenland (2002), and Höfler (2005). In research, counterfactual causality is the basis for the use of control groups (Rychetnik et al., 2004).

The idea of a counterfactual causal effect originated with the 18th century philosopher David Hume, who stated that "we may define a cause to be an object followed by another . . . where, if the first object had not been, the second never had existed." A perhaps even more profound quote from Hume might be that "all arguments concerning existence are founded on the relation of cause and effect." The counterfactual concept of causation and the role of randomization were introduced to statistics by Neyman (1923) and Fisher (1926).

Let me illustrate basic concepts by formulating a simple setting for an RCT with a binary treatment and a continuous outcome (e.g., blood pressure or cholesterol) using counterfactuals. Let Z denote a treatment indicator, equal to 1 if an active treatment is assigned and 0 if a control treatment or placebo is assigned. We suppose that, at each treatment level Z, there exists a counterfactual outcome $Y(Z)$ for a subject. Here, $Y(1)$ and $Y(0)$ are never observed simultaneously because it is impossible to both treat and not treat a single individual at the same time so that treatment effects cannot be calculated for individual subjects. One assignment of treatments is chosen and only the value under that assignment, either $Y(1)$ or $Y(0)$, is observed. A treatment effect on a single subject is *conceptually well defined* as the unobservable quantity, $Y(1)–Y(0) = \tau$. (More realistically, an alternative stochastic view is more viable; the unknown true treatment effect can be defined as $E\{Y(1)\}-E\{Y(0)\} \equiv \mu_1 - \mu_0 = \tau$, where E denotes expectation.) If τ is nonzero, the treatment would then have a causal effect on the outcome. In addition, it can be assumed that there is a counterfactual (say, binary) dose at each treatment level, $D(Z)$. In reality, however, we are only able to see $d=Z*D(1)+(1-Z)*D(0)$ and $y=d*Y(1)+(1-d)*Y(0)$. See Bang and Davis (2007) for details on construction of different treatment effect estimators using the observables.

Confusion between causation and association is one of the biggest problems in most health-related reports, especially sensational findings covered by the news media and major controversies within scientific communities. The word *cause* is severely abused, misused, or misunderstood (Meister, 2007). To determine whether the association between a factor and an outcome may be causal, Hill (1965) proposed the following set of considerations:

- Strength
- Consistency
- Specificity
- Temporality
- Biological gradient
- Plausibility
- Coherence
- Experiment
- Analogy

Although these considerations, frequently called *causal criteria* mistakenly (Phillips and Goodman, 2004), have had enormous influence on epidemiologic thinking, Hill expressed his ambivalence about their usefulness by saying, "None of my nine viewpoints can bring indisputable evidence for or against the cause-and-effect hypothesis, and none can be required as a *sine qua non.*" Actually, *temporality* (i.e., the cause must precede the effect) is a *sine qua non* for causality, whereas the other conditions are neither necessary nor sufficient for determining whether an observed association is causal (Rothman and Greenland, 1998). Rothman and Greenland (2005) concluded that there are no causal criteria in epidemiology by saying that "[c]ausal inference in epidemiology is better viewed as an exercise in measurement of an effect rather than as a criterion-guided process for deciding whether an effect is present or not."

1.2.2 Bias and Confounding

Selection bias and *confounding* are the two major threats to the internal validity of observational studies. Actually, they are closely related concepts because confounding can cause selection bias. These possibilities should always be checked or considered as possible alternative explanations for the observed results.

Selection bias occurs when there is a different probability of a unit or individual being chosen to participate in a study or assigned to a treatment condition, and the characteristics of that individual are confounded with treatment outcomes. If selection biases are not taken into account, then any conclusions drawn may be wrong and certainly are not generalizable. Selection biases or pre-treatment differences are of two distinct types: those that have been accurately measured (measured confounders), called *overt biases*, and those that have not been measured (unmeasured confounders) but are suspected to exist, called *hidden biases*. Removing overt biases and addressing uncertainty about hidden biases are central methodological issues in observational studies. Overt biases can be removed by statistical techniques, while hidden biases can be addressed partly in study design; see Rosenbaum (2005) for more details. (The pitfalls of non-random or defective random samples and lack of control groups are well-documented in elementary texts [Aliaga and Gunderson, 1998].)

Confounding/confounder can lead to the erroneous conclusion that an association between the dependent variable (or outcome) and the independent variable (e.g., treatment/exposure) is causal. If the parameter of interest (e.g., risk ratio or difference or odds ratio) cannot be validly estimated without data on another variable, then that variable is a confounder. Unfortunately, but understandably, confounding and confounder are difficult concepts. Various definitions for them exist, but most definitions available in the literature are descriptions of properties. Indeed, their definitions seem to evolve. See Miettinen and Cook (1981), Robins and Morgenstern (1987), and Greenland et al. (1999) for more rigorous and deeper discussions on this issue.

Let me give some real-life examples of confounding/confounders. Alcohol drinkers die at higher rates from lung cancer than non-drinkers. Drinking causes liver cancer, but it is not known to cause lung cancer. What explains this association? The confounder may be smoking: drinkers smoke more, and smoking causes lung cancer. In order to elucidate the possible effect of drinking on lung cancer, we can compare drinkers and non-drinkers within levels of smoking. In another example, gray hair appears to be a risk factor for heart disease. If age is unknown, a gray-haired man is more likely to have a heart attack than a man without gray hair. However, if two men are the same age, but only one has gray hair, it is not likely that the gray-haired man will be at elevated risk. The initial association is spurious because gray hair, a proxy for age, is no longer an independent risk factor when age is added to the model (Brotman et al., 2005; Gotto, 2007). In a third example, there appeared to be a positive correlation between population growth and the number of storks in Oldenberg, Germany, in 1930–1939, but we would find it hard to believe that shooting storks would decrease the birth rate of humans! In this case, the third variable might be time (Box et al., 1978; Davidian, 1998).

In general, confounding is a complex process in which multiple (known and unknown) factors affect the outcome, so standard statistical approaches, such as those used in regression or stratification, may not fully resolve this issue. Moreover, strictly speaking, there is no statistical test for confounding, although many believe there is. Pearl (2000) argues that confounding variables cannot be defined in terms of statistical notions alone; some causal assumptions are necessary.

1.2.3 Replicability and Type I Error

Replicability (i.e., Hill's *consistency*) is a very important scientific concept for RCTs as well as for observational studies; essentially it means that the findings of a particular study are expected to occur again if the same hypothesis was tested in another study. Chance alone cannot explain this expectation. *Association* is a powerful word and should be reserved for something more than a change that could be accounted for by chance (Dunn, 2004). A scientific finding that cannot be replicated should be immediately discredited. The importance of replicability can never be overemphasized. Results that are *significant* or *predictive* without being replicable will misinform the public, lead to needless expenditures of time and resources, and provide no service to the investigators or to science.

The literature on the replicability of observational studies is mixed (Benson and Hartz, 2002; Ioannidis, 2005). Austin et al. (2006) demonstrated that the search for significance takes the investigator into uncharted territory. Indeed, modeling, the search for significance, the preference for novelty, ignoring multiple testing, confusion between association and causation, and lack of interest in assumptions—these norms generate a flood of nonreproducible results (Freedman, 2008; Breslow, 2003). Given that we currently have too many research findings, often with low credibility, replication and rigorous evaluation become as important as, or more important than, discovery (Ioannidis, 2006). A prudent motto for health care researchers who want to establish themselves as experts in observational studies appears to be replicate or perish or validate or perish, rather than publish or perish.

While some analyses of observational data are specified *a priori*, others need to be developed on a *post hoc* basis—that is, during the actual data analysis (Gelman and Hill, 2006). No analysis is truly prospective if it is retrospectively constructed in light of the data. Findings based on the primary hypotheses are much stronger than those emerging from secondary analyses or discovered through *post hoc* analyses, because the universe of possible secondary analyses is so large. There are an exceedingly large number of associated and correlated factors, compared with true causes. Post hoc arguments about biological plausibility must be viewed with some skepticism, since the human imagination seems capable of developing a rationale for most findings, however unanticipated (Ware, 2003).

Because even the most carefully designed observational study could have weaknesses and ambiguities, replication is necessary. When attempting to replicate findings, one should try to estimate actual treatment effects without repeating biases that might have affected the original study (Rosenbaum, 2005). Lindsay and Ehrenberg (1993) argue that "repetitions need not and should not be mere repetitions." Rather, they state that repetitions "can be designed to extend the scope of previous results, so as to lead to more powerful empirical generalizations." The strength of evidence comes from the fact that the same result is obtained despite the differences in conditions. These authors suggest some strategies for the design of replicated studies.

Throughout this chapter, I emphasize the importance of cause. However, a different perspective on cause would be useful to readers. Taleb (2001) and Lund (2007) argue that society needs to be more cognizant of randomness. Society wants to identify a cause for every occurring event. Is an extra hurricane or two this year really due to El Niño and/or global warming? Are the two less murders your city had this year attributable more to the new police patrol car (the newspaper headline) or to less severe domestic disputes (randomness)? Although we seek causes whenever we can, some phenomena may be explained by randomness and/or extreme events with nonzero probabilities.

1.3 Study Design

All science must begin with observation. Science is only concerned with objects or events that are observable, either directly or indirectly. Much epidemiologic, biomedical, economic, and social science research is observational. A lot of what we know—or think we know—comes from observational studies that serve a wide range of purposes, on a continuum from the discovery of new findings to the confirmation or refutation of previous findings (Vandenbroucke et al., 2007; Freedman, 2008). Some studies are basically exploratory and raise interesting hypotheses that tentatively account for the observation, while others pursue clearly defined hypotheses in available data. In yet another type of study, the collection of new data is carefully planned on the basis of an existing hypothesis (von Elm et al., 2007).

Cohort, cross-sectional, and case-control designs (and some hybrid designs such as nested case-control and case-cohort) are the typical designs covering most observational studies, including genetic studies. In *cohort studies*, subjects that have a particular common exposure (the cohort) are identified and outcomes are observed over time. In *case-control designs*, subjects are identified by whether or not they have the outcome of interest. Then a comparison of the groups with respect to exposures or some other attribute is made. In *cross-sectional studies*, the exposure and outcome information is assessed simultaneously at a single point in time. Because these and other observational or epidemiologic study designs are discussed in standard textbooks and numerous papers, they are not reviewed here.

As outlined in Figure 1.1, observational studies generally rank below RCTs in a hierarchy of evidence. However, full consensus has not yet been reached on this hierarchy, in part because an inadequate RCT is not necessarily superior to a well-conducted observational study.

Of particular note, bias and confounding are not affected by sample size. While large sample sizes provide real advantages in the accurate and powerful detection of association, one should not get too excited about their ability to help identify causality. Indeed, with a very large sample size, a small effect estimate can yield a very low *p*-value, making many researchers claim cause and effect. Study design can be much more important than *p*-values in this context. If you hear a news release or read an article claiming that A causes B, remember that the design of the study in question can be much more important than the number of the participants and the magnitude of the association. If the report comes from an analysis of a nonrandomized study, it is wise not to simply accept the finding without scrutiny and to wait for more evidence.

No amount of fancy statistical analysis can help an experiment that was conducted without attention to key issues such as study design, potential sources of variation, and confounding. Also, design and statistical analysis should go hand in hand (Davidian, 1998).

Figure 1.1 Hierarchy of study designs and scientific evidence

Total Evidence	Establish causality
Meta-analysis of RCTs*	↑
RCTs	
Cohort studies	
Case-control studies	
Cross-sectional studies	
Ecologic studies	
Case series and reports	Generate hypotheses

*assuming that publication bias is minimal or absent.

1.4 Methods

1.4.1 Methodological Issues and Considerations

Standard statistical procedures generally lead to satisfactory results when subjects are properly randomized, implying that the treatments and the risk factors are not subject to selection bias and confounding. The goal of the research endeavor in comparative observational studies is unbiased estimation of treatment effects (or bias reduction, when unbiased estimation is unachievable), so that valid inferences can be drawn. The limitations of standard statistical controls in observational studies have been documented (Christenfeld et al., 2004; Petitti and Freedman, 2005; Freedman and Petitti, 2005). Before introducing some novel methods, however, we must say that to the best of our knowledge there is no optimal or universally applicable causal method. (Of particular note, the theme of the 7th International Conference on Health Policy Statistics in 2008, "Striving for Consensus on Methods," was heavily influenced by discussions of competing or discrepant causal methods.)

Moreover, the sort of partial corrections that we often end up getting can be equally misleading because they may represent *advanced statistical modeling*, rather than unquestionable improvements. For example, these corrections can be used to reconfirm the wrong or problematic analysis and thus the false conclusion. To illustrate, if the odds ratio for a treatment is 0.9 in the standard analysis, but it is reduced to 0.5 in the causal analysis, then most researchers would probably conclude that bias has been eliminated or decreased by the causal model and that this new, supposedly correct or improved, analysis has shown the treatment to be beneficial. However, what if the odds ratio is 0.9 in both analyses? Shall we simply blame the method or unmeasured confounders or declare that 0.9 is the true estimate? Interpretation of causal results is not simple at all.

Although using RCTs as the gold standard approach for confirmatory analyses provides the strongest evidence achievable in clinical research, the use of observational studies to replace or supplement RCTs can be useful, if not mandatory, because of the aforementioned limitations inherent in RCTs. Nevertheless, inferring causality from observational studies is conceptually and methodologically difficult or even impossible when participant characteristics known to be relevant to outcomes were not (or could not be) collected or when an understanding of underlying mechanisms is lacking (leading to unmeasured confounders and/or misspecification of statistical models, which can produce biased estimates of effects). It is also important to note that randomization resolves the issues of selection bias and confounding but not of model misspecification.

Because choosing and implementing an appropriate causal inference methodology is not straightforward, many researchers still analyze observed data by relatively simple standard statistical procedures and draw their conclusions from these analyses. It is ideal to analyze RCTs as RCTs and observational studies as observational studies. The analysis of treatment effects in longitudinal observational studies becomes more difficult because of additional complexities due to the dynamic nature of associations among variables (i.e., treatment, confounders, and outcome) over time. Just like real-life stories, observational studies can take on a number of qualitatively and quantitatively different scenarios. In the absence of a uniform analysis solution, each specific scenario requires a tailored approach depending on data structure and availability, treatment operation/mechanism, and assumptions needed. The key components of observational data analyses can be:

- causal knowledge
- identification of the best-suited approach for the given data
- proper adaptation of the approach to the specific situation at hand
- thorough assumption checking, along with a rigorous sensitivity analysis

Paradigmatic shifts must be undertaken in moving from traditional statistical analysis to causal analysis of multivariate data (Pearl, 2000).

Over the last two decades at least, the development of methodologies for establishing causality using observational data has been an active research area in a variety of scientific disciplines, including (bio)statistics, epidemiology, econometrics, and social sciences. By virtue of recent advances in statistical techniques, causal methods for observed data have become more promising than ever before. If causality can be inferred from observational or secondary data analysis, resources can be saved. Today, obtaining consistent or comparable results from RCTs and observational studies is being emphasized. This combination may lead to definite conclusions about treatment effectiveness.

1.4.2 Statistical Methods

In many applications, the following rules are suggested:

- Rule #1: Define your research question. Do not even collect data until the scientific questions are well-formulated!
- Rule #2: Consider the possibility that an RCT or its variant would be more appropriate for your objectives than an observational study, where group randomized trial (Cornfield, 1978; Hannan, 2006), quasi-randomized trial (Shadish et al., 2002) and practical clinical trial (Tunis et al., 2003; MacPherson, 2004) can be an option. In terms of causal inference of treatment/exposure effect, experimentation trumps observation and design trumps analysis (Petitti, 1998; Rubin, 2008).
- Rule #3: When an RCT is not an option and an observational study will be conducted, choose a suitable design and statistical methods that are appropriate for observational research carefully with proper understanding of the scientific context of the study.

Commonly used statistical tools for observational data are summarized here:

Propensity score (PS)

The PS is the conditional probability of receiving the treatment rather than the control, given the observed covariates. This single summary score can be used to control many variables and is often called the *balancing score*. It can be used for stratification (i.e., sub-classification), model-based adjustment, matching, or a combination of these techniques (Rosenbaum and Rubin, 1983).

Instrumental variable (IV)

An IV is a factor that is associated with the exposure but not with the outcome (see Chapter 6). For example, the price of cigarettes can affect the likelihood of smoking in expectant mothers, but there is no reason to believe that it directly affects the child's birthweight (Greenland, 2000; Wunsch, 2007; Moffitt, 2003). Thus, IVs can change an individual's exposure and, through and only through this effect, also the outcome of interest (Wright, 1928; Angrist et al., 1996).

Marginal structural model (MSM) and structured nested model (SNM)

MSMs generate a pseudo-population via inverse treatment probability weighting, so that potential confounders are no longer confounders. This mimics an RCT. MSMs can also be used to estimate the causal effect of a time-dependent exposure in the presence of time-dependent confounders that are themselves affected by previous exposure in longitudinal studies. SNMs are an alternative to MSMs and estimate the parameters through the method of *g*-estimation (Robins, 1999; Robins et al., 2000).

In the following chapters of this book, these and other approaches for analyses of observational data are presented in detail. Specifics on implementing various PS-based adjustments are provided in Chapters 2 through 5. IV analyses are presented in Chapter 6. Longitudinal naturalistic data approaches that address time-dependent confounding and the switching of treatments over time, such as MSM and SNM, are described in Chapters 8 through 11. Each chapter demonstrates how SAS can be utilized to implement common and newly developed methods for addressing the complexities of observational data. SAS was selected as the analysis software tool in this text because it is a commonly used tool for statistical analysis by a wide variety of researchers and has the flexibility to handle the complexity of such methods. While pre-set procedures for many of these statistical methods do not exist, the code presented in each chapter may allow for relatively easy implementation of these approaches.

Both the characterization of and methodology for handling selection bias and confounding can vary substantially by disciplinary tradition. In the social sciences and economics, IV-based approaches dominate. Identifying IVs is a key to success, but it is not always clear how to recognize such variables. In contrast, in public health and medicine (e.g., epidemiology and biostatistics), selection bias is typically viewed in terms of confounders, and prevailing methods are geared toward making proper adjustments via explicit use of observed confounders, as in PS and MSM methods (Hogan and Lancaster, 2004). Statisticians, epidemiologists, and econometricians are often interested in similar topics, but they often use different languages to interpret and discuss their results, which can create a barrier to mutual communication. Some researchers try to assist in bridging this gap by defining key terms in these fields (Imlach Gunasekara et al., 2008).

Recently, some attempts have been made to address specific treatment scenarios such as optimal dynamic or adaptive treatment (Murphy, 2003; Moodie et al., 2007) and nonrandomized concomitant/adjunctive treatment in longitudinal RCTs (Wu et al., 2008). Further research is currently under way.

1.4.3 Importance of Sensitivity Analysis

Even after novel methods are applied, some questions and doubts usually remain: Can we believe causal estimates? How sure are we? Is any hidden bias still unaccounted for? If unobserved confounders had been measured and adjusted for in the analysis, would conclusions about treatment effects have meaningfully changed?

Because causal inference entails making assumptions that are either testable or untestable with observed data, the plausibility and/or verification of assumptions are critical. In practice, we cannot expect any assumptions to hold precisely. *No unmeasured confounders* and *existence and identification of IVs* are extremely strong assumptions. Indeed, the untestable *absence of unmeasured confounders* assumption is what makes economists reluctant to adopt methods based on PS or MSM, causing them to rely instead on IV methods for causal inference in common economic settings. On the other hand, some epidemiologists question whether IV is just an epidemiologist's dream (Hernán and Robins, 2006), and even economists advise caution (Heckman, 1995).

The magnitude of bias depends on the degree of deviation from an assumed model, but the size of the deviation may be addressed in specialized sensitivity analyses. Since the first formal sensitivity analysis to detect hidden bias was published by Cornfield et al. (1959), various methodological strategies have been proposed to appraise sensitivity quantitatively. Individual methods are not discussed here. Particularly, Brumback et al. (2004) illustrated the importance of sensitivity analysis even after applying a state-of-the-art method to the data by Hernán et al. (2002) through the reanalysis of the same data. Their reanalysis was somewhat sensitive to unmeasured confounding, thus providing an alarming message that it is legitimate to reasonably doubt the validity and credibility of any causal estimates. A good attitude for health care researchers would be to avoid reliance on only one approach. While comprehensive sensitivity analyses are not typically performed, they should be a key component of all causal analyses.

Another source of bias is model misspecification. Because causal modeling is vulnerable to more than one type of model misspecification, doubly robust estimation has been suggested. See Chapter 4, Lunceford and Davidian (2004), and Bang and Robins (2005).

1.5 Some Guidelines for Reporting

Reporting is the last step in research. Transparent reporting is the best assurance of scientific quality and is crucial for assessing the validity of studies. It facilitates synthesis of the findings for evidence-based recommendations. Often, the reporting of observational research is not detailed and clear enough to enable evaluation of the strengths and weaknesses of the investigation, including study design, conduct, and analysis. Transparent reporting is particularly critical in observational research due to potential biases, the making of extra assumptions, and the need for sensitivity analyses. Because inadequacies are common, some recommendations and guidelines have been suggested to ensure quality. Researchers may want to familiarize themselves with the following international collaborative initiatives proposed by teams of epidemiologists, statisticians, researchers, and journal editors for the conduct of observational studies and the dissemination of results:

- Transparent Reporting of Evaluations with Nonrandomized Designs (TREND) (http://www.trend-statement.org/)
- STrengthening the Reporting of OBservational studies in Epidemiology (STROBE) (http://www.strobe-statement.org/) (von Elm et al., 2007)
- Good epidemiological practice: proper conduct in epidemiologic research (http://www.ieatemp.com/pdfs/GEPNov07.pdf)

These guidelines may be regarded as the observational study counterparts of the CONsolidated Standards Of Reporting Trials (CONSORT) statement for RCTs (http://www.consort-statement.org/) (Begg et al., 1996; Moher et al., 2001).

Other important guidelines include the following:

- Meta-analysis Of Observational Studies in Epidemiology (MOOSE) (Stroup et al., 2000)
- Guidelines for pharmacoepidemiology evaluation and practices (http://www.pharmacoepi.org/resources/guidelines_08027.cfm)
- Guidelines for pharmacoeconomics (http://www.ispor.org/workpaper/adpanel/index.asp)
- Guidelines for drug, device, and vaccine research (http://www.rcnrx.com/ISPE guidelines_for_good_epidemiology.htm)

Because meta-analyses of observational studies are more prone to publication bias (within or across studies) and other biases than are those involving RCTs, it is particularly important to perform sensitivity analyses (Rosenthal, 1979; Duval and Tweedie, 2000; Copas and Shi, 2000) and to interpret the results appropriately (Shapiro, 2004; Young and Bang, 2004; Phillips, 2004; Fisher et al., 2007). The potential roles of meta-analysis of observational studies in the drug development and regulatory process are also discussed (Berlin and Colditz, 1999; Temple, 1999).

We should remember, however, that all of these statements are general guidelines and do not suggest specific statistical methods for data analysis, perhaps because analyses of observational studies are highly complex, analytic methods are advanced, and/or we still need to strive for consensus on methods. It is hoped that this book will aid in bringing greater understanding and consistent application of appropriate statistical methods for naturalistic data.

Acknowledgments

Support for the author's contribution to this project came from the Weill Cornell Medical College Clinical and Translational Science Award (NIH UL1-RR024996). The author teaches a course titled "Statistical Methods for Observational Data" at Weill Cornell Medical College. The author wants to thank Paula Trushin, Stan Young, Varsha Shah, Yolanda Barron, the editors of this book, and two anonymous reviewers for reading the manuscript and providing valuable comments. Also, the author wants to thank Sander Greenland, Jay Kaufman, and Michael Oakes for intellectual conversations and scholastic advice on various topics in observational studies.

References

Aliaga, M., and B. Gunderson. 1998. *Interactive Statistics*. Upper Saddle River, New Jersey: Prentice Hall.

Angrist, J. D., G. W. Imbens, and D. B. Rubin. 1996. "Identification of causal effects using instrumental variables." *Journal of the American Statistical Association* 91: 444–455.

Austin, P. C., M. M. Mamdani, D. N. Juurlink, and J. E. Hux. 2006. "Testing multiple statistical hypotheses resulted in spurious associations: a study of astrological signs and health." *Journal of Clinical Epidemiology* 59: 964–969.

Bang, H., and C. E. Davis. 2007. "On estimating treatment effects under non-compliance in randomized clinical trials: are intent-to-treat or instrumental variables analyses perfect solutions?" *Statistics in Medicine* 26: 954–964.

Bang, H., and J. M. Robins. 2005. "Doubly robust estimation in missing data and causal inference models." *Biometrics* 61: 962–972.

Begg, C., M. Cho, S. Eastwood, et al. 1996. "Improving the quality of reporting of randomized controlled trials. The CONSORT statement." The *Journal of the American Medical Association* 276 (8): 637–639.

Benson, K., and A. J. Hartz. 2002. "A comparison of observational studies and randomized, controlled trials." *New England Journal of Medicine* 342: 1878–1886.

Berlin, Jesse A., and Graham A. Colditz. 1999. "The role of meta-analysis in the regulatory process for foods, drugs, and devices." The *Journal of the American Medical Association* 281 (9): 830–834.

Box, G. E. P., W. G. Hunter, and J. S. Hunter. 1978. *Statistics for Experimenters: An Introduction to Design, Data Analysis, and Model Building*. New York: John Wiley & Sons, Inc.

Breslow, N. E. 2003. "Are statistical contributions to medicine undervalued?" *Biometrics* 59: 1–8.

Brotman, D. J., E. Walker, M. S. Lauer, and R. G. O'Brien. 2005. "In search of fewer independent risk factors." *Archives of Internal Medicine* 165: 138–145.

Brumback, B.A., M. A. Hernán, S. J. Haneuse, and J. M. Robins. 2004. "Sensitivity analyses for unmeasured confounding assuming a marginal structural model for repeated measures." *Statistics in Medicine* 23: 749–767.

Christenfeld, N. J. S., R. P. Sloan, D. Carroll, and S. Greenland. 2004. "Risk factors, confounding, and the illusion of statistical control." *Psychosomatic Medicine* 66 (6): 868–875.

Cochran, W. G. 1965. "The planning of observational studies of human populations (with discussion)." *Journal of the Royal Statistical Society, Series A (Statistics in Society)* 128: 234–266.

Concato, J., N. Shah, and R. I. Horwitz. 2000. "Randomized, controlled trials, observational studies, and the hierarchy of research designs." The *New England Journal of Medicine* 342: 1887–1892.

Copas, J. B. and J. Q. Shi. 2000. "Metaanalysis, funnel plots and sensitivity analysis." *Biostatistics* 1: 247–262.

Cornfield, J. 1978. "Randomization by group: a formal analysis." *American Journal of Epidemiology* 108: 100–102.

Cornfield, J., W. Haenszel, E. C. Hammond, et al. 1959. "Smoking and lung cancer: recent evidence and a discussion of some questions." *Journal of the National Cancer Institute* 22 (1): 173–203.

Davidian, M. 1998. "ST 501, Experimental Statistics for Biological Sciences I Lecture Notes." Available at http://www4.stat.ncsu.edu/~davidian/511notes.pdf.

Dunn, J. D. December 22, 2004. "EPA junk science on air pollution deaths." Available at http://www.acsh.org/printVersion/hfaf_printNews.asp?newsID=479.

Duval, S. J., and R. L. Tweedie. 2000. "Trim and fill: a simple funnel plot-based method of testing and adjusting for publication bias in meta-analysis." *Biometrics* 56: 455–463.

Fisher, J.C., H. Bang, and S. H. Kapiga. 2007. "The association between HIV infection and alcohol use: a systematic review and meta-analysis of African studies." *Sexually Transmitted Diseases* 34: 856–863.

Fisher, R. A. 1926. "The arrangement of field experiments." *Journal of the Ministry of Agriculture of Great Britain* 33: 503–513.

Freedman, D. A. 2008. "Oasis or mirage?" *Chance* 21 (1): 59–61.

Freedman, D. A., and D. A. Petitti. 2005. "Hormone replacement therapy does not save lives: comments on the women's health initiative." *Biometrics* 61: 918–920.

Funk, M. J., D. Westreich, M. Davidian, and C. Wiesen. 2007. "Introducing a SAS Macro for Doubly Robust Estimation." SAS Global Forum 2007. Paper 189–2007.

Gelman, A., and J. Hill. 2006. *Data Analysis Using Regression and Multilevel/Hierarchical Models*. New York: Cambridge University Press.

Gotto, A. M. 2007. "Role of C-reactive protein in coronary risk reduction: focus on primary prevention." *American Journal of Cardiology* 99: 718–725.

Greenland, S. 2000. "An introduction to instrumental variables for epidemiologists." *International Journal of Epidemiology* 29: 722–729.

Greenland, S., J. M. Robins, and J. Pearl. 1999. "Confounding and collapsibility in causal inference." *Statistical Science* 14 (1): 29–46.

Grimes, D. A., and K. F. Schulz. 2002. "Bias and causal associations in observational research." The *Lancet* 359: 248–252.

Hannan, P. J. 2006. "Experimental social epidemiology: Controlled community trials." In *Methods in Social Epidemiology*, 341–369. Edited by J. M. Oakes and J. S. Kaufman. San Francisco: Jossey-Bass/Wiley.

Heckman, J. J. September 1995. "Instrumental variables: a cautionary tale." NBER Working Paper No. T0185. Available at http://ssrn.com/abstract=225094.

Hernán, M. A., B. A. Brumback, and J. M. Robins. 2002. "Estimating the causal effect of zidovudine on CD4 count with a marginal structural model for repeated measures." *Statistics in Medicine* 21: 1689–1709.

Hernán, M. A., and J. M. Robins. 2006. "Instruments for causal inference: an epidemiologist's dream?" *Epidemiology* 17 (4): 360–372.

Hill, A. B. 1965. "The environment and disease: association or causation?" *Proceedings of the Royal Society of Medicine* 58: 295–300.

Höfler, M. 2005. "The Bradford Hill considerations on causality: a counterfactual perspective." *Emerging Themes in Epidemiology* 2 (11).

Hogan, J. W., and T. Lancaster. 2004. "Instrumental variables and inverse probability weighting for causal inference from longitudinal observational studies." *Statistical Methods in Medical Research* 13: 17–48.

Imlach Gunasekara, F., K. Carter, and T. Blakely. 2008. "Glossary for econometrics and epidemiology." *Journal of Epidemiology & Community Health* 62 (10): 858–861.

Ioannidis, J. P. A. 2005. "Contradicted and initially stronger effects in highly cited clinical research." The *Journal of the American Medical Association* 294: 218–228.

Ioannidis, J. P. A. 2006. "Evolution and translation of research findings: from bench to where?" *PLoS Clinical Trials* 1 (7): e36.

Levi, M., G. K. Hovingh, S. C. Cannegieter, M. Vermeulen, H. R. Büller, and F. R. Rosendaal. 2008. "Bleeding in patients receiving vitamin K antagonists who would have been excluded from trials on which the indication for anticoagulation was based." *Blood* 111 (9): 4471–4476.

Lindsay R.M., and A. S. C. Ehrenberg. 1993. "The design of replicated studies." The *American Statistician* 47: 217–228.

Little, R. J., and D. B. Rubin. 2000. "Causal effects in clinical and epidemiological studies via potential outcomes: concepts and analytical approaches." *Annual Review of Public Health* 21: 121–145.

Lunceford, J. K., and M. Davidian. 2004. "Stratification and weighting via the propensity score in estimation of causal treatment effects: a comparative study." *Statistics in Medicine* 23: 2937–2960.

Lund, R. 2007. "Revenge of the white swan." The *American Statistician* 61: 189–191.

MacPherson, H. 2004. "Pragmatic clinical trials." *Complementary Therapies in Medicine* 12 (2–3): 136–140.

Maldonado, G., and S. Greenland. 2002. "Estimating causal effects." *International Journal of Epidemiology* 31: 422–429.

Meister, K. 2007. "Distinguishing association from causation: a backgrounder for journalists." Available at http://www.acsh.org/publications/pubID.1629/pub_detail.asp.

Miettinen, O. S., and E. F. Cook. 1981. "Confounding: essence and detection." *American Journal of Epidemiology* 114: 593–603.

Moffitt, R. 2003. "Causal analysis in population research: an economist's perspective." *Population and Development Review* 29: 448–458.

Moher, D., K. F. Schulz, and D. Altman. 2001. "The CONSORT statement: revised recommendations for improving the quality of reports of parallel group randomized trials." The *Journal of the American Medical Association* 285 (15): 1987–1991.

Moodie, E. E. M., T. S. Richardson, and D. A. Stephens. 2007. "Demystifying optimal dynamic treatment regimes." *Biometrics* 63: 447–455.

Murphy, S. A. 2003. "Optimal dynamic treatment regimes." *Journal of the Royal Statistical Society, Series B (Statistical Methodology)* 65: 331–366.

Neyman, J. 1923. "On the application of probability theory to agricultural experiments." From *Essay on Principles*. Section 9, translated in *Statistical Science* (1990) 5: 465–480.

Park, J., H. Bang, and I. Cañette. 2008. "Blinding in clinical trials, time to do it better." *Complementary Therapies in Medicine* 16 (3): 121–123.

Pearl, J. 2000. *Causality: Models of Reasoning and Inference*. New York: Cambridge University Press.

Petitti, D. B. 1998. "Hormone replacement therapy and heart disease prevention: experimentation trumps observation." The *Journal of the American Medical Association* 280 (7): 650–652.

Petitti, D. B., and D. A. Freedman. 2005. "Invited commentary: how far can epidemiologists get with statistical adjustment?" *American Journal of Epidemiology* 162: 415–418.

Phillips, C. V. 2004. "Publication bias *in situ*." *BMC Medical Research Methodology* 4: 20.

Phillips, C. V., and K. J. Goodman. 2004. "The missed lessons of Sir Austin Bradford Hill." *Epidemiologic Perspectives and Innovations* 1: 3.

Rimm, A. A., and M. Bortin. 1978. "Clinical trials as a religion." *Biomedicine: The European Journal of Clinical and Biological Research* 28: 60–63.

Robins, J. M. 1999. "Marginal structural models versus structural nested models as tools for causal inference." In *Statistical Models in Epidemiology: The Environment and Clinical Trials*. Edited by M. E. Halloran and D. Berry. *IMA* 116: 95–134. New York: Springer-Verlag.

Robins, J. M., and H. Morgenstern. 1987. "The foundations of confounding in epidemiology." *Computers and Mathematics with Applications* 14: 869–916.

Robins, J. M., M. A. Hernán, and B. Brumback. 2000. "Marginal structural models and causal inference in epidemiology." *Epidemiology* 11: 550–560.

Rose, G. 2001. "Sick individuals and sick populations." *International Journal of Epidemiology* 30: 427–432.

Rosenbaum, P. R. 2005. "Observational Study." In *Encyclopedia of Statistics in Behavioral Science* 3: 1451–1462. Edited by B. S. Everitt and D. C. Howell. Chichester: John Wiley & Sons, Ltd.

Rosenbaum, P. R., and D. B. Rubin. 1983. "The central role of the propensity score in observational studies for causal effects." *Biometrika* 70: 41–55.

Rosenthal, R. 1979. "The file drawer problem and tolerance for null results." *Psychological Bulletin* 86: 638–641.

Rothman, K. J., and S. Greenland. 1998. *Modern Epidemiology*. 2d ed. Philadelphia: Lippencott-Raven.

Rothman, K. J., and S. Greenland. 2005. "Causation and causal inference in epidemiology." *American Journal of Public Health* 95: S144–150.

Roy-Byrne, P. P., C. D. Sherbourne, M. G. Craske, et al. 2003. "Moving treatment research from clinical trials to the real world." *Psychiatric Services* 54 (3): 327–332.

Rubin, D. B. 1978. "Bayesian inference for causal effects: the role of randomization." *Annals of Statistics* 6: 34–58.

Rubin, D. B. 2007. "The design versus the analysis of observational studies for causal effects: parallels with the design of randomized trials." *Statistics in Medicine* 26: 20–36.

Rubin, D. B. 2008. "For objective causal inference, design trumps analysis." *Annals of Applied Statistics* 2: 808–840.

Rychetnik, L., P. Hawe, E. Waters, A. Barratt, and M. Frommer. 2004. "A glossary for evidence based public health." *Journal of Epidemiology and Community Health* 58 (4): 538–545.

Shadish, W. R., T. D. Cook, and D. T. Campbell. 2002. *Experimental and Quasi-Experimental Designs for Generalized Causal Inference*. Boston: Houghton-Mifflin.

Shapiro, S. 2004. "Looking to the 21st century: have we learned from our mistakes, or are we doomed to compound them?" *Pharmacoepidemiology and Drug Safety* 13 (4): 257–265.

Stroup, D. F., J. A. Berlin, S. C. Morton, et al. 2000. "Meta-analysis of observational studies in epidemiology (MOOSE): a proposal for reporting." The *Journal of the American Medical Association* 283: 2008–2012.

Taleb, N. N. 2001. *Fooled by Randomness: The Hidden Role of Chance in Life and in the Markets*. New York: Random House.

Temple, R. 1999. "Meta-analysis and epidemiologic studies in drug development and postmarketing surveillance." The *Journal of the American Medical Association* 281: 841–844.

Tunis, S. R., D. B. Stryer, and C. M. Clancy. 2003. "Practical clinical trials: increasing the value of clinical research for decision making in clinical and health policy." The *Journal of the American Medical Association* 290: 1624–1632.

Vandenbroucke, J. P., E. von Elm, D. G. Altman, P. C. Gøtzsche, C. D. Mulrow, et al. 2007. "Strengthening the reporting of observational studies in epidemiology (STROBE): explanation and elaboration." *PLoS Medicine* 4 (10): e297.

von Elm, E., D. G. Altman, M. Egger, S. J. Pocock, P. C. Gøtzsche, et al. 2007. "The strengthening the reporting of observational studies in epidemiology (STROBE) statement: guidelines for reporting observational studies." *PLoS Medicine* 4 (10): e296.

Ware, J. H. 2003. "The national emphysema treatment trial—how strong is the evidence?" The *New England Journal of Medicine* 348: 2055–2056.

Wright, P. G. 1928. *The Tariff on Animal and Vegetable Oils*. New York: Macmillan.

Wu, C. O., X. Tian, and H. Bang. 2008. "A varying-coefficient model for the evaluation of time-varying concomitant intervention effects in longitudinal studies." *Statistics in Medicine* 27: 3042–3056.

Wunsch, G. 2007. "Confounding and control." *Demographic Research* 16: 97–120.

Young, S. S., H. Bang, and D. Kennedy. 2004. "The file-drawer problem, revisited/response." *Science* 306: 1133–1134.

Part 2

Cross-Sectional Selection Bias Adjustment

balance across covariates between the treatments being compared. Specific methods for assessing the balance produced by propensity adjustment are described in Section 2.5.

Last, sensitivity analyses are critical. Producing causal inferences from observational data requires assumptions beyond those in randomized research (e.g., no unmeasured confounders, positivity), and such assumptions should be examined. For instance, while one cannot ever prove there are no missing confounders, one can consider running an analysis that may relax this assumption, such as an instrumental variable analysis (as described in Chapter 6). However, to obtain unbiased estimates with an instrumental variable, several other strong conditions must hold (Hernán and Robins, 2006b). Another option is quantifying the sensitivity of the results to unmeasured confounding (Schneeweiss, 2006; see also Section 2.6.1). Examination of the propensity distribution for each treatment group can aid in assessing positivity (positive probability for selection of each treatment for any combination of covariates). Sensitivity surrounding the covariate balance within treatment groups can be assessed by using methods such as propensity score matching, which can provide superior balance but with the potential tradeoff of a reduced sample (Austin et al., 2007a).

In summary, a quality propensity score stratification or regression analysis involves more than simply estimating the propensity score and running an adjusted model. Quality analyses include an assessment of the balance produced by the propensity score, assessment of statistical assumptions, sensitivity analyses, and transparency in reporting. Transparency is important as a reader should be able to understand the quality of the analyses that were performed, knowing what decisions were made, when they were made, and why.

2.5 Evaluation of Propensity Scores

In the report of a randomized study, a table comparing the distribution of the most important pretreatment assignment covariates between treatment and control groups is usually shown in order to assess if randomization was effective. Because the objective of propensity scores is to create a quasi-randomized experiment from a non-randomized observational study, a similar approach can be performed to assess if the quasi-randomization was achieved. As discussed in Section 2.3, the key assessment of the success of the propensity score adjustment is demonstrating that the propensity score produced balance between the treatments for comparisons.

There are multiple approaches to assessing the balance produced by a propensity model. Austin and Mamdani (2006) and Austin (2008) provide a nice summary of methods. At a high level the methods include the following:

1. assessment of standardized differences of each covariate between treatment groups
2. assessment of the propensity score distribution
3. comparison of distributions of the covariates between treatments
4. assessment of goodness-of-fit statistics

More specifically, for propensity score stratification analyses, because the treatment comparisons are ultimately made within each propensity score stratum, the focus is on assessing balance within strata. Three common approaches for propensity score stratification balance assessment are the use of two-way ANOVA modeling for each covariate, within-strata standardized differences for each covariate, and within-strata side-by-side box plots of the propensity score and covariate distributions.

Rosenbaum and Rubin (1984) proposed a two-way ANOVA (or logistic regression for binary covariates), with each covariate as the dependent variable and a model including treatment, propensity score strata, and the interaction of treatment and propensity score strata. This approach detects differences in mean covariate values between the treatment groups that are both consistent across strata (significance of the treatment factor) and not consistent (significance of the interaction term). This approach corresponds to standard baseline comparison tables commonly used in randomized controlled trials and is thus readily accepted.

Standardized differences are defined here as the difference in means between the two groups divided by a measure of the standard deviation of the variable. Standardized differences can be computed for both continuous and binary covariates (Austin, 2008). Computation of the standardized differences for all covariates allows for an assessment, on a common scale, of differences in means between treatment groups within each quintile. One can then identify the specific covariates with the largest residual imbalance after propensity adjustment. As a rule of thumb, standardized differences greater than 0.10 indicate an imbalance that might require further investigation (Austin and Mamdani, 2006).

As opposed to standardized differences, which assess differences in means, box plots can be used to investigate differences in the distributions of a covariate or the propensity score between the treatment groups. If balancing is achieved, one would expect that the distributions of propensity scores for treated and control groups within each quintile are similar (Austin and Mamdani, 2006). Also, by investigating the overall distribution of the propensity scores, one can detect if there are different ranges for the two treatment groups that might indicate a violation of the positivity assumption. Recall that positivity (positive probability for either treatment group being selected regardless of the combination of the covariates) is a key assumption for causal inference. If box plots identify nonoverlapping regions (i.e., patients in one group have propensity scores in a given range but patients in the other group do not), this should result in further investigation by the researcher. For instance, sensitivity analyses without patients in nonoverlapping regions should be conducted.

As mentioned previously, these balance diagnostics may suggest the need for modification of the propensity model or other sensitivity analyses. For instance, one can modify the propensity model by adding or deleting covariates, adding interaction terms, or adding nonlinear terms for the continuous covariates.

For propensity score regression analyses, fewer methods have been developed for assessing balance. The assumption for analysis here is that patients in both treatment groups who have the same propensity score will have similar distributions of the covariates. Two approaches have been proposed for propensity regression analyses: weighted conditional standardized differences and quantile regression. The standardized differences approach corresponds to assessments for propensity stratification and matching analyses. Standardized differences are estimated at each value of the propensity score and averaged across the observed distribution of propensity scores. Quantile regression assesses the distribution of the covariates for patients in each treatment group with the same propensity score. We demonstrate here the assessment of the weighted standardized differences—given its similarity to methods used for other propensity based analyses. We also recommend assessing the distribution of propensity scores in this situation as well—to avoid positivity assumption violations. In addition, when propensity score regression is used with propensity score strata as the covariate, the methods for assessing balance in the stratification analysis could be utilized.

Output from Program 2.2

```
                    Response Profile

            Ordered                        Total
              Value          tx        Frequency

                  1          A                96
                  2          _B               96

           Probability modeled is tx='A'.

              The LOGISTIC Procedure

                Odds Ratio Estimates

                                Point          95% Wald
Effect                       Estimate      Confidence Limits

gender 0 vs 1                   1.111        0.528        2.342
spouse Yes vs _No               0.875        0.471        1.623
work   Yes vs _No               1.330        0.719        2.462
age                             0.981        0.960        1.003
phq1                            0.919        0.868        0.973
```

The next step in the analysis is to evaluate the balance produced by our a priori selected propensity model—and to make any adjustments necessary to improve the balance prior to assessing the outcome variable. However, as we are demonstrating here the use of multiple propensity approaches, for simplicity we first present the analysis with our preselected model using each approach. Then we follow with the assessment of the propensity adjustment and sensitivity analyses.

To estimate treatment effect by stratification on propensity score, one can estimate a regression model for treatment effect for each quintile and then pool the five estimates into one. Nevertheless, if the outcome is binary as remission, one can estimate the pooled estimate by using the Mantel-Haenszel approach. PROC FREQ (see Program 2.3) was used to obtain the difference in treatment effect on remission stratified by propensity score.

Two approaches were used to estimate treatment effects by regression adjusting for propensity score. First, a logistic regression model with remission as the dependent variable and treatment and quintiles of propensity score as independent variables was fitted. Second, the same model was fitted but included propensity scores as a continuous covariate, instead of a categorical variable for the propensity score (the quintiles). The two models were fitted by using PROC LOGISTIC (see Program 2.3).

Output from Program 2.3 shows the unadjusted odds ratios (ORs) of treatment effect on remission and the corresponding estimated ORs by using the three different propensity score methods presented. The apparent superiority of treatment A vs. B from the unadjusted analysis disappeared once baseline imbalances were taking into account by the propensity score estimates. The three estimates of treatment effect from the different propensity scores were highly consistent as summarized in Table 2.3.

Table 2.3 Summary of Estimated Odds Ratios

	Odds Ratio	95% CI	*P*-value
Unadjusted	1.89	(1.06, 3.36)	.030
PS Stratified	1.50	(0.82, 2.75)	.178
PS Regression (categorical)	1.54	(0.83, 2.86)	.173
PS Regression (continuous)	1.44	(0.78, 2.65)	.247

The interaction between treatment and propensity score was also assessed in each case. Though there is considerable numeric variation in group differences across strata, these differences were not statistically significant (p-values > 0.10). Kurth and colleagues (2006) provide an example of issues to consider when the treatment effect varies by propensity score.

Program 2.3 Computing Treatment Effects

```
/* This section of code computes 1) the unadjusted treatment effects,
2) the treatment effects by stratifying on propensity scores, 3) the
treatment effects by regression adjusting for quintiles of propensity
scores, and 4) the treatment effects by regression adjusting for
propensity scores as a continuous covariate */

/* unadjusted treatment effects*/
TITLE 'UNADJUSTED ESTIMATE';
PROC LOGISTIC DATA=ADOS3;
CLASS TX;
MODEL  REMISSION = TX;
RUN;

/* treatment effects by stratifying on propensity scores*/
TITLE 'STRATIFYING ON PROPENSITY SCORES ESTIMATE';
PROC FREQ DATA=ADOS3;
TABLE QUINTILES_PS*TX*REMISSION / NOCOL CMH ;
RUN;

/* treatment effects by regression adjusting for quintiles of
propensity scores*/
TITLE 'REGRESSION ADJUSTING FOR QUINTILES OF PROPENSITY SCORES
ESTIMATE';
PROC LOGISTIC DATA=ADOS3;
CLASS TX QUINTILES_PS;
MODEL  REMISSION = TX QUINTILES_PS;
RUN;

/* treatment effects by regression adjusting for propensity score as
a continuous covariate*/
TITLE 'REGRESSION ADJUSTING FOR PROPENSITY SCORES AS A CONTINUOUS
COVARIATE ESTIMATE';
PROC LOGISTIC DATA=ADOS3;
CLASS TX;
MODEL  REMISSION = TX PS;
RUN;
```

Output from Program 2.3

```
                         UNADJUSTED ESTIMATE
                           Response Profile

                    Ordered                          Total
                      Value       remission      Frequency

                          1       Yes                  105
                          2       _No                   87

                 Probability modeled is remission='Yes'.

                    Type 3 Analysis of Effects

                                          Wald
                Effect         DF     Chi-Square     Pr > ChiSq

                tx              1         4.6882         0.0304

                     Odds Ratio Estimates

                              Point          95% Wald
          Effect            Estimate      Confidence Limits

         tx A  vs _B         1.889        1.062        3.359

             STRATIFYING ON PROPENSITY SCORES ESTIMATE
    Cochran-Mantel-Haenszel Statistics (Based on Table Scores)

   Statistic     Alternative Hypothesis    DF        Value       Prob
 ---------------------------------------------------------------------
       1         Nonzero Correlation        1       1.8177     0.1776
       2         Row Mean Scores Differ     1       1.8177     0.1776
       3         General Association        1       1.8177     0.1776

          Estimates of the Common Relative Risk (Row1/Row2)

 Type of Study      Method                 Value      95% Confidence Limits
 ---------------------------------------------------------------------------
 Case-Control       Mantel-Haenszel       1.5036       0.8215        2.7520
   (Odds Ratio)     Logit                 1.5187       0.8063        2.8606

    REGRESSION ADJUSTING FOR QUINTILES OF PROPENSITY SCORES ESTIMATE
                         Response Profile

                  Ordered                          Total
                  Value       remission        Frequency

                      1       Yes                    105
                      2       _No                     87

               Probability modeled is remission='Yes'.

                    Type 3 Analysis of Effects
                                         Wald
           Effect              DF     Chi-Square     Pr > ChiSq

           tx                   1         1.8561         0.1731
           quintiles_ps         4        16.3637         0.0026
```

(continued)

Output from Program 2.3 *(continued)*

```
                    Odds Ratio Estimates
                                 Point              95% Wald
      Effect                      Estimate         Confidence Limits

      tx              A  vs  _B      1.539          0.828          2.863
      quintiles_ps 0 vs 4            0.186          0.067          0.518
      quintiles_ps 1 vs 4            0.198          0.074          0.535
      quintiles_ps 2 vs 4            0.608          0.222          1.667
      quintiles_ps 3 vs 4            0.446          0.166          1.197

REGRESSION ADJUSTING FOR PROPENSITY SCORES AS A CONTINUOUS COVARIATE ESTIMATE
                         Response Profile

                Ordered                              Total
                  Value       remission          Frequency

                      1       Yes                      105
                      2       _No                       87

                Probability modeled is remission='Yes'.

                      Type 3 Analysis of Effects

                                          Wald
                 Effect         DF     Chi-Square      Pr > ChiSq

                 tx              1         1.3428          0.2465
                 ps              1        14.7809          0.0001

                          Odds Ratio Estimates

                                    Point              95% Wald
                 Effect           Estimate         Confidence Limits

                 tx A   vs  _B       1.436         0.779          2.648
                 ps                153.900        11.808       >999.999
```

Prior to analyzing the outcome data, one should evaluate whether balancing the baseline characteristics was achieved by the propensity scores. Program 2.4 displays the SAS code for assessing the quality of the propensity score adjustment for the stratification approach (two-way models, within-quintile strata box plots, and within-quintile strata standardized differences) and for the regression approach (weighted standardized differences).

Macro GEN1 (see Program 2.4) runs the two-way models (Rosenbaum and Rubin, 1984) to assess covariate imbalance after propensity stratification. PROC GENMOD is used for the two-way models because it can handle continuous and binary covariates as outcome measures. The GEN1 macro is run to assess each possible confounder. The summary listing displays the test statistics and p-values for both the treatment effect and the treatment by propensity strata interaction. For comparison, the unadjusted treatment effect is also included. For each covariate, one can see the reduction in imbalance produced by the propensity scoring (smaller test statistics and larger p-values). There was no indication of significant residual imbalance. However, the significance of the covariate differences is a function (among other things) of the sample size—and thus the ability to detect differences in this sample may be limited.

PROC BOXPLOT in Program 2.4 produces box plots of the propensity score distributions for each treatment group within each propensity stratum. The within-strata box plots showed general agreement, with potential exceptions of strata 1 and 5. However, assessment of treatment by strata interaction in the analysis model did not suggest differential results in these strata. The box plot can also be used to assess the distributions of each continuous covariate by treatment group within each propensity score stratum. The box plots of the baseline PHQ1 variable are provided in the output.

Macro GEN2 computes standardized differences for the unadjusted sample (without propensity scoring), averaged across propensity scores (adjusted) and within each propensity score stratum. The standardized differences are output to a data set so that summaries, listings, or box plots of the standardized differences can easily be created. Four of the five unadjusted standardized differences were greater than 0.10, while all of the standardized differences averaged over the strata were small. However, within-propensity score strata demonstrated many standardized differences greater than 0.10. While such differences are not greater than chance (as indicated by the two-way models), this does show the difficulty in producing and assessing balance with relatively small samples within each stratum. Balance in the propensity score does not necessarily mean balance in each individual covariate. Because of this, we examined other propensity models, including interactions as well as term removal. A model with significant two-way interactions and two-way interactions involving the PHQ1 term reduced the standardized differences, though modest imbalances were still noted in strata 1 and 5. Ultimately, variables other than PHQ1 did not appear strongly related to outcome, and the various models did not affect the outcome. One possible sensitivity analysis here would be to consider a propensity score matching analysis in order to obtain greater balance (see Chapter 3).

Macro GEN3 computes the weighted standardized differences for assessing covariate balance in a propensity score regression analysis. Output data sets from PROC GENMOD are used to compute the standardized differences and the MEANS procedure is used to summarize the data set with results from all the covariates. Both age and PHQ1 have standardized differences slightly greater than 0.1, indicating further assessment might be warranted. Adding these variables to the regression model as a sensitivity analysis once again did not result in any differences in the final results (OR=1.47; p=.235).

For this analysis, we assumed that there were no missing data for the covariate values, no dropouts, and no treatment changes (from A to B or from B to A) during the three months of the study. Chapter 5 covers computation of the propensity scores with missing covariate data, and Chapters 8 through 11 discuss methods used to address issues found in longitudinal naturalistic data.

In conclusion, various sensitivity analyses were all supportive of the initial analysis results. Thus, while unadjusted results suggested treatment differences, the propensity adjusted techniques revealed that the differences between treatments A and B on remission were not statistically significant.

Program 2.4 Evaluating Balance Produced by Propensity Score

```
/* This section of code evaluates the balance produced by the
propensity score by 1) summarizing the distribution of the propensity
scores via box plots, 2) running two-way models to compare the
balance of covariates before and after adjustment, and 3) computing
standardized treatment differences for each covariate before and
after adjustment.   */

/*1.  assessing balance between covariates by treatment and quintiles
of propensity scores by box plots*/
```

```
PROC FORMAT;
     VALUE BPF    1 = 'Q1-A'
                  2 = 'Q1-B'
                  3 = 'Q2-A'
                  4 = 'Q2-B'
                  5 = 'Q3-A'
                  6 = 'Q3-B'
                  7 = 'Q4-A'
                  8 = 'Q4-B'
                  9 = 'Q5-A'
                 10 = 'Q5-B';
RUN;

DATA ADOS4;
  SET ADOS3;
  LABEL BP='QUINTILE-TREATMENT';
  FORMAT BP BPF.;

  IF TX=1 AND QUINTILES_PS=0 THEN BP=1;
    ELSE IF TX=0 AND QUINTILES_PS=0 THEN BP=2;
    ELSE IF TX=1 AND QUINTILES_PS=1 THEN BP=3;
    ELSE IF TX=0 AND QUINTILES_PS=1 THEN BP=4;
    ELSE IF TX=1 AND QUINTILES_PS=2 THEN BP=5;
    ELSE IF TX=0 AND QUINTILES_PS=2 THEN BP=6;
    ELSE IF TX=1 AND QUINTILES_PS=3 THEN BP=7;
    ELSE IF TX=0 AND QUINTILES_PS=3 THEN BP=8;
    ELSE IF TX=1 AND QUINTILES_PS=4 THEN BP=9;
    ELSE IF TX=0 AND QUINTILES_PS=4 THEN BP=10;
RUN;

PROC SORT DATA=ADOS4;
BY BP;
RUN;

TITLE 'Distribution of propensity scores by quintiles and treatment';
PROC BOXPLOT DATA=ADOS4;
  PLOT PS*BP;
RUN;
TITLE 'Distribution of Baseline PHQ1 by quintiles and treatment';
PROC BOXPLOT DATA=ADOS4;
  PLOT PHQ1*BP;
RUN;

*********************************************************;
* MACRO GEN1 assesses balance produced by a propensity    *;
* stratification adjustment via a two-way model approach  *;
* (Rosenbaum and Rubin, 1984). A data set with the test   *;
* statistics and p-values for the treatment effect and the*;
*  treatment by ps strata is produced.                    *;
* INPUT VARIABLES:                                        *;
*    VAR - covariate to be evaluated                      *;
*    DST - NOR for normal, BIN for binary variables       *;
*    LNK - ID for normal, LOGIT for binary variables      *;
*********************************************************;

%MACRO GEN1(VAR,DST,LNK);
```

```
  * Run main effect and ps-adjusted models using GENMOD,
    output parameter estimates to data sets for compilation*;
 PROC GENMOD DATA = ADOS3 DESCENDING;
   CLASS TX;
   MODEL &VAR = TX / DIST = &DST LINK = &LNK TYPE3;
   ODS OUTPUT TYPE3 = TEST1;
   TITLE2 'TESTING FOR COVARIATE BALANCE: WITHOUT PS';
   TITLE3 "VAR: &VAR"; RUN;

 PROC GENMOD DATA = ADOS3 DESCENDING;
   CLASS TX QUINTILES_PS;
   MODEL &VAR = TX QUINTILES_PS TX*QUINTILES_PS / DIST =
                &DST LINK = &LNK TYPE3;
   LSMEANS TX / DIFF;
   ODS OUTPUT TYPE3 = TEST2;
   ODS OUTPUT LSMEANS = TESTL1;
   TITLE2 'TESTING FOR COVARIATE BALANCE: WITH PS';
   TITLE3 "VAR: &VAR"; RUN;

 DATA TEST1;
   SET TEST1;
   OVAR = "&VAR";
   DUM = 1;
   PVAL_TX_UNADJ = PROBCHISQ;
   TSTAT_TX_UNADJ = CHISQ;
   TSTATDF_TX_UNADJ = DF;
   KEEP DUM OVAR TSTAT_TX_UNADJ TSTATDF_TX_UNADJ PVAL_TX_UNADJ;

 DATA TEST2A;
   SET TEST2;
   IF SOURCE = 'tx';
   OVAR = "&VAR";
   DUM=1;
   PVAL_TX_ADJ = PROBCHISQ;
   TSTAT_TX_ADJ = CHISQ;
   TSTATDF_TX_ADJ = DF;
   KEEP DUM OVAR TSTAT_TX_ADJ TSTATDF_TX_ADJ PVAL_TX_ADJ;
 DATA TEST2B;
   SET TEST2;
   IF SOURCE = 'tx*QUINTILES_PS';
   OVAR = "&VAR";
   DUM=1;
   PVAL_TXPS_ADJ = PROBCHISQ;
   TSTAT_TXPS_ADJ = CHISQ;
   TSTATDF_TXPS_ADJ = DF;
   KEEP DUM OVAR TSTAT_TXPS_ADJ TSTATDF_TXPS_ADJ PVAL_TXPS_ADJ;

  PROC SORT DATA = TEST1; BY DUM; RUN;
  PROC SORT DATA = TEST2A; BY DUM; RUN;
  PROC SORT DATA = TEST2B; BY DUM; RUN;

 DATA BPP_&VAR;
   MERGE TEST1 TEST2A TEST2B;
   BY DUM;

%MEND GEN1;


* Call GEN1 macro to assess balance for each covariate and summarize
  output in single data set*;
  ODS LISTING CLOSE;
```

```
%GEN1(GENDER, BIN, LOGIT); RUN;
%GEN1(SPOUSE, BIN, LOGIT); RUN;
%GEN1(WORK, BIN, LOGIT); RUN;
%GEN1(AGE, NOR, ID); RUN;
%GEN1(PHQ1, NOR, ID); RUN;

 ODS LISTING;

DATA BPP_ALL;
  SET BPP_GENDER BPP_SPOUSE BPP_WORK BPP_AGE BPP_PHQ1;

PROC PRINT DATA = BPP_ALL;
  VAR OVAR TSTAT_TX_UNADJ PVAL_TX_UNADJ TSTAT_TX_ADJ
      PVAL_TX_ADJ PVAL_TXPS_ADJ;
  TITLE 'PROPENSITY STRAT. BALANCE ASSESSMNT: 2-WAY MODELS';
  TITLE2 'TEST STATISTICS (TSTAT) AND PVALUES (PVAL) FOR
         MODELS WITHOUT PROPENSITY';
  TITLE3 'ADJUSTMENT (UANDJ) AND WITH PROPENSITY ADJUSTMENT
         (ADJ)'; RUN;


***********************************************************;
* MACRO STRATA is called by MACRO GEN2 and computes the   *;
* standardized differences for a given subgroup (quintile)*;
* of the data.                                            *;
*   Input Variables:                                      *;
*        DATAIN - analysis data set                       *;
*        DATOUT - output data set containing standardized *;
*                 differences                             *;
*        STRN - strata number                             *;
***********************************************************;

%MACRO STRAT(DATIN,DATOUT,STRN);

  DATA ONE;
    SET &DATIN;
    IF QUINTILES_PS = &STRN;

  DATA ONE_A ONE_B;
    SET ONE;
    IF TX = 1 THEN OUTPUT ONE_A;
    IF TX = 0 THEN OUTPUT ONE_B;

  DATA ONE_A;
    SET ONE_A;
    MN_A_&STRN = MN;
    SD_A_&STRN = SD;
    NUM_A_&STRN = NUM;
    DUMM = 1;
    KEEP MN_A_&STRN SD_A_&STRN NUM_A_&STRN DUMM;

  DATA ONE_B;
    SET ONE_B;
    MN_B_&STRN = MN;
    SD_B_&STRN = SD;
    NUM_B_&STRN = NUM;
    DUMM = 1;
    KEEP MN_B_&STRN SD_B_&STRN NUM_B_&STRN DUMM;
  * This step merges the summary stats for each treatment and
    computes the pooled variances and then the standardized
    difference. For binary data variances a percentage value
    between .05 and .95 is used to avoid infinite values. *;
```

```
 DATA &DATOUT;
   MERGE ONE_A ONE_B;
   BY DUMM;
   MN_DIFF_&STRN = MN_A_&STRN - MN_B_&STRN;
   MN2_A_&STRN = MAX(MN_A_&STRN,.05); MN2_A_&STRN =
     MIN(MN2_A_&STRN,.95);
   MN2_B_&STRN = MAX(MN_B_&STRN,.05); MN2_B_&STRN =
      MIN(MN2_B_&STRN,.95);
   IF &BNRY = 0 THEN SD_DIFF_&STRN = SQRT( 0.5*(
      SD_A_&STRN**2 + SD_B_&STRN**2 ));
   IF &BNRY = 1 THEN SD_DIFF_&STRN = SQRT( (MN2_A_&STRN*(1-
      MN2_A_&STRN) + MN2_B_&STRN*(1-MN2_B_&STRN)) / 2 );
   STDDIFF_&STRN = MN_DIFF_&STRN / SD_DIFF_&STRN;

 %MEND STRAT;


**********************************************************;
* MACRO GEN2 computes the standardized differences for a  *;
*  given covariate within each propensity score strata    *;
*  (by calling the MACRO STRAT), unadjusted in the full   *;
*  sample (without propensity scoring), and averaging     *;
*  across the propensity score strata (adjusted)          *;
* INPUT VARIABLES:                                        *;
*    VAR  - covariate to be evaluated                     *;
*    BNRY - enter 1 for binary covariate, 0 for continuous*;
**********************************************************;

%MACRO GEN2(VAR,BNRY);

* Generate summary statistics for entire sample using PROC SUMMARY
  and then compute the standardized difference for the unadjusted
  full sample      *;

 PROC SUMMARY DATA = ADOS3;
   CLASS TX;
   VAR &VAR;
   OUTPUT OUT=SSTAT MEAN=MN STD=SD N=NUM;

 DATA SSTAT1;
   SET SSTAT;
   IF TX = 1;
   MEAN_A = MN;
   SD_A = SD;
   N_A = NUM;
   DUMM = 1;
 DATA SSTAT2;
   SET SSTAT;
   IF TX = 0;
   MEAN_B = MN;
   SD_B = SD;
   N_B = NUM;
   DUMM = 1;

  PROC SORT DATA = SSTAT1; BY DUMM; RUN;
  PROC SORT DATA = SSTAT2; BY DUMM; RUN;

 DATA SSTATF;
   MERGE SSTAT1 SSTAT2;
   BY DUMM;
   MN_DIFF = MEAN_A - MEAN_B;
   SDP = SQRT( ( (SD_A**2) + (SD_B**2) ) / 2 );
   MEAN_A2 = MAX(MEAN_A,.05); MEAN_A2 = MIN(MEAN_A2,.95);
```

```
    MEAN_B2 = MAX(MEAN_B,.05); MEAN_B2 = MIN(MEAN_B2,.95);
    IF &BNRY = 1 THEN SDP = SQRT( (MEAN_A2*(1-MEAN_A2) +
      MEAN_B2*(1-MEAN_B2)) / 2 );
    STDDIFF_UNADJ = MN_DIFF / SDP;
    OVAR = "&VAR";
    KEEP OVAR DUMM MN_DIFF SDP STDDIFF_UNADJ;

   * Generate summary statistics for each propensity strata
     using PROC SUMMARY and then compute the standardized
     difference for each strata using STRAT macro  *;

  PROC SORT DATA = ADOS3; BY QUINTILES_PS; RUN;

  PROC SUMMARY DATA = ADOS3;
    BY QUINTILES_PS;
    CLASS TX;
    VAR &VAR;
    OUTPUT OUT=PSSTAT MEAN=MN STD=SD N=NUM;

  DATA PSSTAT;
    SET PSSTAT;
    IF TX = ' ' THEN DELETE;

  %STRAT(PSSTAT,SD0,0); RUN;
  %STRAT(PSSTAT,SD1,1); RUN;
  %STRAT(PSSTAT,SD2,2); RUN;
  %STRAT(PSSTAT,SD3,3); RUN;
  %STRAT(PSSTAT,SD4,4); RUN;

  DATA MRG;
    MERGE SD0 SD1 SD2 SD3 SD4;
    BY DUMM;
    ADJ_DIFF = (MN_DIFF_0 + MN_DIFF_1 + MN_DIFF_2 + MN_DIFF_3
      + MN_DIFF_4) / 5;


   * Create final data set with standardized differences from
     unadjusted, adjusted, and within each quintile approach.
     The unadjusted SD is used here rather than a pooled
     within SD across strata to provide a direct comparison
     with the unadjusted standardized difference. *;

  DATA FINAL_&VAR;
    MERGE MRG SSTATF;
    BY DUMM;
    STDDIFF_ADJ = ADJ_DIFF / SDP;
    KEEP OVAR STDDIFF_UNADJ STDDIFF_ADJ  STDDIFF_0 STDDIFF_1
         STDDIFF_2 STDDIFF_3 STDDIFF_4 ;

%MEND GEN2;

  * Compute the standardized difference for each covariate by
    running GEN2 macro and then compile results into a single data
    set for summarizing. *;

%GEN2(GENDER,1); RUN;
%GEN2(SPOUSE,1); RUN;
%GEN2(WORK,1); RUN;
%GEN2(AGE,0); RUN;
%GEN2(PHQ1,0); RUN;
```

```
DATA FINAL;
  SET FINAL_GENDER FINAL_SPOUSE FINAL_WORK FINAL_AGE
      FINAL_PHQ1;

PROC PRINT DATA = FINAL;
  VAR OVAR STDDIFF_UNADJ STDDIFF_ADJ STDDIFF_0 STDDIFF_1
      STDDIFF_2 STDDIFF_3 STDDIFF_4;
  TITLE 'STANDARDIZED DIFFERENCES BEFORE PS ADJUSTMENT
    (STAND DIFF UNADJ), AFTER PS ';
  TITLE2 ' ADJUSTMENT AVERAGING ACROSS STRATA
    (STAND DIFF ADJ), AND WITHIN EACH PS';
  TITLE3 ' QUINTILE (STDDIFF_0 ... STDIFF_4)'; RUN;


*************************************************************;
* MACRO GEN3 assesses the balance produced by a propensity*;
*  scoring for a propensity score regression analysis.     *;
*  Weighted standardized differences (Austin, 2007a) are   *;
*  produced for a given covariate.                         *;
* INPUT VARIABLES:                                         *;
*    DVAR - covariate to be evaluated                      *;
*    BNR - enter 1 for binary variable, 0 for continuous   *;
*    DST - NOR for normal, BIN for binary variables        *;
*    LNK - ID for normal, LOGIT for binary variables       *;
*************************************************************;

%MACRO GEN3(DVAR,BNR,DST,LNK);

* Run the two-way model and output parameter estimates *;

PROC GENMOD DATA = ADOS3;
  CLASS TX;
  MODEL &DVAR = TX PS TX*PS / DIST = &DST LINK = &LNK TYPE3;
  LSMEANS TX / DIFF;
  ODS OUTPUT PARAMETERESTIMATES = TEST11;
  ODS OUTPUT MODELFIT = TEST111;
  TITLE2 'TESTING FOR COVARIATE BALANCE: WITH PS'; RUN;

DATA TRT_EST (KEEP = DUM TRT0_EST) PS_EST (KEEP = DUM
  PS_EST) TRTPS_EST (KEEP = DUM TRT0PS_EST) INTRCPT_EST
  (KEEP = DUM INTRCPT_EST);
  SET TEST11;
  DUM = 1;
  IF PARAMETER = 'tx' AND LEVEL1 = 'A' THEN DO;
    TRT0_EST = ESTIMATE;
   OUTPUT TRT_EST;
  END;
  IF PARAMETER = 'PS' THEN DO;
    PS_EST = ESTIMATE;
   OUTPUT PS_EST;
  END;
  IF PARAMETER = 'PS*tx' AND LEVEL1 = 'A' THEN DO;
    TRT0PS_EST = ESTIMATE;
   OUTPUT TRTPS_EST;
  END;
  IF PARAMETER = 'Intercept' THEN DO;
    INTRCPT_EST = ESTIMATE;
   OUTPUT INTRCPT_EST;
  END;
```

```
DATA TEST111;
  SET TEST111;
  IF CRITERION = 'Deviance';
  SIGHAT = SQRT(VALUEDF);
  DUM = 1;
  KEEP DUM SIGHAT;

DATA EST;
  MERGE TEST111 TRT_EST PS_EST TRTPS_EST INTRCPT_EST;
  DUM = 1;
  KEEP TRT0_EST PS_EST TRT0PS_EST INTRCPT_EST SIGHAT DUM;

 * Merge parameter estimates with analysis data to allow computation
   of predicted values for each patient.   *;

DATA ADOS3;
  SET ADOS3;
  DUM = 1;

PROC SORT DATA = ADOS3; BY DUM; RUN;
PROC SORT DATA = EST; BY DUM; RUN;

DATA ALL;
  MERGE ADOS3 EST;
  BY DUM;
   * For each observation, compute the predicted value assuming each
     treatment group *;
  PRED0 = INTRCPT_EST + TRT0_EST + PS_EST*PS +
          TRT0PS_EST*PS;
  PRED1 = INTRCPT_EST + PS_EST*PS;
      * Compute the standardized difference for continuous and binary
covariates *;
  IF &BNR = 0 THEN DO;
    TRTDIFF = TRT0_EST + TRT0PS_EST*PS;
    STDDIFF = ABS(TRT0_EST + TRT0PS_EST*PS) / SIGHAT;
  END;
  IF &BNR = 1 THEN DO;
    PRED0B = EXP(PRED0) / (1 + EXP(PRED0));
    PRED1B = EXP(PRED1) / (1 + EXP(PRED1));
    TRTDIFF = PRED0B - PRED1B;
    STDDIFF = ABS( TRTDIFF / SQRT( (PRED0B*(1-PRED0B) +
              PRED1B*(1-PRED1B)) / 2  ) );
  END;

DATA OUT_&DVAR;
  SET ALL;
  STDDIFF_&DVAR = STDDIFF;
  KEEP AGE PHQ1 GENDER SPOUSE WORK PS STDDIFF_&DVAR;

%MEND GEN3;


* Call GEN3 macro for each covariate to compute the weighted
  standardized differences and then combine the results into a
  single data set for reporting. *;

ODS LISTING CLOSE;
%GEN3(GENDER, 1, BIN, LOGIT); RUN;
%GEN3(SPOUSE, 1, BIN, LOGIT); RUN;
%GEN3(WORK, 1, BIN, LOGIT); RUN;
%GEN3(AGE, 0, NOR, ID); RUN;
%GEN3(PHQ1, 0, NOR, ID); RUN;
```

```
ODS LISTING;

DATA REGSTD;
  SET OUT_GENDER OUT_SPOUSE OUT_WORK OUT_AGE OUT_PHQ1;

PROC MEANS DATA = REGSTD N MEAN STD MIN MAX;
  VAR STDDIFF_GENDER STDDIFF_SPOUSE STDDIFF_WORK
      STDDIFF_AGE STDDIFF_PHQ1;
  TITLE 'Assessing Propensity Score Balance for PS
     Regression Analyses';
  TITLE2 'Summary of Weighted Standardized Differences for
     all covariates'; RUN;
```

Output from Program 2.4

PROPENSITY STRATIFICATION BALANCE ASSESSMENT: 2-WAY MODELS
TEST STATISTICS (TSTAT) AND PVALUES (PVAL) FOR MODELS WITHOUT PROPENSITY ADJUSTMENT (UANDJ) AND WITH PROPENSITY ADJUSTMENT (ADJ)

Obs	OVAR	TSTAT_ TX_UNADJ	PVAL_TX_ UNADJ	TSTAT_ TX_ADJ	PVAL_TX_ ADJ	PVAL_ TXPS_ADJ
1	GENDER	0.52574	0.46840	0.75414	0.38517	0.43693
2	SPOUSE	0.36448	0.54603	0.12642	0.72217	0.91679
3	WORK	1.83639	0.17537	0.26352	0.60771	0.39002
4	AGE	1.55113	0.21297	0.00735	0.93168	0.55912
5	PHQ1	8.47659	0.00360	0.38192	0.53658	0.38868

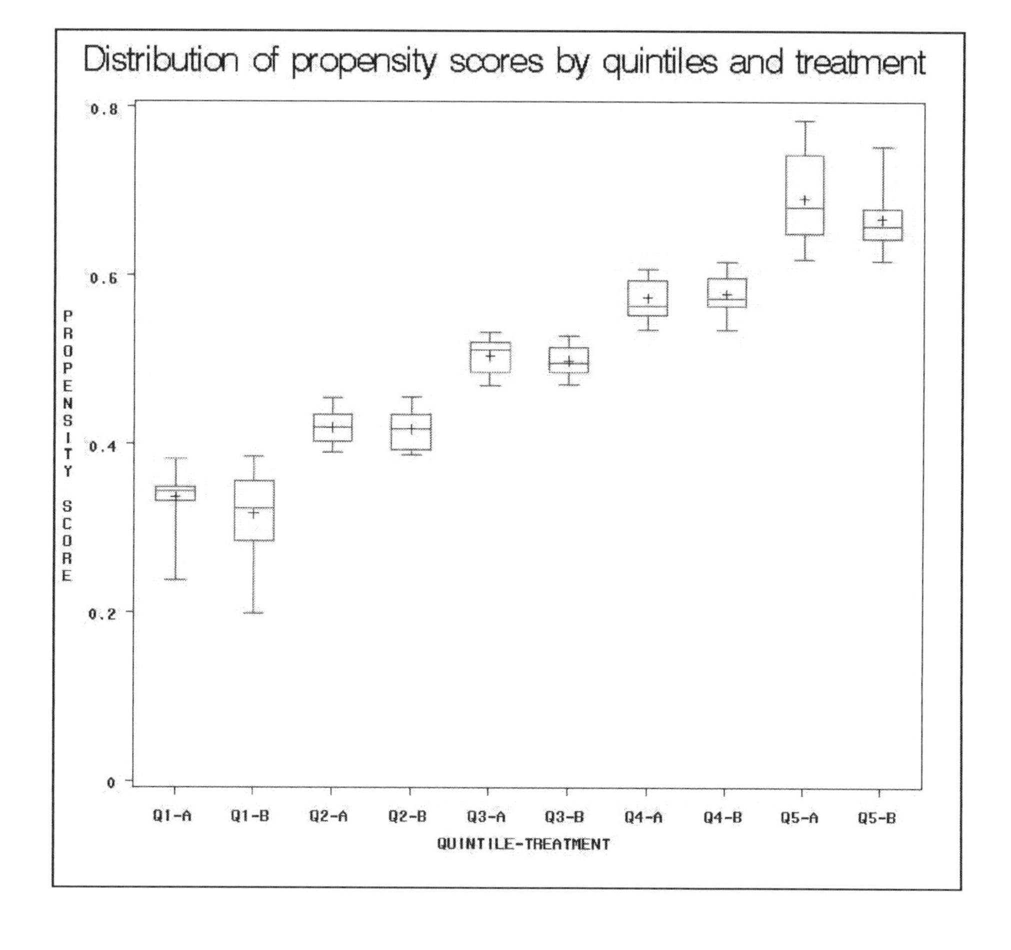

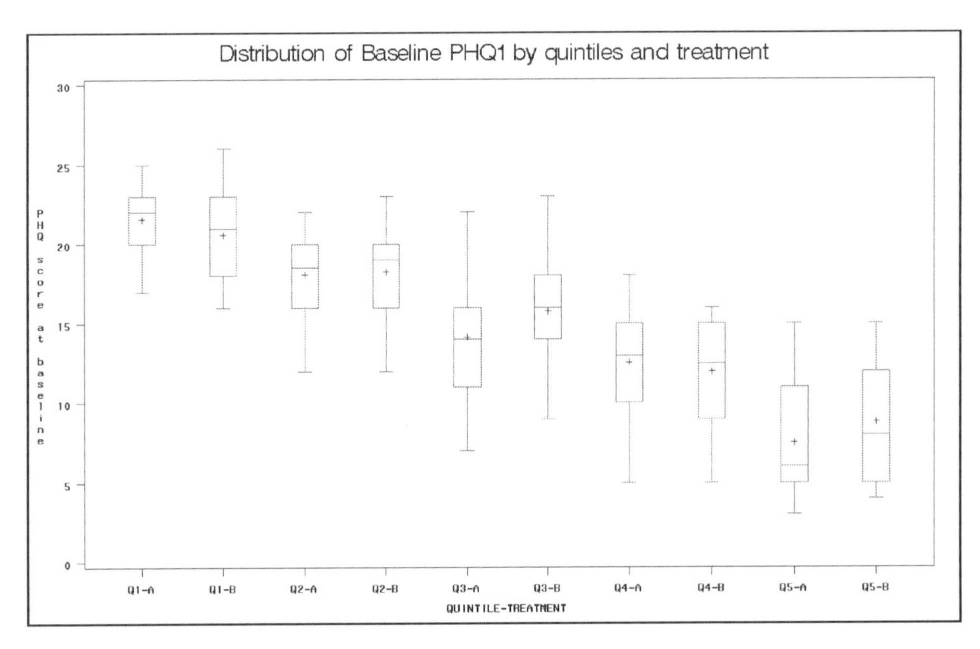

STANDARDIZED DIFFERENCES BEFORE PS ADJUSTMENT (STAND_DIFF_UNADJ), AFTER PS ADJUSTMENT AVERAGING ACROSS STRATA (STAND_DIFF_ADJ), AND WITHIN EACH PS QUINTILE (STDDIFF_0 ... STDIFF_4)

Obs	OVAR	STDDIFF_ UNADJ	STDDIFF_ ADJ	STDDIFF_ 0	STDDIFF_ 1	STDDIFF_ 2	STDDIFF_ 3	STDDIFF_ 4
1	GENDER	-0.10472	-0.027202	-0.27458	0.09386	0.15247	-0.30824	0.34522
2	SPOUSE	-0.08720	-0.038501	-0.12512	-0.23010	0.08454	0.14960	-0.11032
3	WORK	0.19633	0.084570	0.47314	-0.28228	-0.01852	0.43424	-0.17660
4	AGE	-0.17919	-0.012030	-0.41389	-0.11483	0.36707	0.12328	-0.10241
5	PHQ1	-0.42270	-0.055802	0.35965	-0.03898	-0.42395	0.16759	-0.35988

Summary of Weighted Standardized Differences for all covariates

The MEANS Procedure

Variable	N	Mean	Std Dev	Minimum	Maximum
STDDIFF_GENDER	192	0.0176960	0.0129160	0.000075936	0.0660873
STDDIFF_SPOUSE	192	0.0520099	0.0343423	0.000088147	0.1374309
STDDIFF_WORK	192	0.0167626	0.0052507	0.0042665	0.0233658
STDDIFF_AGE	192	0.1976337	0.1329724	0.0018827	0.5687586
STDDIFF_PHQ1	192	0.1702790	0.1142801	0.0039389	0.4802105

2.8 Summary

This chapter presents the stratification and regression methods for conducting a propensity score analysis. We have demonstrated how these analyses are conducted and discussed how to assess the quality of the propensity adjustment, the sensitivity analyses, and the differences from classical regression modeling. Finally, we have illustrated the details of the methods using SAS code applied to data from an observational study. In summary, propensity scores are a valuable approach for estimating the causal effects of exposures in naturalistic data.

Acknowledgments

The authors gratefully acknowledge the help of Josep Maria Haro.

References

Austin P. C., and M. M. Mamdani. 2006. "A comparison of propensity score methods: a case-study estimating the effectiveness of post-AMI statin use." *Statistics in Medicine* 25(12): 2084–106.

Austin P. C., P. Grootendorst, and G. M. Anderson. 2007a. "A comparison of the ability of different propensity score models to balance measured variables between treated and untreated subjects: a Monte Carlo study." *Statistics in Medicine* 26(4): 734–53.

Austin P. C., P. Grootendorst, S. T. Normand, and G. M. Anderson. 2007b. "Conditioning on the propensity score can result in biased estimation of common measures of treatment effect: a Monte Carlo study." *Statistics in Medicine* 26: 754–768.

Austin, P. C. 2008. "Goodness-of-fit diagnostics for the propensity score model when estimating treatment effects using covariate adjustment with the propensity score." *Pharmacoepidemiology and Drug Safety* 17(12): 1202–1217.

Braitman, L. E., and P. R. Rosenbaum. 2002. "Rare outcomes, common treatments: analytic strategies using propensity scores." *Annals of Internal Medicine* 137(8): 693–695.

Brookhart , M. A., S. Schneeweiss, K. J. Rothman, R. J. Glynn, J. Avorn, and T. Stürmer. 2006. "Variable selection for propensity score models." *American Journal of Epidemiology* 163(12): 1149–1156.

Cadarette, S. M., J. N. Katz, M. A. Brookhart, T. Stürmer, M. R. Stedman, and D. H. Solomon. 2008. "Relative effectiveness of osteoporosis drugs for preventing nonvertebral fracture." *Annals of Internal Medicine* 148(9): 637–646.

Cepeda, M. S., R. Boston, J. T. Farrar, and B. L. Strom. 2003. "Comparison of logistic regression versus propensity score when the number of events is low and there are multiple confounders." *American Journal of Epidemiology* 158(3): 280–287.

Cochran, W. G. 1968. "The effectiveness of adjustment by subclassification in removing bias in observational studies." *Biometrics* 24: 295–313.

D'Agostino, Jr., R. B., and R. B. D'Agostino, Sr. 2007. "Estimating treatment effects using observational data." The *Journal of the American Medical Association* 297(3): 314–316.

D'Agostino, R. B. 1998. "Propensity score methods for bias reduction in the comparison of a treatment to a non-randomized control group." *Statistics in Medicine* 17 (19): 2265–2281.

Grimes D. A., and K. F. Schulz. 2002. "An overview of clinical research: the lay of the land." The *Lancet* 359: 57–61.

Haro, J. M., S. Kontodimas, M. A. Negrin, M. D. Ratcliffe, D. Suarez, and F. Windmeijer. 2006. "Methodological aspects in the assessment of treatment effects in observational health outcomes studies." *Applied Health Economics & Health Policy* 5 (1): 11–25.

Hernán, M. A. 2004. "A definition of causal effect for epidemiological research." *Journal of Epidemiology and Community Health* 58 (4): 265–271.

Hernán, M. A., and J. M. Robins. 2006a. "Estimating causal effects from epidemiological data." *Journal of Epidemiology and Community Health* 60 (7): 578–586. (a)

Hernán, M. A., and J. M. Robins. 2006b. "Instruments for causal inference: an epidemiologist's dream?" *Epidemiology* 17(4): 360–372.

Imbens, G. W. 2000. "The role of the propensity score in estimating dose-response functions." *Biometrika* 87 (3): 706–710.

Joffe, M. M., and P. R. Rosenbaum. 1999. "Invited commentary: propensity scores." *American Journal of Epidemiology* 150(4): 327–333.

Kurth, T., A. M. Walker, R. J. Glynn, K. A. Chan, et al., 2006. "Results of multivariable logistic regression, propensity matching, propensity adjustment, and propensity-based weighting under conditions of nonuniform effect." *American Journal of Epidemiology* 163(3): 262–270.

Lunceford, J. K., and M. Davidian. 2004. "Stratification and weighting via the propensity score in estimation of causal treatment effects: a comparative study." *Statistics in Medicine* 23 (19): 2937–2960.

Martens, E.P., W. R. Pestman, A. D. Boer, S. V. Belitser, and O. H. Klungel. 2008. "Systematic differences in treatment effect estimates between propensity score methods and logistic regression." *International Journal of Epidemiology* 37(5): 1142–1147.

McCandless, L. C., P. Gustafson, and A. Levy. 2007. "Bayesian sensitivity analysis for unmeasured confounding in observational studies." *Statistics in Medicine* 26: 2331–2347.

McKee, M., A. Britton, N. Black, K. McPherson, et al. 1999. "Interpreting the evidence: choosing between randomised and non-randomised studies." *British Medical Journal* 319: 312–315.

Rosenbaum, P. R. 2002. *Observational Studies*. New York: Springer-Verlag.

Rosenbaum, P. R., and D. B. Rubin. 1983. "The central role of the propensity score in observational studies for causal effects." *Biometrika* 70 (1): 41–55.

Rosenbaum, P. R., and D. B. Rubin. 1984. "Reducing bias in observational studies using subclassification on the propensity score." *Journal of the American Statistical Association* 79: 516–524.

Rothwell, P. M. 2005. "Testing individuals 1: external validity of randomised controlled trials: "to whom do the results of this trial apply?" The *Lancet* 365(9453): 82–93.

Rubin, D. B. 2007. "The design versus the analysis of observational studies for causal effects: parallels with the design of randomized trials." *Statistics in Medicine* 26: 20–36.

Schneeweiss, S. 2006. "Sensitivity analysis and external adjustment for unmeasured confounders in epidemiologic database studies of therapeutics." *Pharmacoepidemiology and Drug Safety* 15 (5): 291–303.

Senn, S. , E. Graf, and A. Caputo. 2007. "Stratification for the propensity score compared with linear regression techniques to assess the effect of treatment or exposure." *Statistics in Medicine* 26 (30): 5529–5544.

Setoguchi, S., S. Schneeweiss, M. A. Brookhart, R. J. Glynn, and E. F. Cook. 2008. "Evaluating uses of data mining techniques in propensity score estimation: a simulation study." *Pharmacoepidemiology and Drug Safety* 17(6): 546–555.

Shah, B. R., A. Laupacis, J. E. Hux, and P. C. Austin. 2005. "Propensity score methods gave similar results to traditional regression modeling in observational studies: a systematic review." *Journal of Clinical Epidemiology* 58(6): 550–9.

Stürmer, T., M. Joshi, R. J. Glynn, J. Avorn, K. J. Rothman, and S. Schneeweiss. 2006. "A review of the application of propensity score methods yielded increasing use, advantages in specific settings, but not substantially different estimates compared with conventional multivariable methods." *Journal of Clinical Epidemiology* 59 (5): 437.e1–437.e24.

Stürmer, T., S. Schneeweiss, J. Avorn, and R. J. Glynn. 2005. "Adjusting effect estimates for unmeasured confounding with validation data using propensity score calibration." *American Journal of Epidemiology* 162: 279–289.

Weitzen, S. , K. L. Lapane, A. Y. Toledano, A. L. Hume, and V. Mor. 2004. "Principles for modeling propensity scores in medical research: a systematic literature review." *Pharmacoepidemiology and Drug Safety* 13 (12): 841–853.

Weitzen, S., K. L. Lapane, A. Y. Toledano, A. L. Hume, and V. Mor. 2005. "Weaknesses of goodness-of-fit tests for evaluating propensity score models: the case of the omitted confounder." *Pharmacoepidemiology and Drug Safety* 14 (4): 227–238.

Woo, M. J., J. P. Reiter, and A. F. Karr. 2008. "Estimation of propensity scores using generalized additive models." *Statistics in Medicine* 27(19): 3805–3816.

Chapter 3

Propensity Score Matching for Estimating Treatment Effects

Peter C. Austin
Maria Chiu
Dennis T. Ko
Ron Goeree
Jack V. Tu

Abstract

Propensity score matching entails forming matched sets of treated and untreated subjects who have a similar propensity score value. The most common implementation of propensity score matching is 1:1 or pair matching, in which matched pairs of treated and untreated subjects with similar propensity score values are formed. The estimation of the treatment effect is then done in the resultant matched sample. In this chapter, we discuss

- estimating the propensity score
- forming matched sets of subjects
- assessing the similarity of baseline characteristics between treated and untreated subjects in the matched sample
- estimating the effect of treatment on outcomes in the matched sample

3.1 Introduction

The focus of this chapter is propensity score matching. Propensity score matching entails the formation of matched sets of treated and untreated subjects with similar values of the propensity score. Estimation of the effects of treatment on outcomes is done in the matched sample consisting of all propensity score matched sets.

Treatment selection bias arises in observational studies because treatment allocation is not random. Instead, treatment assignment may be influenced by subject and provider characteristics. Therefore, treated subjects can differ systematically from untreated subjects in both observed and unobserved baseline characteristics. Propensity score matching is increasingly being used, particularly in the medical literature, to eliminate confounding due to measured covariates when estimating treatment effects in the presence of treatment selection bias.

This chapter is divided into sections as follows:

- Section 3.2 discusses estimation of the propensity score.
- Section 3.3 discusses methods for forming propensity score matched sets of treated and untreated subjects.
- Section 3.4 reviews methods for assessing the comparability of treated and untreated subjects in the propensity score matched sample.
- Section 3.5 discusses methods for estimating the effect of treatment in the propensity score matched sample.
- Section 3.6 describes sensitivity analyses for studies that employ propensity score matching.
- Section 3.7 compares propensity score matching to other methods of using the propensity score for estimating treatment effects.
- Section 3.8 illustrates the application of propensity score matching using SAS in a large sample of patients undergoing coronary percutaneous intervention (PCI) with either a bare-metal stent (BMS) or a drug-eluting stent (DES).

3.2 Estimating the Propensity Score

The propensity score is the probability of treatment assignment conditional on observed baseline characteristics (Rosenbaum and Rubin, 1983a). The propensity score model is the statistical model that relates measured baseline covariates to the probability of treatment assignment. In medical research, the propensity score is usually estimated using a logistic regression model. Although less commonly encountered, probit regression or classification and regression trees can also be employed for estimating the propensity score. When you are using logistic regression, a dichotomous variable denoting receipt of the treatment is regressed on measured baseline characteristics. Importantly, outcome variables and variables that may be modified by the treatment and that are in the causal pathway are not included in the propensity score model. Only variables that are measured at baseline, prior to exposure, should be considered for inclusion in the propensity score model.

Because the propensity score is defined as a subject's probability of treatment assignment conditional on measured baseline characteristics, it is natural to consider including in the propensity score model only those variables that influence treatment assignment. However, recent research into variable selection for propensity score models suggests that other sets of variables should be considered for inclusion in the propensity score model (Austin et al., 2007a). One can consider four categories of variables for inclusion in the propensity score model:

- Baseline covariates that affect treatment assignment.
- Baseline covariates that affect both treatment assignment and outcome. These variables are the true confounders of the treatment outcome relationship (Rothman and Greenland, 1998).
- Baseline covariates that affect the outcome. These have been referred to as the potential confounders (Austin et al., 2007a).
- All measured baseline variables, regardless of their effect on treatment and outcome.

Including only the true confounders or the potential confounders in the propensity score model has been shown to result in the formation of a larger number of propensity score matched pairs, thus resulting in estimates of treatment effect with greater precision (Austin et al., 2007a). Including only those variables that affect treatment selection or all measured variables (including those that do not affect the outcome) resulted in the formation of fewer propensity score matched pairs. Furthermore, including either the potential or true confounders in the propensity score model did not result in an increase in the residual systematic differences in prognostically important covariates between treated and untreated subjects in the propensity score matched sample compared to including the variables that affect treatment assignment.

An advantage of including all potential confounders in the propensity score model is that the outcome predictors are likely to be relatively consistent across different jurisdictions and regions. Therefore, the existing medical literature may be used to identify baseline characteristics that affect the outcome. In contrast, factors influencing treatment assignment may vary across jurisdictions and regions, since treatment assignment can be influenced by health policy, insurance coverage, local availability, physician and patient preferences, and national regulations, all of which may vary regionally. A disadvantage of including only the potential or true confounders in the propensity score model is that a separate propensity score model may be required for each outcome. In contrast, including only the predictors of treatment assignment in the propensity score model allows one to use the same propensity score model for multiple outcomes.

3.3 Forming Propensity Score Matched Sets

Propensity score matching entails the formation of sets of treated and untreated subjects with similar propensity scores. A matched set is a set of at least one treated subject and at least one untreated subject with similar propensity score values. The most commonly used approach to propensity score matching in the medical literature is to form pairs of treated and untreated subjects with similar propensity scores. This approach is the focus of this section. At the end of this section, we briefly describe alternative approaches for propensity score matching.

Propensity score matching typically involves the formation of pairs of treated and untreated subjects with a similar propensity score. The most commonly used method for the formation of these pairs is *greedy matching* using calipers of a specified width (Rosenbaum, 1995). This method is so named because, for a given treated subject, the closest untreated subject within the specified caliper distance is selected for matching to this treated subject, even if the untreated subject would better have served as a match for a different treated subject.

In this approach, a treated subject is randomly selected, and the untreated subject with the closest propensity score that lies within a fixed distance (the propensity score caliper) of the treated subject's propensity score is selected for matching. If multiple untreated subjects have propensity scores that are equally close to that of the treated subject, then one of these untreated subjects is selected at random. If no untreated subjects have propensity scores that lie within the caliper distance of the treated subject, then that treated subject is not included in the propensity score matched sample. Similarly, unmatched untreated subjects are excluded from the propensity score matched sample.

In matching without replacement, once an untreated subject has been matched to a treated subject, that untreated subject is not available for consideration as a match for subsequent treated subjects. Therefore, when matching without replacement is employed, the final propensity score matched sample consists of unique subjects. Although matching without replacement is almost always used in practice in the medical literature, matching with replacement is also possible. When using matching with replacement, a single untreated subject may be matched to multiple treated subjects. Matching with replacement may allow for a greater use of the available data. However, variance estimation can be more complex due to the inclusion of the same untreated subject in multiple matched pairs (Hill and Reiter, 2006).

An alternative to greedy matching is optimal matching (Rosenbaum, 1995), where matched pairs are formed to minimize the total difference in propensity scores between matched treated and untreated subjects. Optimal matching appears to be rarely used in the medical literature. This may be related either to the computational complexity of this method for large data sets or to the limited awareness of the existence of this method.

Recent systematic reviews have shown that a wide range of calipers have been used for propensity score matching in the medical literature (Austin, 2007a; Austin, 2008; Austin, 2008d). The choice of calipers may affect the variance bias trade off: increasing the width of the caliper can result in the matching of more dissimilar subjects. This can result in greater bias in estimating the treatment effect due to greater systematic differences between treated and untreated subjects in the matched sample. However, it can also result in the formation of a larger number of matched pairs, thus increasing the precision of the estimated treatment effect. Conversely, decreasing the width of the calipers used can result in the matching of more similar subjects, and thus eliminate a greater degree of the bias in the estimated treatment effect. However, it may also result in the formation of fewer matched pairs, thus decreasing the precision of the estimated treatment effect.

In a large number of applied studies, researchers used calipers of a predetermined width that appeared to be independent of the distribution of the propensity score. For instance, researchers have used calipers of width 0.1, 0.05, 0.03, 0.02, 0.01, 0.005, and 0.001 on the probability scale (Austin 2007a; Austin 2008a; Austin 2008b). A limitation to the choice of these calipers is that the caliper width appears to have been selected on an ad hoc basis. They did not appear to have been selected based on the distribution of the estimated propensity scores. An alternative approach that has greater theoretical justification is to match subjects on the logit of the propensity score using a caliper width that is defined as a proportion of the standard deviation of the logit of the propensity score. In this way, one is using the distribution of the propensity score to influence the width of the calipers used for matching. In the medical literature, researchers have used calipers of width 0.6 and 0.2 of the standard deviation of the logit of the propensity score (Austin and Mamdani, 2006; Austin et al., 2007a; Normand et al., 2001). The use of this approach is motivated by a study that examined the reduction in bias when matching on a single normally distributed confounding variable (Cochran and Rubin, 1973). Rosenbaum and Rubin extended this result to matching on the propensity score (1985). They determined the reduction in bias when using matching on the logit of the propensity score using calipers that were defined as a proportion of the standard deviation of the logit of the propensity score. Recent research has found that matching on the logit of the propensity score using calipers of width 0.2 of the standard deviation of the logit of the propensity score resulted in estimates of treatment effect with lower mean squared error compared to other methods that are commonly used in the medical literature (Austin, 2009a).

Until now in this section, we have focused on matching only on the propensity score. One can also require that subjects are matched on both the propensity score and a small number of baseline covariates. This approach can be employed for two reasons. First, you can use this approach if there are factors that are strongly prognostic of the outcome and you want to ensure that these factors are equally balanced between treated and untreated subjects in the propensity score matched sample. The rationale for this approach is similar to that for stratified randomization within randomized controlled trials. Second, you can use this approach if you want to pursue subsequent subgroup analyses (subject to the caveats of the limitations of subgroup analyses) (Freemantle, 2001; Rothwell, 2005; Austin et al., 2006). Conducting subgroup analyses without forcing both subjects within a matched pair to lie within the same subgroup can result in a violation of the matched nature of the propensity score matched sample. By forcing agreement on the subgroup variables, the members of each matched pair will belong to the same subgroup. For instance, if one matched only on the propensity score, then the sex of the subjects would be balanced between treated and untreated subjects in the matched sample. However, individual matched pairs could consist of one male treated subject and one female untreated subject. Examining the effect of treatment in subgroups defined by the sex of the subject would result in these matched pairs being broken, with one subject from the matched pair lying within each subgroup. As a result, the distribution of baseline characteristics between treated and untreated subjects might no longer hold within a given subgroup. An adverse consequence of matching on both the propensity score and a limited number of covariates is that it might result in fewer matched sets being formed compared to matching on the propensity score alone.

While one-to-one matching without replacement is the most commonly implemented method of propensity score matching in the literature, other methods exist. Many-to-one matching, in which each treated subject is matched to multiple untreated subjects, can also be employed. An advantage of this method is that it may enable a greater proportion of the sample to be used. Given a rare exposure, pair matching on the propensity score would result in only a minority of the subjects being included in the matched sample. For instance, if only 10% of the sample were exposed to the treatment, then pair matching would result in at most 20% of the original sample being included in the propensity score matched sample. However, if each treated subject was matched to multiple untreated subjects, a greater proportion of the sample could be included in the matched sample. This may allow for greater precision when estimating treatment effects. For instance, if each untreated subject were matched to up to four untreated subjects, then up to 50% of the original sample could be included in the propensity score matched sample. As another alternative, Hansen (2004) has described full matching, in which all subjects are included. Full matching results in matched sets containing variable numbers of treated and untreated subjects. See Rosenbaum (1995) and Hansen (2004) for further discussion of these methods.

3.4 Assessing Balance in Baseline Characteristics

Rosenbaum and Rubin (1983a) demonstrated that in strata matched on the true propensity score, treatment assignment is independent of measured baseline characteristics. Therefore, the true propensity score is a balancing score: the distribution of measured baseline variables will be similar between treated and untreated subjects within stratum matched on the true propensity score.

In observational studies, the propensity score must be estimated using the observed study data. The test of whether the propensity score model has been adequately specified is an empirical one: whether observed baseline covariates are balanced between treated and untreated subjects in the matched sample. Ho and colleagues (2007) refer to this as the propensity score tautology: "We know we have a consistent estimate of the propensity score when matching on the propensity score balances the raw covariates." In other words, Ho and colleagues are suggesting that one has adequately specified the propensity score model when, after matching on the estimated propensity score, the distribution of measured baseline covariates is similar between treated and untreated subjects. Therefore, the appropriateness of the specification of the propensity score is assessed by examining the degree to which matching on the estimated propensity score has resulted in a matched sample in which the distribution of measured baseline covariates is similar between treated and untreated subjects.

Imai and colleagues (2008) discuss appropriate statistical methods for assessing balance in matched samples. Importantly, they criticize the use of significance testing to assess balance in baseline covariates as being inappropriate for two reasons. First, they suggest that balance is a property of a sample and not of a hypothetical superpopulation about which one wishes to make inferences. Second, significance testing is confounded with sample size. The matched sample will have a smaller sample size than the initial sample. Therefore, the use of significance testing to assess balance may result in misleading conclusions solely due to the decreased statistical power to detect imbalance in baseline covariates. See Hansen (2008) for a dissenting argument against these criticisms of using significance testing to assess balance.

Reflecting the prescription of Imai and colleagues, we describe a variety of sample-specific methods for assessing the comparability of treated and untreated subjects. These methods include standardized differences, side-by-side box plots, quantile-quantile plots, and non-parametric density estimates to compare the distribution of measured baseline covariates between treated and untreated subjects. We then describe sample-specific methods that are inappropriate for assessing the adequacy of the specification of the propensity score model. For a more in-depth discussion of balance diagnostics when propensity score matching is used, see Austin (2009b).

Many researchers have used the standardized difference to assess balance between treated and untreated subjects in propensity score matched samples (Rosenbaum and Rubin, 1985; Normand et al., 2001; Austin and Mamdani, 2006; Austin et al., 2007a). For continuous covariates, the standardized difference is defined as:

$$d = \frac{\left|\bar{x}_{treatment} - \bar{x}_{control}\right|}{\sqrt{\frac{s^2_{treatment} + s^2_{control}}{2}}}$$

where $\bar{x}_{treatment}$ and $\bar{x}_{control}$ denote the sample mean of the covariate in treated and untreated subjects, and $s^2_{treatment}$ and $s^2_{control}$ are the sample standard deviations of the covariate in the treated and untreated subjects, respectively (Flury and Riedwyl, 1986). For dichotomous covariates, the standardized difference is defined as:

$$d = \frac{|\hat{p}_T - \hat{p}_C|}{\sqrt{\frac{\hat{p}_T(1-\hat{p}_T) + \hat{p}_C(1-\hat{p}_C)}{2}}}$$

where $\hat{p}_T$ and $\hat{p}_C$ denote the prevalence of the dichotomous covariate in treated and untreated subjects, respectively. The standardized difference is typically defined without the use of absolute values. The sign of the standardized difference then denotes the direction of the difference in means. Because we are usually not interested in the direction of the difference, we have used the absolute value of the difference in the numerator. The standardized difference is the absolute difference in sample means divided by an estimate of the pooled standard deviation (not the standard error) of the variable (the standardized difference should not be confused with *z*-scores, which contain an estimate of the standard error in the denominator). It represents the difference in means between the two groups in units of standard deviation (Flury and Riedwyl, 1986). The standardized difference does not depend on the unit of measurement nor is it influenced by sample size. Therefore, it can be used to compare the relative balance of variables measured in different units. It can also be used to compare the balance of a given variable in the initial sample with the balance of the same variable in the propensity score matched sample. Unlike significance testing, where the convention that a *p*-value of less than 0.05 denotes statistical significance, no such universally accepted criterion exists for the use of standardized differences. However, some authors have suggested that standardized differences of less than 0.10 (10%) likely denote a negligible imbalance between treated and untreated subjects (Austin and Mamdani, 2006; Austin et al., 2007a; Normand et al., 2001).

The standardized difference allows one to compare the mean of continuous variables between treated and untreated subjects in the propensity score matched sample. However, conditional on the true propensity score, treated and untreated subjects have the same distribution of measured baseline characteristics. Therefore, not only the mean but the distribution of each continuous variable should be similar between treated and untreated subjects in the propensity score matched sample. It has been suggested that one should compare higher order moments and interactions between variables between treated and untreated subjects (Imai et al., 2008; Ho et al., 2007). Rosenbaum and Rubin (1985) state that if the outcome has a nonlinear relationship with a baseline covariate in each of the two exposure groups, then balancing the mean of that covariate between treated and untreated subjects does not necessarily imply that bias due to that covariate has been eliminated. In such a setting, both the mean and the variance of the covariate in each of the two groups are important. Thus, one should assess the comparability of both the mean and the variance of that covariate between treated and untreated subjects. Furthermore, the use of side-by-side box plots and quantile-quantile plots can be used to compare the distribution of continuous baseline covariates between treated and untreated subjects (Imai et al., 2008; Ho et al., 2007; Austin, 2009b).

The balance diagnostics proposed here are appropriate for pair matching on the propensity score. When many-to-one matching on the propensity score is used, these methods must be modified to account for the possible imbalance in the number of subjects within each matched set. Adaptations for some of these balance diagnostics for many-to-one matching have been described elsewhere (Austin, 2008d). In brief, assume that each matched set consists of one treated subject and at least one untreated subject. Then each treated subject is assigned a weight of one, while each untreated subject is assigned a weight that is the reciprocal of the number of untreated subjects in that matched set. These weights are then incorporated when computing sample-specific measures of balance.

These balance diagnostics are used for comparing the distribution of measured baseline covariates between treated and untreated subjects. However, balance diagnostics based on the distribution of the estimated propensity score in treated and untreated subjects may not be appropriate. It has been shown that the distribution of the estimated propensity score can be similar between treated and untreated subjects despite a misspecified propensity score model (Austin, 2009b). Thus, side-by-side box plots or quantile-quantile plots comparing the distribution of the estimated propensity score in treated and untreated subjects may not serve as appropriate diagnostics of whether the propensity score model has been adequately specified. Appropriate balance diagnostics for the estimated propensity score model consist of comparing the distribution of measured baseline covariates between treated and untreated subjects. While many authors report the Receiver Operating Characteristic (ROC) curve area (equivalent to the c-statistic) of the propensity score model, this information provides no information on whether the propensity score model has been adequately specified or whether important confounders have been omitted from the model (Austin et al., 2007a; Weitzen et al., 2005; Austin, 2009b).

In many applications, the initially specified propensity score model may require modification. Rosenbaum and Rubin (1984) describe an iterative approach to specifying the propensity score model. While Rosenbaum and Rubin's method was illustrated in the context of stratification on the quintiles of the propensity score, one can modify their approach to the context of propensity score matching. Using this approach, an initial propensity score model is specified. Treated and untreated subjects are then matched on the estimated propensity score. The balance in baseline variables between treated and untreated subjects in the propensity score matched sample is then assessed. If there are measured baseline variables that are unbalanced between treated and untreated subjects in the matched sample, and these variables are not in the current propensity score model, then the propensity score model can be modified by including them. If continuous variables that are already in the current propensity score model are unbalanced between treated and untreated subjects in the matched sample, then the propensity score model can be modified by adding higher order terms (for example, quadratic or cubic terms) of these continuous variables (alternatively, one could model these variables using cubic splines). If there are variables that are already in the propensity score model and are unbalanced between treated and untreated subjects in the matched sample, then the initial propensity score model can be modified by including interactions between these variables and other variables that are currently in the propensity score model. See Rosenbaum and Rubin (1984) for an application of this iterative approach.

Remember that in randomized controlled trials (RCTs), randomization will, on average, result in both measured and unmeasured baseline variables being balanced between the treatment arms of the study. Propensity score methods only provide the expectation that measured baseline covariates will be balanced between treated and untreated subjects. They make no claim to balance unmeasured covariates between treated and untreated subjects (Austin et al., 2005, 2007a).

3.5 Estimating the Treatment Effect

Once the propensity score has been estimated, a propensity score matched sample has been created, and the balance in measured baseline variables between treated and untreated subjects has been assessed and found to be acceptable, researchers must estimate the effect of the treatment on the outcome and assess its statistical significance.

The propensity score matched sample does not consist of independent observations. Matched treated and untreated subjects have similar propensity scores. Therefore, their observed baseline covariates come from the same distribution. Thus, matched subjects will, on average, be more similar than randomly selected treated and untreated subjects from the matched sample. In the presence of confounding, some of the baseline covariates are related to the outcome. Therefore, matched subjects are, on average, more likely to have similar outcomes than are randomly selected treated and untreated subjects. Thus, outcomes are not independent within matched pairs, and conventional statistical methods that assume independent observations are not appropriate for estimating treatment effects in propensity score matched samples.

For further information, see Austin (2009c), a paper examining variance estimation in propensity score matched samples. It was shown that accounting for the matched nature of the sample resulted in estimates of standard error that more closely reflected the sampling variability of the treatment effect compared with instances when matching was not taken into account. Furthermore, accounting for the matched nature of the propensity score matched sample tended to result in type I error rates that were closer to the advertised level and confidence intervals with coverage rates closer to the nominal level, compared with instances where matching was not accounted for.

In health research, outcomes are typically continuous, dichotomous, or time-to-event in nature. We discuss appropriate statistical methods for each of these families of outcomes in the subsequent subsections.

3.5.1 Continuous Outcomes

When the outcome variable is continuous, the treatment effect can be measured by the differences in means between treated and untreated subjects. The statistical significance of the difference in means can be assessed using a paired *t*-test. When the response variables are non-normally distributed, then the difference between treated and untreated subjects within propensity score matched pairs may be more likely to be normally distributed than the raw responses themselves. Therefore, a one-sample *t*-test on the differences may still be appropriate. In the event that the paired differences are still strongly non-normal, then a paired nonparametric test, such as the Wilcoxon Signed Ranks test, may be employed (Conover, 1999).

3.5.2 Dichotomous Outcomes

When the outcome variable is dichotomous, there are several options for metrics with which to quantify the effect of treatment on outcomes. In randomized controlled trials with dichotomous outcomes, risk differences and relative risks are frequently reported. Indeed, some clinical journals require that the number needed to treat (NNT—the reciprocal of the absolute risk reduction) be reported for any randomized clinical trial with dichotomous outcomes (http://resources.bmj.com/bmj/authors/types-of-article/research. Site accessed February 5, 2009). Because matching on the propensity score can be expected to eliminate all or most of the observed systematic differences between treated and untreated subjects, one can report risk differences and relative risks by comparing outcomes directly between treated and untreated subjects in the matched sample. Agresti and Min (2004) describe appropriate statistical methods for constructing confidence intervals and assessing the statistical significance of risk differences and relative risks in matched samples. For instance, the statistical significance of differences in proportions (risk differences or absolute risk reduction) can be assessed using McNemar's test for paired binary data. In a matched sample, let us use the following definitions:

- Let a denote the number of matched pairs in which both the treated and untreated subjects experience the event of interest.
- Let b denote the number of matched pairs in which the treated subject does not experience the event of interest, while the untreated subject does experience the event.
- Let c denote the number of matched pairs in which the treated subject experiences the event of interest, while the untreated subject does not experience the event.

- Let d denote the number of matched pairs in which both the treated and untreated subjects do not experience the event (defining d helps visualize the 2x2 table for outcomes within matched pairs. However, d is not used in any of the computations described here).

Then the relative risk is estimated by $(a+c)/(a+b)$. The asymptotic variance of the log-relative risk is estimated by $(b+c)/(a+b)(a+c)$ (Agresti and Min, 2004). A z-test can be constructed by taking the ratio of the log-relative risk and its asymptotic standard error.

In randomized controlled trials, some authors have recommended conducting adjusted analyses in which the effect of exposure on the outcome is adjusted for possible residual imbalance in important prognostic variables that are measured at baseline (Senn, 1994; Senn, 1989; Rothman, 1977). This approach can be implemented in the propensity score matched sample. Logistic regression models, estimated using generalized estimating equation (GEE) methods, can be used to determine the effect of the treatment on outcomes after adjusting for residual imbalance in measured baseline variables. The use of GEE methods allows one to account for the potential homogeneity of outcomes within propensity score matched pairs (Diggle et al., 1994).

Regression adjustment can be useful in small samples in which prognostically important baseline covariates may be imbalanced between treated and untreated subjects in the matched sample. A limitation of this method is that, when the outcome is dichotomous, the measure of treatment effect is the odds ratio, rather than the relative risk or risk difference. The use of the odds ratio has been discouraged as a measure of effect in prospective studies for several reasons (Newcombe, 2006). Prior research has shown that propensity score methods can result in biased estimation of conditional odds ratios (Austin et al., 2007b), while risk differences and relative risks do not suffer from this effect (Rosenbaum and Rubin, 1983a; Austin, 2008c). Furthermore, propensity score methods can result in suboptimal inferences about marginal odds ratios (Austin, 2007b). For these reasons, using odds ratio as a measure of treatment effect in propensity score matched studies is discouraged.

Because propensity score matching tends to reduce much of the systematic differences between treated and untreated subjects, subsequent regression adjustment within the matched sample may not be necessary. When outcomes are dichotomous, investigators are encouraged to report absolute risk reductions, relative risks, and numbers needed to treat, rather than odds ratios. Several authors in clinical journals have suggested that these measures of effect are of greater clinical relevance compared to the odds ratio (Schechtman, 2002; Cook and Sackett, 1995; Jaeschke et al., 1995; Sinclair and Bracken, 1994).

3.5.3 Time-to-Event Outcomes

When the outcome is a time-to-event outcome with possible censoring, then multiple options are present for the analysis. Differences in survival between treated and untreated subjects in the propensity score matched sample can be compared using Kaplan-Meier survival curves. However, conventional tests such as the log-rank test are not appropriate for testing the statistical significance of the difference in survival curves. Klein and Moeschberger (1997) have proposed a test that is appropriate for comparing survival curves that arise from matched data. We describe this test briefly. Let D_1 denote the number of matched pairs in which the treated subject experiences the event first, while D_2 denotes the number of matched pairs in which the untreated subject experiences the event first. The test statistic is $\frac{D_1 - D_2}{\sqrt{D_1 + D_2}}$, which has a standard normal distribution under the null hypothesis and the number of matched pairs is large. Note that data from matched pairs where one of the paired observations is censored will not contribute to the test statistic if the censored observation occurs at an earlier time point than the observed event. The test is analogous to McNemar's test for correlated binary proportions. As an alternative to non-parametric analyses, Cummings and colleagues (2003) have suggested that in matched cohort studies, one can use Cox proportional hazards models that stratify on the matched sets. In the context of propensity score matching, one can fit a propensity score model that stratifies on the matched pairs (Therneau and Grambsch, 2000). Alternatively, one could fit a Cox proportional hazards model and use a robust variance estimator, as proposed by Lin and Wei (1989), to account for the paired nature of the data.

3.6 Sensitivity Analyses for Propensity Score Matching

Conditioning on the propensity score allows for unbiased estimation of the treatment effect under the assumption that all variables that affect treatment assignment have been measured. Rosenbaum and Rubin developed sensitivity analyses that allow one to determine the potential impact of unmeasured confounding variables on the significance of the observed treatment effect (Rosenbaum and Rubin, 1983b; Rosenbaum, 1995). The sensitivity analyses assume that two subjects have the same vector of observed covariates, and hence the same probability of treatment assignment conditional on the observed covariates. However, their true odds of receiving the treatment differ by a factor of Γ. In the remainder of this section, we use the terminology of Rosenbaum (1995).

Let *i* and *j* denote two subjects in the original sample. Let $x_{[i]}$ and $x_{[j]}$ denote the observed vector of covariates for these two subjects, respectively. Furthermore, let $\pi_{[i]}$ and $\pi_{[j]}$ denote the probability of treatment assignment for these two subjects, respectively. Assume that $x_{[i]} = x_{[j]}$, but that $\pi_{[i]} \neq \pi_{[j]}$. Therefore, despite having the same vector of observed covariates, these two subjects have different probabilities of treatment assignment. Thus, these two subjects may be placed in the same matched pair, despite having different probabilities of receiving the treatment. Assume that

$$\frac{1}{\Gamma} \leq \frac{\pi_{[j]}(1-\pi_{[k]})}{\pi_{[k]}(1-\pi_{[j]})} \leq \Gamma \quad \text{for all } j, k \text{ with } x_{[j]} = x_{[k]} \text{ and with } \Gamma \geq 1$$

Thus, for two subjects with the same observed covariate pattern, the odds of receiving the treatment differ by most Γ (Γ ≥ 1). Rosenbaum (1995) demonstrates that this is equivalent to the following two relationships:

$$\log\left(\frac{\pi_{[j]}}{1-\pi_{[j]}}\right) = \kappa(x_{[j]}) + \gamma u_{[j]}$$

$$0 \leq u_{[j]} \leq 1$$

where $x_{[j]}$ denotes the vector of observed covariates and $u_{[j]}$ denotes an unobserved covariate. This relationship says that the odds of receiving the treatment are related to both the observed covariates and an unobserved covariate. Furthermore, this unobserved covariate takes values that lie between 0 and 1 (therefore, the unobserved covariate can be a binary covariate). The sensitivity analyses proposed by Rosenbaum allow one to determine, for a fixed value of

$\Gamma = \exp(\gamma)$, the range of significance levels for the treatment effect that would be observed had the unobserved covariate been accounted for. In particular, the extremes of this range would be achieved when the unobserved covariate was almost perfectly associated with the outcome. Assume that for a specific value of Γ (say, Γ_0), the extreme right of the range of plausible significance values exceeded 0.05. Then one would conclude that if there was an unmeasured binary variable that increased the odds of exposure by a factor of Γ_0 and if this factor was a near-perfect predictor of the outcome, then accounting for this unmeasured factor would nullify the statistical significance of the observed treatment effect (Rosenbaum, 1995). Rosenbaum provides details on how to estimate the range of significance levels in the context of McNemar's test and the Signed Rank Test.

3.7 Propensity Score Matching Compared with Other Propensity Score Methods

Three propensity score methods were proposed by Rosenbaum and Rubin (1983a) in their initial paper: matching on the propensity score, stratification on the propensity score, and covariate adjustment using the propensity score. In a subsequent paper, Rosenbaum (1987) proposed weighting by the inverse probability of treatment using the propensity score. A limitation to the use of covariate adjustment using the propensity score compared with propensity score matching and stratification on the propensity score is that it requires the assumption that the outcomes regression model has been correctly specified (Rubin, 2004). In contrast, propensity score matching and stratification on the propensity score do not require the specification of an outcomes model to estimate the treatment effect. Additionally, covariate adjustment using the propensity score does not explicitly determine the degree of overlap of the distribution of the propensity score within each treatment group. For instance, there may be no untreated subjects with high propensity scores and no treated subjects with low propensity scores. Including these subjects with low or high propensity scores when using covariate adjustment using the propensity score would result in extrapolating the treatment effect from the area of common support to those areas of the distribution of the propensity that consist only of treated subjects or untreated subjects. Both empirical studies and Monte Carlo simulations have found that propensity score matching eliminates a greater degree of the systematic differences in observed covariates between treated and untreated subjects compared to stratification on the propensity score (Austin and Mamdani, 2006; Austin et al., 2007a; Austin, 2009d). When outcomes are dichotomous, propensity score matching and stratification on the propensity score allow for the estimation of risk differences, relative risks, and numbers needed to treat, while covariate adjustment using the propensity score only allows odds ratio estimation.

3.8 Case Study

In this section, we illustrate these methods using SAS software applied to data from a previously published observational study to examine the safety and efficacy of drug-eluting stents (DES) with that of bare metal stents (BMS) in patients undergoing percutaneous coronary interventions (PCI) (Tu et al., 2007).

3.8.1 Data Sources

The data were obtained from a prospective clinical registry maintained by the Cardiac Care Network of Ontario (CCN) of all patients undergoing invasive cardiac procedures in Ontario, Canada. The registry contains information on patient demographic characteristics, cardiac history, cardiac procedures, and relevant coexisting conditions. The current case study is intended only to illustrate the application of propensity score matching. It is not intended to be a clinical examination of the safety and efficacy of DES, which is a complex question. See Tu and colleagues (2007) for an examination of these clinical issues.

The sample for the current tutorial consisted of 13,338 patients who underwent a PCI with placement of either a DES or a BMS in Ontario between December 1, 2003, and March 31, 2005. Patients could have either a single stent or multiple stents placed during the procedure. However, patients who had stents of both types inserted were excluded from the study. The study subjects and the CCN Cardiac Registry are described in greater detail elsewhere (Tu et al., 2007).

3.8.2 Outcomes and Baseline Covariates

There were three outcomes of interest in the original study: target-vessel revascularization, myocardial infarction, and death. The original study identified 21 baseline characteristics that were associated with these outcomes. These characteristics are the baseline covariates in the current study. Baseline characteristics were compared between patients receiving DES and patients receiving BMS when undergoing PCI. Categorical variables were compared using the chi-squared test, while continuous variables were compared using a *t*-test. Baseline characteristics of DES and BMS patients are reported in Table 3.1.

Table 3.1 Comparison of Baseline Characteristics between DES and BMS Patients in the Original Sample

Variable	BMS (N=8,241)	DES (N=5,097)	P-value
Demographic characteristics			
Age, Mean ± SD	62.64 ± 11.83	61.71 ± 11.54	<.001
Male, N (%)	6,130 (74.4%)	3,568 (70.0%)	<.001
Income quintile, N (%)			0.884
1	1,548 (18.8%)	955 (18.7%)	
2	1,676 (20.3%)	1,012 (19.9%)	
3	1,709 (20.7%)	1,080 (21.2%)	
4	1,775 (21.5%)	1,080 (21.2%)	
5	1,533 (18.6%)	970 (19.0%)	
Cardiac condition or procedure			
Hypertension, N (%)	3,057 (37.1%)	1,858 (36.5%)	0.455
Myocardial infarction, N (%)			<.001
Same day as index PCI	1,128 (13.7%)	378 (7.4%)	
1-7 days before index PCI	1,837 (22.3%)	933 (18.3%)	
8-365 days before index PCI	932 (11.3%)	649 (12.7%)	
None within 365 days before index PCI	4,344 (52.7%)	3,137 (61.5%)	
CCS angina classification, N (%)			<.001
0	616 (7.5%)	326 (6.4%)	
I	397 (4.8%)	285 (5.6%)	
II	1,135 (13.8%)	795 (15.6%)	
III	1,700 (20.6%)	1,336 (26.2%)	
IVA	2,343 (28.4%)	1,288 (25.3%)	
IVB	913 (11.1%)	553 (10.8%)	
IVC	998 (12.1%)	479 (9.4%)	
IVD	139 (1.7%)	35 (0.7%)	

(*continued*)

Table 3.1 *(continued)*

Variable	BMS (N=8,241)	DES (N=5,097)	P-value
Congestive heart failure, N (%)	411 (5.0%)	276 (5.4%)	0.278
Previous coronary artery bypass surgery, N (%)	639 (7.8%)	486 (9.5%)	<.001
PCI > 1 year before index PCI	361 (4.4%)	313 (6.1%)	<.001
Coexisting condition			
Diabetes, N (%)	2,018 (24.5%)	1,937 (38.0%)	<.001
Peripheral vascular disease, N (%)	473 (5.7%)	294 (5.8%)	0.945
Chronic obstructive pulmonary disease, N (%)	435 (5.3%)	203 (4.0%)	<.001
Cerebrovascular disease, N (%)	295 (3.6%)	300 (5.9%)	<.001
Primary cancer, N (%)	87 (1.1%)	48 (0.9%)	0.523
Renal failure requiring dialysis, N (%)	67 (0.8%)	67 (1.3%)	0.005
Index PCI			
Ad hoc PCI, N (%)	4,833 (58.6%)	2,576 (50.5%)	<.001
Stent length (mm), Mean ± SD	24.73 ± 15.27	28.68 ± 16.81	<.001
Stent diameter (mm), Mean ± SD	3.06 ± 0.49	2.76 ± 0.36	<.001
No. of stents per patient, Mean ± SD	1.47 ± 0.81	1.48 ± 0.76	0.959
No. of vessels stented, Mean ± SD	1.12 ± 0.35	1.13 ± 0.35	0.158
ACC-AHA lesion type, N (%)			<.001
A	1,091 (13.2%)	328 (6.4%)	
B1	2,443 (29.6%)	1,320 (25.9%)	
B2	2,966 (36.0%)	1,928 (37.8%)	
C	1,741 (21.1%)	1,521 (29.8%)	

In examining Table 3.1, one observes that the distribution of 14 out of the 21 baseline variables differed significantly between DES and BMS patients. The distribution of age, gender, history of myocardial infarction, CCS angina classification, previous coronary artery bypass graft surgery, PCI over a year prior to index procedure, diabetes, chronic obstructive pulmonary disease, cerebrovascular disease, renal disease requiring dialysis, ad hoc PCI, stent length, stent diameter, and ACC-AHA lesion type differed between the two treatment groups.

3.8.3 Estimating the Propensity Score Model

The initial propensity score was estimated using a logistic regression model that had a dichotomous variable indicating receipt of a DES as the response variable and that contained as predictor variables the 21 baseline variables listed in Table 3.1. Categorical variables with more than two levels were represented using multiple indicator variables (for example, CCS angina classification). The propensity score model was fit using the SAS code in Program 3.1:

Program 3.1 SAS Code for Fitting Propensity Score Model

```
/*************************************************************************/
/* SAS code for estimating propensity score model.                       */
/* Indicator variable denoting receipt of a DES is regressed on baseline */
/* characteristics.                                                      */
/*************************************************************************/

proc logistic descending data=stent_data;
  model des = cov_locancer cov_adhoc cov_age cov_ccnprevacb
   cov_ccnprevptca ccscat_1 ccscat_2 ccscat_3 ccscat_4A ccscat_4B ccscat_4C
   ccscat_4D cov_cerebvd cov_chf prevmi_index prevmi_7days prevmi_1year
   cov_copd cov_diab_2cat cov_dialysis
```

```
    cov_hyperten income2 income3 income4 income5
    lesion_type_B1 lesion_type_B2 lesion_type_C
    cov_male cov_pvd cov_s_lensum cov_s_sizemin cov_vesnum stents;
  output out=out_ps prob=ps xbeta=logit_ps;
  /* Output the propensity score and logit of the propensity score */
run;
```

3.8.4 Propensity Score Matching

Patients were then matched on the logit of the propensity score using a caliper of 0.2 standard deviations of the logit of the propensity score. The Division of Biostatistics at the Mayo Clinic provides a set of SAS macros on its Web site that can be used for propensity score matching (http://mayoresearch.mayo.edu/mayo/research/biostat/sasmacros.cfm)[1]. The %GMATCH macro performs greedy matching, while the %VMATCH macro can be used for optimal matching (these two macros replaced the earlier %MATCH macro that performed both greedy matching and optimal matching). The SAS code for using the %GMATCH macro to form pairs of DES and BMS patients matched on the logit of the propensity score using calipers of width equal to 0.2 of the standard deviation of the logit of the propensity score is shown in Program 3.2.

Program 3.2 SAS Code for Forming Propensity Score Matched Sample

```
/***********************************************************************/
/* Compute standard deviation of the logit of the propensity score     */
/***********************************************************************/

proc means std data=out_ps;
  var logit_ps;
  output out=stddata (keep = std) std=std;
run;

data stddata;
  set stddata;
  std = 0.2*std;
  /* calipers of width 0.2 standard deviations of the logit of PS.     */
run;

/* Create macro variable that contains the width of the caliper for matching */

data _null_;
  set stddata;
  call symput('stdcal',std);
run;

/* Match subjects on the logit of the propensity score.              */
```

[1] These SAS macros were written locally and are maintained by Mayo Clinic staff. They contain the SAS source code, a brief description of the macro's function, and an example of the macro call. Copyright 2005 Mayo Foundations for Medical Education and Research. This software is free software; you can redistribute it and/or modify it under the terms of the GNU General Public License as published by the Free Software Foundation; either version 2 of the License, or (at your option) any later version. These macros are distributed in the hope that they will be useful, but WITHOUT ANY WARRANTY; without even the implied warranty of MERCHANTABILITY or FITNESS FOR A PARTICULAR PURPOSE. See the GNU General Public License for more details. If you use functions from the Mayo Clinic, please acknowledge the original contributor of the material.

```
proc sort data=out_ps;
  by des;
run;

data out_ps;
  set out_ps;
  id=_N_;
run;

%include 'gmatch.sas';

/* The macro %gmatch.sas uses the following parameters:
   Data: the name of the SAS data set containing the treated and untreated subjects.
   Group: the variable identifying treated/untreated subjects.
   Id: the variable denoting subjects' identification numbers.
   Mvars: the list of variables on which one is matching.
   Wts: the list of non-negative weights corresponding to each matching variable.
   Dist: the type of distance to calculate [1 indicates weighted sum (over matching
        variables) of absolute case-control differences].
   Dmaxk: the maximum allowable difference in the matching difference between matched
        treated and untreated subjects.
   Ncontls: the number of untreated subjects to be matched to each treated subject.
   Seedca: the random number seed for sorting the treated subjects prior to matching.
   Seedco: the random number seed for sorting the untreated subjects prior to
          matching.
   Out: the name of a SAS data set containing the matched sample.
   Print: the flag indicating whether the matched data should be printed.   */

%gmatch(
  data = out_ps,
  group = des,
  id = id,
  mvars = logit_ps,
  wts = 1,
  dist = 1,
  dmaxk = &stdcal,
  ncontls = 1,
  seedca = 25102007,
  seedco = 26102007,
  out = matchpairs,
  print = F
);

data matchpairs;
  set matchpairs;
  pair_id = _N_;
run;

/* Create a data set containing the matched BMS patients (untreated subjects) */

data control_match;
  set matchpairs;
  control_id = __IDCO;
  logit_ps = __CO1;
  keep pair_id control_id logit_ps;
run;

/* Create a data set containing the matched DES patients (treated subjects) */

data case_match;
  set matchpairs;
  case_id = __IDCA;
  logit_ps = __CA1;
  keep pair_id case_id logit_ps;
run;

proc sort data=control_match;
  by control_id;
run;
```

```
proc sort data=case_match;
  by case_id;
run;

data exposed;
  set out_ps;
  if des = 1;
  case_id = id;
run;

data control;
  set out_ps;
  if des = 0;
  control_id = id;
run;

proc sort data=exposed;
  by case_id;
run;

proc sort data=control;
  by control_id;
run;

data control_match;
  merge control_match (in=f1) control (in=f2);
  by control_id;
  if f1 and f2;
run;

data case_match;
  merge case_match (in=f1) exposed (in=f2);
  by case_id;
  if f1 and f2;
run;

data long;
  set control_match case_match;
  prop_score = exp(logit_ps) / (exp(logit_ps) + 1);
run;

data wide_des;
  set case_match;

  death_1_yr_des = death_1_yr;
  tvra_time_des = tvra_time;
  tvra_des = tvra;
run;

data wide_bms;
  set control_match;

  death_1_yr_bms = death_1_yr;
  tvra_time_bms = tvra_time;
  tvra_bms = tvra;
run;

proc sort data=wide_des;
  by pair_id;
run;

proc sort data=wide_bms;
  by pair_id;
run;

/* Data set containing outcomes for the matched subjects.              */
/* Each row contains outcomes for the treated and untreated subjects */
/* in the matched pair.                                                */
```

```
data wide_combo;
  merge wide_des (in=f1) wide_bms (in=f2);
  by pair_id;
  if f1 and f2;
run;
```

This resulted in the formation of 3,746 matched pairs of DES and BMS patients. Of the 5,097 DES patients in the initial sample, 3,746 (73.5%) were matched to a BMS patient, while 1,351 (26.5%) DES patients were excluded from the matched sample because an appropriate BMS patient was not identified. Similarly, 4,495 (54.5%) of the BMS patients were excluded from the matched sample. Two SAS data sets containing the matched subjects were constructed. The first (Long) contained one row per subject, while the second (Wide_Combo) contained one row per matched pair.

3.8.5 Assessing Balance in Measured Covariates

We examined the similarity of treated and untreated subjects in the propensity score matched sample. Standardized differences were computed for each of the baseline variables listed in Table 3.1. Program 3.3 shows the SAS code for calculating standardized differences.

Program 3.3 SAS Code for Calculating Standardized Differences between Treated and Untreated Subjects

```
/*************************************************************************/
/* Compute standardized differences for each covariate in the matched sample. */
/*************************************************************************/

proc sort data=long;
  by des;
run;

/*************************************************************************/
/* Macro for computing standardized differences for continuous variables.     */
/*************************************************************************/

%macro cont(var=,label=);

proc means mean stddev data=long noprint;
  var &var;
  by des;
  output out=outmean (keep = des mean stddev) mean = mean stddev=stddev;
run;

data des0;
  set outmean;
  if des = 0;
  mean_0 = mean;
  s_0 = stddev;

  keep mean_0 s_0;
run;

data des1;
  set outmean;
  if des = 1;
  mean_1 = mean;
  s_1 = stddev;

  keep mean_1 s_1;
run;

data newdata;
  length label $ 25;
  merge des0 des1;
```

```
  d = (mean_1 - mean_0)/ sqrt((s_1*s_1 + s_0*s_0)/2);
  d = round(abs(d),0.001);

  label = &label;

  keep d label;
run;

proc append data=newdata base=standiff force;
run;

%mend cont;

/*****************************************************************************/
/* Macro for computing standardized differences for binary variables.        */
/*****************************************************************************/

%macro binary(var=,label=);

proc means mean data=long noprint;
  var &var;
  by des;
  output out=outmean (keep = des mean) mean = mean;
run;

data des0;
  set outmean;
  if des = 0;
  mean_0 = mean;

  keep mean_0;
run;

data des1;
  set outmean;
  if des = 1;
  mean_1 = mean;

  keep mean_1;
run;

data newdata;
  length label $ 25;
  merge des0 des1;

  d = (mean_1 - mean_0)/ sqrt((mean_1*(1-mean_1) + mean_0*(1-mean_0))/2);
  d = round(abs(d),0.001);

  label = &label;

  keep d label;
run;

proc append data=newdata base=standiff force;
run;

%mend binary;

%cont(var=cov_age,label="Age");
%cont(var=cov_s_lensum,label="Length of stents");
%cont(var=cov_s_sizemin,label="Stent diameter");
%cont(var=stents,label="Number of stents");
%cont(var=cov_vesnum,label="Number of vessels");

%binary(var=cov_male,label="Male sex");
%binary(var=income1,label="Income 1");
%binary(var=income2,label="Income 2");
%binary(var=income3,label="Income 3");
%binary(var=income4,label="Income 4");
```

```
%binary(var=income5,label="Income 5");
%binary(var=cov_hyperten,label="Hypertension");
%binary(var=prevmi_none,label="Previous MI: none within 365 days of index PCI");
%binary(var=prevmi_index,label="Previous MI: same day as index PCI");
%binary(var=prevmi_7days,label="Previous MI: 1-7 days before index PCI");
%binary(var=prevmi_1year,label="Previous MI: 8-365 days before index PCI");
%binary(var=ccscat_0,label="CCS Class 0");
%binary(var=ccscat_1,label="CCS Class I");
%binary(var=ccscat_2,label="CCS Class II");
%binary(var=ccscat_3,label="CCS Class III");
%binary(var=ccscat_4A,label="CCS Class IVA");
%binary(var=ccscat_4B,label="CCS Class IVB");
%binary(var=ccscat_4C,label="CCS Class IVC");
%binary(var=ccscat_4D,label="CCS Class IVD");
%binary(var=cov_diab_2cat,label="Diabetes");
%binary(var=cov_chf,label="CHF");
%binary(var=cov_pvd,label="PVD");
%binary(var=cov_copd,label="COPD");
%binary(var=cov_cerebvd,label="Cerebrovascular disease");
%binary(var=cov_1ocancer,label="Primary cancer");
%binary(var=cov_dialysis,label="Renal disease requiring dialysis");
%binary(var=cov_ccnprevacb,label="Previous CABG surgery");
%binary(var=cov_ccnprevptca,label="PCI > 1 year before index PCI");
%binary(var=cov_adhoc,label="Ad hoc procedure");
%binary(var=lesion_type_A,label="Lesion Type A");
%binary(var=lesion_type_B1,label="Lesion Type B1");
%binary(var=lesion_type_B2,label="Lesion Type B2");
%binary(var=lesion_type_C,label="Lesion Type C");


proc print data=standiff;
  title 'Standardized differences in propensity score matched sample';
run;
```

Output from Program 3.3

```
Standardized differences in propensity score matched sample

        Obs    label                                            d

          1    Age                                          0.006
          2    Length of stents                             0.014
          3    Stent diameter                               0.003
          4    Number of stents                             0.004
          5    Number of vessels                            0.005
          6    Male sex                                     0.009
          7    Income 1                                     0.006
          8    Income 2                                     0.007
          9    Income 3                                     0.005
         10    Income 4                                     0.013
         11    Income 5                                     0.007
         12    Hypertension                                 0.016
         13    Previous MI: none within 365 days of index PCI  0.004
         14    Previous MI: same day as index PCI           0.012
         15    Previous MI: 1-7 days before index PCI       0.017
         16    Previous MI: 8-365 days before index PCI     0.005
         17    CCS Class 0                                  0.001
         18    CCS Class I                                  0.010
         19    CCS Class II                                 0.018
         20    CCS Class III                                0.031
         21    CCS Class IVA                                0.013
         22    CCS Class IVB                                0.010
         23    CCS Class IVC                                0.020
         24    CCS Class IVD                                0.014
         25    Diabetes                                     0.011
         26    CHF                                          0.011
```

(continued)

Output from Program 3.3 (*continued*)

```
     27      PVD                                                    0.019
     28      COPD                                                   0.010
     29      Cerebrovascular disease                                0.018
     30      Primary cancer                                         0.003
     31      Renal disease requiring dialysis                       0.008
     32      Previous CABG surgery                                  0.014
     33      PCI > 1 year before index PCI                          0.012
     34      Ad hoc procedure                                       0.013
     35      Lesion Type A                                          0.019
     36      Lesion Type B1                                         0.026
     37      Lesion Type B2                                         0.011
     38      Lesion Type C                                          0.003
```

Table 3.2 reports the baseline characteristics of DES and BMS patients in the propensity score matched sample, along with the associated standardized differences in both the matched sample and the initial sample.

Table 3.2 Standardized Differences of Baseline Covariates in Original and Matched Sample

Variable	BMS (N=3,746)	DES (N=3,746)	Standardized difference (matched sample)	Standardized difference (original unmatched sample)
		Demographic characteristics		
Age, Mean ± SD	62.33 ± 11.67	62.26 ± 11.57	0.006	0.080
Male, N (%)	2,657 (70.9%)	2,672 (71.3%)	0.009	0.098
Income quintile 1, N (%)	722 (19.3%)	713 (19.0%)	0.006	0.001
Income quintile 2, N (%)	754 (20.1%)	765 (20.4%)	0.007	0.012
Income quintile 3, N (%)	772 (20.6%)	780 (20.8%)	0.005	0.011
Income quintile 4, N (%)	799 (21.3%)	779 (20.8%)	0.013	0.009
Income quintile 5, N (%)	699 (18.7%)	709 (18.9%)	0.007	0.011
		Cardiac condition or procedure		
Hypertension	1,356 (36.2%)	1,384 (36.9%)	0.016	0.013
Previous MI: None within 365 days of index PCI	2,200 (58.7%)	2,207 (58.9%)	0.004	0.179
Previous MI: same day as index PCI	329 (8.8%)	342 (9.1%)	0.012	0.199
Previous MI: 1-7 days before index PCI	753 (20.1%)	727 (19.4%)	0.017	0.098
Previous MI: 8-365 days before index PCI	464 (12.4%)	470 (12.5%)	0.005	0.044
CCS angina class 0	259 (6.9%)	258 (6.9%)	0.001	0.042
CCS angina class I	213 (5.7%)	204 (5.4%)	0.010	0.035
CCS angina class II	573 (15.3%)	549 (14.7%)	0.018	0.052
CCS angina class III	853 (22.8%)	902 (24.1%)	0.031	0.133
CCS angina class IVA	1,019 (27.2%)	998 (26.6%)	0.013	0.071
CCS angina class IVB	422 (11.3%)	410 (10.9%)	0.010	0.007

(*continued*)

Table 3.2 *(continued)*

Variable	BMS (N=3,746)	DES (N=3,746)	Standardized difference (matched sample)	Standardized difference (original unmatched sample)
CCS angina class IVC	371 (9.9%)	394 (10.5%)	0.020	0.087
CCS angina class IVD	36 (1.0%)	31 (0.8%)	0.014	0.088
Congestive heart failure	193 (5.2%)	202 (5.4%)	0.011	0.019
Previous coronary artery bypass surgery	338 (9.0%)	323 (8.6%)	0.014	0.064
PCI > 1 year before index PCI	201 (5.4%)	211 (5.6%)	0.012	0.080
Coexisting condition				
Diabetes	1,215 (32.4%)	1,196 (31.9%)	0.011	0.299
Peripheral vascular disease	225 (6.0%)	208 (5.6%)	0.019	0.001
Chronic obstructive pulmonary disease	176 (4.7%)	168 (4.5%)	0.010	0.061
Cerebrovascular disease	184 (4.9%)	199 (5.3%)	0.018	0.112
Primary cancer	39 (1.0%)	40 (1.1%)	0.003	0.011
Renal failure requiring dialysis	40 (1.1%)	43 (1.1%)	0.008	0.050
Index PCI				
Ad hoc PCI	2,006 (53.6%)	2,030 (54.2%)	0.013	0.164
Stent length (mm)	26.17 ± 16.68	26.40 ± 15.00	0.014	0.249
Stent diameter (mm)	2.83 ± 0.39	2.84 ± 0.36	0.003	0.678
No. of stents per patient	1.45 ± 0.76	1.45 ± 0.76	0.004	0.001
No. of vessels stented	1.13 ± 0.36	1.13 ± 0.35	0.005	0.025
ACC-AHA lesion type: A	280 (7.5%)	299 (8.0%)	0.019	0.222
ACC-AHA lesion type: B1	1,105 (29.5%)	1,061 (28.3%)	0.026	0.083
ACC-AHA lesion type: B2	1,421 (37.9%)	1,441 (38.5%)	0.011	0.038
ACC-AHA lesion type: C	940 (25.1%)	945 (25.2%)	0.003	0.204

The estimated propensity score ranged from 0.0138 to 0.9587 in DES patients and from 0.0138 to 0.9610 in BMS patients. Figure 3.1 compares the distribution of the propensity scores between DES and BMS patients in both the original sample and the matched sample. Figure 3.1 depicts non-parametric density estimates of the distribution of the propensity score in both DES and BMS patients. The upper panel is in the original (unmatched) sample, while the lower panel is in the matched sample. The distribution of the propensity score appears to be essentially identical between DES and BMS patients in the matched sample. The top panel of Figure 3.1 demonstrates that the range of propensity scores is similar between DES and BMS patients. Therefore, for each DES patient, there was a BMS patient with a comparable propensity score.

Figure 3.1 Distribution of the Propensity Score in Treated (DES) and Untreated (BMS) Subjects

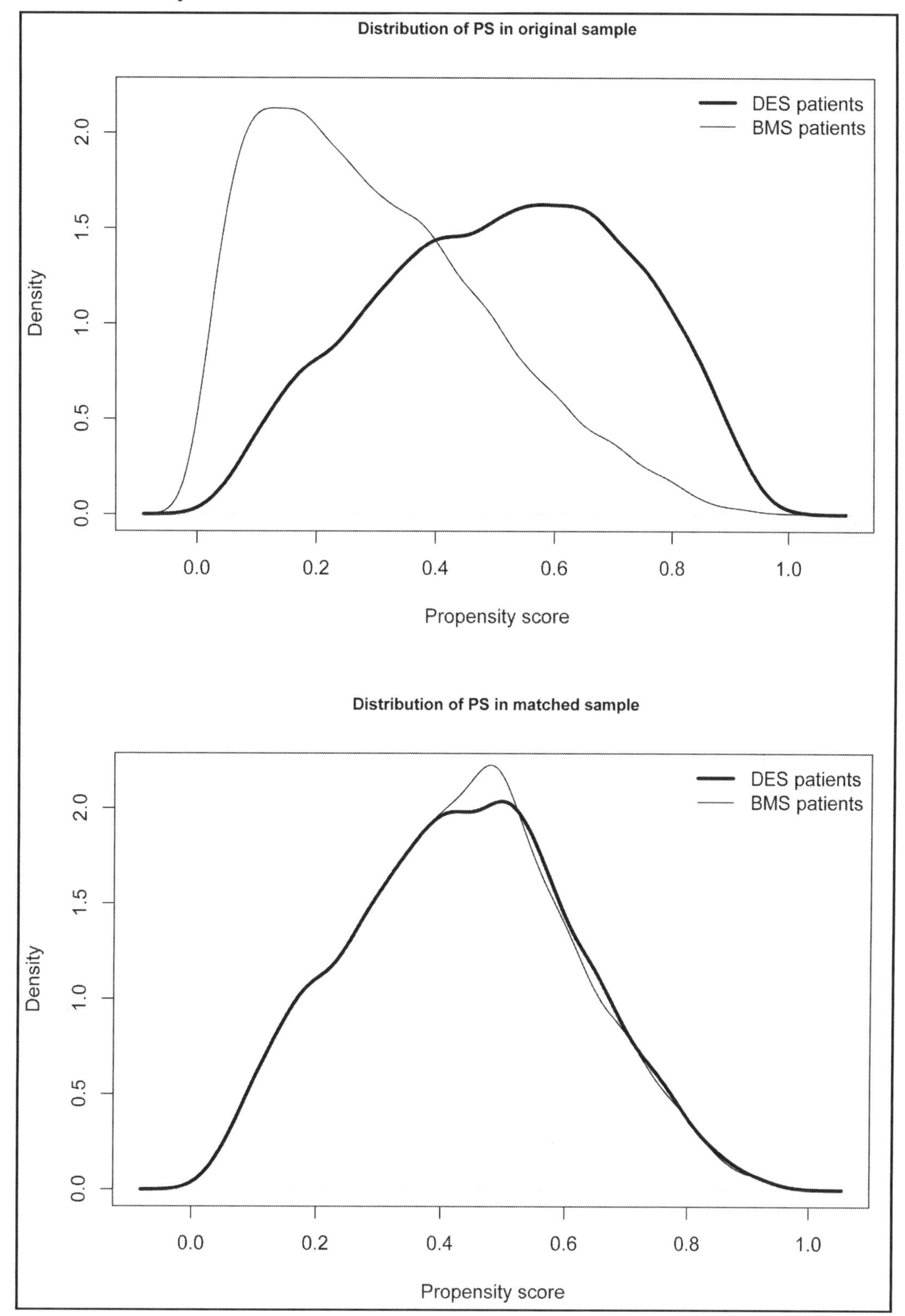

Because the standardized differences were all small in the matched sample (standardized differences ≤ 0.031), the initial propensity score model was not modified. The largest standardized difference in the matched sample was 0.031 (CCS angina class III; prevalence of 22.8% vs. 24.1% in BMS and DES patients, respectively). By comparison, the largest standardized difference in the original (unmatched) sample was 0.678 (for the variable denoting stent diameter). The mean stent diameters in the original (unmatched) sample were 3.06 mm and 2.76 mm in BMS and DES patients, respectively.

Graphical balance diagnostics for comparing the distribution of measured baseline covariates between the two treatment groups are not presented here. Statistical software with high-level graphics can optimize the presentation of quantile-quantile plots of baseline covariates in the matched sample and other methods of comparing the distribution of baseline covariates between treated and untreated subjects in the propensity score matched sample.

3.8.6 Effect of Exposure on Outcomes

In this case study, we considered two outcomes: a safety outcome and an efficacy outcome. The safety outcome we considered was a dichotomous outcome, death within 1 year of the index PCI procedure. In the matched sample, there were 5 matched pairs in which both subjects died within 1 year of the procedure, 3,516 matched pairs in which neither subject died within 1 year of the procedure, 138 matched pairs in which the BMS patient died and the DES patient did not die, and 87 matched pairs in which the DES patient died and the BMS patient did not die. The 1-year mortality rates in the DES and BMS patients were 2.46% and 3.82%, respectively. According to McNemar's test, the 1-year mortality rates were significantly different between the two treatment groups (P = 0.0008 using the exact version of McNemar's test). The relative risk of 1-year mortality for DES patients compared to BMS patients was 0.64. The 95% confidence interval, computed using methods appropriate for matched data, was (0.50, 0.83). The SAS code for estimating the statistical significance of the effect of treatment on mortality (as measured using the risk difference) appears in Program 3.4.

Program 3.4 SAS Code for Estimating Effect of Treatment on Dichotomous Outcomes

```
proc freq data=wide_combo;
  exact agree;
  tables death_1_yr_bms*death_1_yr_des /nopercent agree;
  title "McNemar's test for comparing risk of death within 1 year of
    procedure";
run;
```

Output from Program 3.4

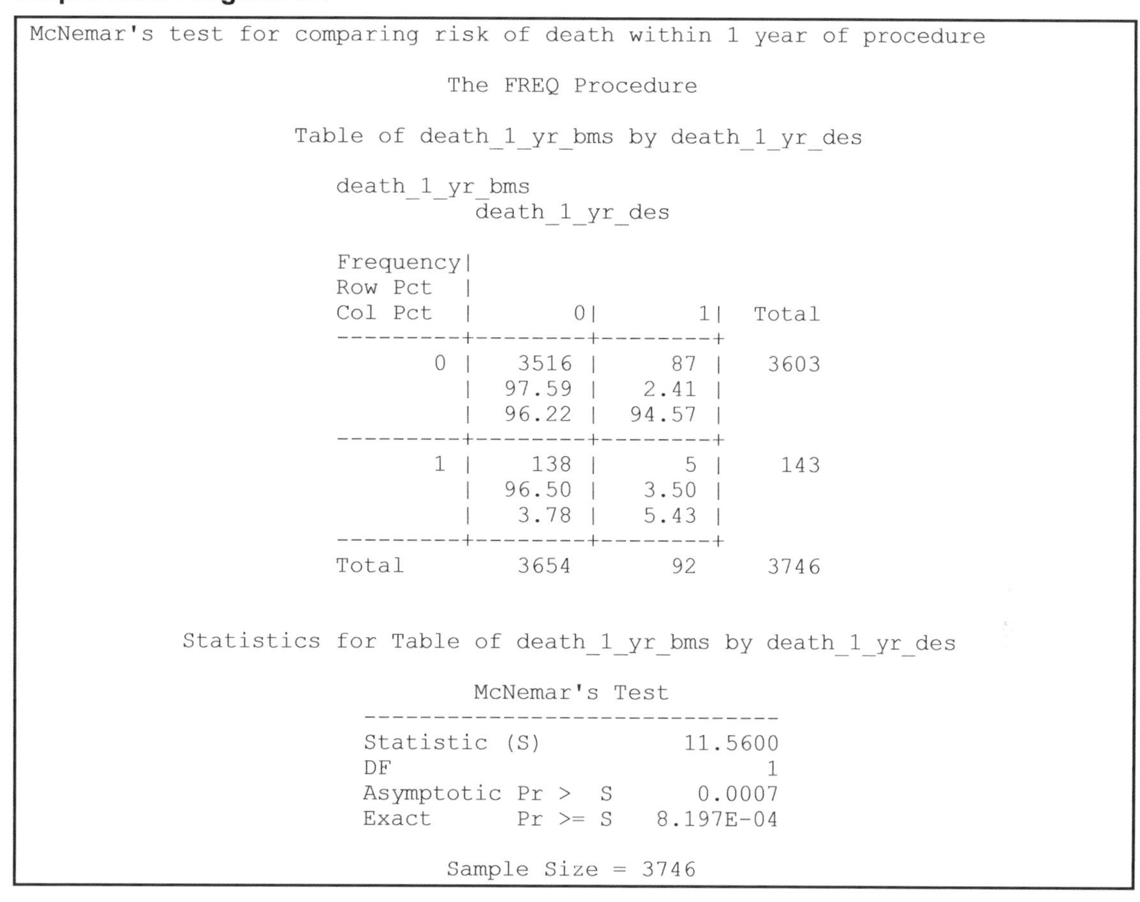

```
McNemar's test for comparing risk of death within 1 year of procedure

                         The FREQ Procedure

            Table of death_1_yr_bms by death_1_yr_des

              death_1_yr_bms
                        death_1_yr_des

              Frequency|
              Row Pct  |
              Col Pct  |       0|       1|  Total
              ---------+--------+--------+
                     0 |   3516 |     87 |   3603
                       |  97.59 |   2.41 |
                       |  96.22 |  94.57 |
              ---------+--------+--------+
                     1 |    138 |      5 |    143
                       |  96.50 |   3.50 |
                       |   3.78 |   5.43 |
              ---------+--------+--------+
              Total        3654       92     3746

       Statistics for Table of death_1_yr_bms by death_1_yr_des

                          McNemar's Test
               ------------------------------
               Statistic (S)          11.5600
               DF                           1
               Asymptotic Pr >  S      0.0007
               Exact      Pr >= S   8.197E-04

                        Sample Size = 3746
```

We conducted a sensitivity analysis to determine the sensitivity of the observed effect of treatment on mortality to unmeasured confounders. There were 225 discordant pairs. Of these, 138 were pairs in which the BMS patient died and the DES patient did not. For a given value of Γ, Rosenbaum (1995) defines the following two proportions: $p^{+} = \Gamma/(1+\Gamma)$ and $p^{-} = 1/(1+\Gamma)$. Then, the bounds for the significance of the treatment effect if the unmeasured confounder were taken into account are as follows:

$$2 \times \sum_{a=138}^{225} \binom{225}{a} (p^{+})^{a} (1-p^{+})^{225-a} \geq 2 \times prob(T \geq 138 \mid m) \geq 2 \times \sum_{a=138}^{225} \binom{225}{a} (p^{-})^{a} (1-p^{-})^{225-a}$$

where T is McNemar's statistic and m denotes the observed data. The exact boundaries of the significance levels can be determined for different values of Γ using the following SAS code in Program 3.5.

Program 3.5 SAS Code for Examining the Sensitivity of the Propensity Score Matched Analysis to an Unmeasured Confounding Variable

```
data gamma;
  do gamma_init = 0 to 5;
    gamma = 1 + gamma_init/20;
    p_plus = gamma/(1 + gamma);
    p_neg = 1/(1 + gamma);

    p_upper = 2*(1 - probbnml(p_plus,225,137) );
    p_lower = 2*(1 - probbnml(p_neg,225,137) );
    output;
  end;
run;

proc print data=gamma noobs;
  var gamma p_plus p_neg p_lower p_upper;
  title "Sensitivity analysis for McNemar's test";
run;
```

Output from Program 3.5

```
                  Sensitivity analysis for McNemar's test

   gamma       p_plus       p_neg         p_lower       p_upper

    1.00      0.50000     0.50000     .000819738     0.000820
    1.05      0.51220     0.48780     .000206443     0.002869
    1.10      0.52381     0.47619     .000049244     0.008434
    1.15      0.53488     0.46512     .000011232     0.021289
    1.20      0.54545     0.45455     .000002469     0.047026
    1.25      0.55556     0.44444     .000000527     0.092418
```

If there was an unmeasured binary variable that increased the odds of exposure by no more than 20%, the statistical significance of the observed treatment effect would be at most 0.047. However, if there was an unmeasured binary variable that increased the odds of exposure by 25%, and if this variable was almost perfectly associated with mortality, then the significance level of the treatment effect could be as large as 0.092.

The efficacy outcome we considered was a time-to-event outcome: time to total vessel revascularization. Figure 3.2 depicts the Kaplan-Meier survival curves in each of the two treatment arms of the study. Survival free of total vessel revascularization was better in the DES group than it was in the BMS group. The difference between the survival curves was significant, according to the test proposed by Klein and Moeschberger (1997) ($P < 0.0001$). The SAS code for assessing the difference between the survival curves is shown in Program 3.6.

Figure 3.2 Kaplan-Meier Survival Curves in PS-Matched Sample: Time to Target Vessel Revascularization

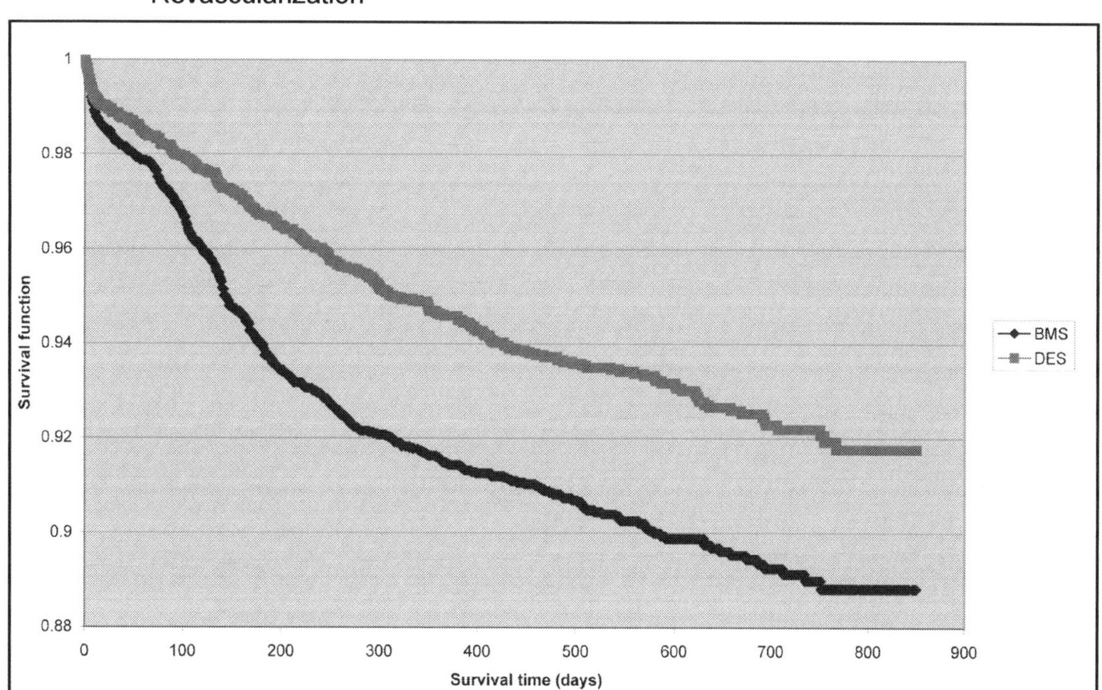

Program 3.6 SAS Code for Comparing the Kaplan-Meier Survival Curves between DES and BMS Patients in the Propensity Score Matched Sample

```
data long;
  set long;
  if des = 1 then stent = "DES";
    else stent = "BMS";
run;

proc lifetest data=long outsurv=kmdata_tvra notable;
  time tvra_time*tvra(0);
  strata stent;
   /* 'tvra_time' denotes time to total vessel revascularization */
   /* 'tvra' is the censoring indicator: 1 indicates that the event
       occurred, while   */
   /* 0 indicates that the subject has been censored.           */
   /* 'stent' denotes the exposure group: DES vs. BMS.          */
  title 'Kaplan-Meier survival curves for DES and BMS patients';
run;

data km_compare;
  set wide_combo;
  if (tvra_time_des < tvra_time_bms) and (tvra_des = 0) then delete;
  if (tvra_time_bms < tvra_time_des) and (tvra_bms = 0) then delete;
 /* Delete pairs in which the shorter of the two observation times */
 /* is for a subject who is censored.                              */

  if (tvra_time_des < tvra_time_bms) and (tvra_des = 1) then D1 = 1;
    else D1 = 0;
```

```
  if (tvra_time_bms < tvra_time_des) and (tvra_bms = 1) then D2 = 1;
    else D2 = 0;
run;
proc means sum data=km_compare noprint;
  var D1 D2;
  output out=km_stat (keep = D1 D2) sum = D1 D2;
run;

data km_stat;
  set km_stat;
  z = (D1 - D2)/sqrt(D1 + D2);
  /* Test statistic for comparing K-M curves from matched sample */

  p_value = 2*(1 - probnorm(abs(z)));
run;

proc print data=km_stat;
  var D1 D2 z p_value;
  title 'Comparing K-M survival curve from matched sample';
run;
```

Output from Program 3.6

```
Comparing K-M survival curve from matched sample

                    Obs      D1       D2          z            p_value

                      1     222      336     -4.82600     .000001393
```

A Cox proportional hazards model was fit to the matched sample. The model contained exposure status as the sole predictor variable, stratified on the matched pairs. The hazard ratio for DES compared to BMS was 0.661 (95% CI = [0.558, 0.783]) ($P < 0.0001$). When a univariate Cox proportional hazards model was fit and a robust variance estimate was obtained, the associated hazards ratio was 0.683 (95% CI = [0.582, 0.800]) ($P < 0.0001$). The SAS code for each of these survival regression models is provided in Program 3.7.

Program 3.7 SAS Code for Fitting Cox Proportional Hazards Models in the Propensity Score Matched Sample

```
/* Cox proportional hazards model stratifying on matched pairs */

proc phreg data=long nosummary;
  model tvra_time*tvra(0) = des/ties=exact rl;
  strata pair_id;
  title 'Cox proportional hazards model stratifying on matched sets';
run;

/* Cox proportional hazards model with robust standard errors to */
/* account for clustering in matched pairs.                      */

proc phreg data=long covs(aggregate);
  model tvra_time*tvra(0) = des/ties=exact rl;
  id pair_id;
  title 'Cox proportional hazards model with robust standard errors';
run;
```

Output from Program 3.7

```
Cox proportional hazards model stratifying on matched sets

                         The PHREG Procedure

                          Model Information

                  Data Set                      WORK.LONG
                  Dependent Variable            tvra_time
                  Censoring Variable            tvra
                  Censoring Value(s)            0
                  Ties Handling                 EXACT


                Number of Observations Read         7492
                Number of Observations Used         7492


                         Convergence Status

            Convergence criterion (GCONV=1E-8) satisfied.


                        Model Fit Statistics

                                 Without          With
                Criterion      Covariates    Covariates

                -2 LOG L          773.552       750.097
                AIC               773.552       752.097
                SBC               773.552       756.532


                Testing Global Null Hypothesis: BETA=0

        Test                 Chi-Square        DF      Pr > ChiSq

        Likelihood Ratio        23.4551         1          <.0001
        Score                   23.2903         1          <.0001
        Wald                    22.9594         1          <.0001


               Analysis of Maximum Likelihood Estimates

                     Parameter      Standard
    Variable    DF    Estimate         Error    Chi-Square    Pr > ChiSq

    des          1    -0.41443       0.08649       22.9594        <.0001

               Analysis of Maximum Likelihood Estimates

                             Hazard      95% Hazard Ratio
               Variable       Ratio     Confidence Limits

               des            0.661      0.558        0.783
```

Output from Program 3.7 *(continued)*

```
Cox proportional hazards model with robust standard errors

                        The PHREG Procedure

                         Model Information

                Data Set                    WORK.LONG
                Dependent Variable          tvra_time
                Censoring Variable          tvra
                Censoring Value(s)          0
                Ties Handling               EXACT

              Number of Observations Read          7492
              Number of Observations Used          7492

         Summary of the Number of Event and Censored Values

                                                  Percent
              Total        Event     Censored     Censored

               7492          623         6869        91.68


                         Convergence Status

          Convergence criterion (GCONV=1E-8) satisfied.

                       Model Fit Statistics

                              Without            With
              Criterion     Covariates      Covariates

              -2 LOG L       10307.321       10284.920
              AIC            10307.321       10286.920
              SBC            10307.321       10291.354


              Testing Global Null Hypothesis: BETA=0

         Test                         Chi-Square       DF     Pr > ChiSq

         Likelihood Ratio                22.4017        1         <.0001
         Score (Model-Based)             22.3257        1         <.0001
         Score (Sandwich)                22.1856        1         <.0001
         Wald (Model-Based)              22.0567        1         <.0001
         Wald (Sandwich)                 22.1776        1         <.0001


              Analysis of Maximum Likelihood Estimates

                     Parameter    Standard   StdErr
     Variable   DF    Estimate       Error    Ratio   Chi-Square   Pr > ChiSq

     des         1    -0.38187     0.08109    0.997      22.1776       <.0001

Cox proportional hazards model with robust standard errors

                        The PHREG Procedure

              Analysis of Maximum Likelihood Estimates

                           Hazard       95% Hazard Ratio
              Variable      Ratio       Confidence Limits

              des           0.683       0.582         0.800
```

3.9 Summary

Three recent systematic reviews found that propensity score matching was poorly implemented in the medical literature overall between 1996 and 2003 (Austin, 2008b) and, in a more recent era, in the cardiovascular surgery literature between 2004 and 2006 (Austin, 2007a) and in the general cardiology literature between 2004 and 2006 (Austin, 2008d). Indeed, in the first review of 47 articles, it was found that only two studies conducted all aspects of propensity score matching correctly, while in the second review it was found that none of the 60 articles examined conducted all of the statistical analyses correctly. Similar findings were observed in the third review. Common errors included employing inappropriate methods for assessing the balance of measured baseline covariates between treated and untreated subjects in the propensity score matched sample and failing to account for the matched nature of the sample when estimating the variance of the treatment effect. Furthermore, many studies did not provide sufficient detail on how the propensity score matched pairs were formed, thereby limiting the ability of other researchers to replicate the study methods.

In this chapter, we have discussed and illustrated the use of propensity score matching for estimating causal treatment effects. In particular, there are four important components to properly conducting an analysis using propensity score matching. First, specify the propensity score model. Second, create matched sets of treated and untreated subjects by matching on the propensity score. Fully report how the propensity score matched sample was formed. This allows other researchers to replicate your study methods and thereby confirm the findings of your study. Third, assess whether matching on the propensity score has resulted in a matched sample in which the distribution of measured baseline covariates are similar between treated and untreated subjects. Investigators should employ sample-specific methods for assessing the similarity of the distribution of measured covariates between treated and untreated subjects. The first three steps may need to be repeated iteratively until an acceptable balance between treated and untreated subjects has been achieved. Finally, statistical methods that account for the matched nature of the propensity score matched sample should be employed for estimating the treatment effect and its statistical significance.

Acknowledgments

The Institute for Clinical Evaluative Sciences (ICES) and the PATH Research Institute are supported in part by a grant from the Ontario Ministry of Health and Long-Term Care (MOHLTC). The opinions, results, and conclusions are those of the authors, and no endorsement by the Ministry of Health and Long-Term Care or by the Institute for Clinical Evaluative Sciences is intended or should be inferred. Dr. Austin is supported in part by a Career Investigator award from the Heart and Stroke Foundation of Ontario. Dr. Ko is supported in part by a Clinician Scientist award from the Heart and Stroke Foundation of Ontario. Dr. Tu is supported by a Tier 1 Canada Research Chair in Health Services Research and a Career Investigator award from the Heart and Stroke Foundation of Ontario. The authors wish to acknowledge the Ontario Health Technology Advisory Committee (OHTAC) for funding support for the comparative stent study in Ontario. The authors acknowledge that the clinical registry data used in this chapter are from the Cardiac Care Network of Ontario and its member hospitals. The Cardiac Care Network of Ontario serves as an advisory body to the MOHLTC and is dedicated to improving the quality, efficiency, access, and equity in the delivery of the continuum of adult cardiac services in Ontario, Canada. The Cardiac Care Network of Ontario is funded by the MOHLTC.

References

Agresti, A., and Y. Min. 2004. "Effects and non-effects of paired identical observations in comparing proportions with binary matched-pairs data." *Statistics in Medicine*. 23: 65–75.

Austin, P. C. 2007a. Propensity-score matching in the cardiovascular surgery literature from 2004 to 2006: a systematic review and suggestions for improvement." *Journal of Thoracic and Cardiovascular Surgery* 134: 1128–1135.

Austin, P. C. 2007b. "The performance of different propensity score methods for estimating marginal odds ratios." *Statistics in Medicine* 26: 3078–3094.

Austin, P. C. 2008a. "Assessing balance in baseline covariates when using many-to-one propensity-score matching." *Pharmacoepidemiology and Drug Safety* 17: 1218–1225.

Austin, P. C. 2008b. "A critical appraisal of propensity-score matching in the medical literature between 1996 and 2003." *Statistics in Medicine* 27 (12): 2037–2049.

Austin, P. C. 2008c. "The performance of different propensity-score methods for estimating relative risks. *Journal of Clinical Epidemiology* 61 (6): 537–545.

Austin, P. C. 2008d. "Primer on statistical interpretation or methods report card on propensity-score matching in the cardiology literature from 2004 to 2006: A systematic review." *Circulation: Cardiovascular Quality and Outcomes* 1(1): 62–67.

Austin, P. C. 2009a. "Some methods of propensity-score matching had superior performance to others: results of an empirical investigation and Monte Carlo simulations." *Biometrical Journal* 51: 171–184.

Austin, P.C. 2009b. "Balance diagnostics for comparing the distribution of baseline covariates between treatment groups in propensity-score matched samples." *Statistics in Medicine* 28: 3083-3107.

Austin, P.C. 2009c. "Type 1 Error Rates, Coverage of Confidence Intervals, and Variance Estimation in Propensity-score Matched Analyses." *The International Journal of Biostatistics* 5: Article 13. DOI: 10.2202/1557-4679.1146.

Austin, P.C. 2009d. "The relative ability of different propensity-score methods to balance measured covariates between treated and untreated subjects in observational studies." *Medical Decision Making* 29:661-677.

Austin, P. C., and M. M. Mamdani. 2006. "A comparison of propensity score methods: a case-study estimating the effectiveness of post-AMI statin use." *Statistics in Medicine*. 25: 2084–2106.

Austin, P. C., M. M. Mamdani, D. N. Juurlink, and J. E. Hux. 2006. "Testing multiple statistical hypotheses resulted in spurious associations: a study of astrological signs and health." *Journal of Clinical Epidemiology* 59: 964–969.

Austin, P. C., M. M. Mamdani, T. A. Stukel, G. M. Anderson, and J. V. Tu. 2005. "The use of the propensity score for estimating treatment effects: administrative versus clinical data." *Statistics in Medicine*. 24: 1563–1578.

Austin, P. C., P. Grootendorst, and G. M. Anderson. 2007a. "A comparison of the ability of eifferent propensity score models to balance measured variables between treated and untreated subjects: a Monte Carlo study." *Statistics in Medicine* 26: 734–753.

Austin, P. C., P. Grootendorst, S. L. T. Normand, and G. M. Anderson. 2007b. "Conditioning on the propensity score can result in biased estimation of common measures of treatment effect: a Monte Carlo study." *Statistics in Medicine* 26: 754–768.

Cochran, W. G., and D. B. Rubin. 1973. "Controlling bias in observational studies: a review." *Sankhya Series A* 35: 417–446.

Conover, W. J. 1998. *Practical Nonparametric Statistics*. 3d ed. New York: John Wiley & Sons, Inc.

Cook, R. J., and D. L. Sackett. 1995. "The number needed to treat: a clinically useful measure of treatment effect." *British Medical Journal* 310: 452–454.

Cummings, P., B. McKnight, and S. Greenland. 2003. "Matched cohort methods for injury research." *Epidemiologic Reviews* 25: 43–50.

Diggle, P. J., K. Y. Liang, S. L. Zeger, and P. Heagerty. 1994. *Analysis of Longitudinal Data*. Oxford: Oxford University Press.

Flury, B. K., and H. Riedwyl. 1986. "Standard distance in univariate and multivariate analysis." *The American Statistician* 40: 249–251.

Freemantle, N. 2001. "Interpreting the results of secondary end points and subgroup analyses in clinical trials: should we lock the crazy aunt in the attic?" *British Medical Journal* 322: 989–991.

Hansen, B.B. 2004. "Full matching in an observational study of coaching for the SAT." *Journal of the American Statistical Association* 99: 609–618.

Hansen, B. B. 2008. "The essential role of balance tests in propensity-matched observational studies: comments on 'A critical appraisal of propensity-score matching in the medical literature between 1996 and 003'." *Statistics in Medicine* 27: 2050–2054.

Hill, J., and J. P. Reiter. 2006. "Interval estimation for treatment effects using propensity score matching." *Statistics in Medicine* 25: 2230–2256.

Ho, D. E., K. Imai, G. King, and E. A. Stuart. 2007. "Matching as nonparametric preprocessing for reducing model dependence in parametric causal inference." *Political Analysis* 15: 199–236.

Imai, K., G. King, and E. A. Stuart. 2008. "Misunderstandings between experimentalists and observationalists about causal inference." *Journal of the Royal Statistical Society, Series A (Statistics in Society)* 171: 481–502.

Jaeschke, R., G. Guyatt, H. Shannon, S. Walter, D. Cook, and N. Heddle. 1995. "Basic statistics for clinicians: 3. Assessing the effects of treatment: measures of association." *Canadian Medical Association Journal* 152 (3): 351–357.

Klein, J. P., and M. L. Moeschberger. 1997. *Survival Analysis: Techniques for Censored and Truncated Data*. New York: Springer-Verlag.

Lin, D. 1989. "Goodness-of-fit tests and robust statistical inference for the Cox proportional hazards model." *Journal of the American Statistical Association* 84: 1074–1078.

Newcombe, R. G. 2006. "A deficiency of the odds ratio as a measure of effect size." *Statistics in Medicine* 25: 4235–40.

Normand, S. T., M. B. Landrum, E. Guadagnoli, et al. 2001. "Validating recommendations for coronary angiography following acute myocardial infarction in the elderly: a matched analysis using propensity scores." *Journal of Clinical Epidemiology* 54(4): 387–98.

Rosenbaum, P. R. 1987. "Model-based direct adjustment." *The Journal of the American Statistical Association* 82: 387–394.

Rosenbaum, P. R. 1995. *Observational Studies*. New York: Springer-Verlag.

Rosenbaum, P. R., and D. B. Rubin. 1983a. "The central role of the propensity score in observational studies for causal effects." *Biometrika* 70: 41–55.

Rosenbaum, P. R., and D. B. Rubin. 1983b. "Assessing sensitivity to an unobserved binary covariate in an observational study with binary outcome." *Journal of the Royal Statistical Society, B (StatisticalMethodology)* 45: 212–218.

Rosenbaum, P. R., and D. B. Rubin. 1984. "Reducing bias in observational studies using subclassification on the propensity score." *Journal of the American Statistical Association* 79: 516–524.

Rosenbaum, P. R., and D. B. Rubin. 1985. "Constructing a control group using multivariate matched sampling methods that incorporate the propensity score." *The American Statistician* 39: 33–38.

Rothman, K. J. 1977. "Epidemiologic methods in clinical trials." *Cancer* 39 (S4): 1771–1775.

Rothman, K. J., and S. Greenland. 1998. *Modern Epidemiology*. Philadelphia, PA: Lippincott Williams & Wilkins.

Rothwell, P. M. 2005. "Treating individuals 2: Subgroup analysis in randomised controlled trials: importance, indications, and interpretation." The *Lancet* 365: 176–186.

Rubin, D. B. 2004. "On principles for modeling propensity scores in medical research." *Pharmacoepidemiology and Drug Safety* 13(12): 855–857.

Schechtman, E. 2002. "Odds ratio, relative risk, absolute risk reduction, and the number needed to treat—which of these should we use?" *Value in Health* 5(5): 431–436.

Senn, S. 1994. "Testing for baseline balance in clinical trials." *Statistics in Medicine* 13: 1715–1726.

Senn, S. J. 1989. "Covariate imbalance and random allocation in clinical trials." *Statistics in Medicine* 8: 467–475.

Sinclair, J. C., M. B. Bracken. 1994. "Clinically useful measures of effect in binary analyses of randomized trials." *Journal of Clinical Epidemiology* 47(8): 881–889.

Therneau, T. M., and P. M. Grambsch. 2001. *Modeling Survival Data: Extending the Cox Model*. New York: Springer-Verlag.

Tu, J. V., J. Bowen, M. Chiu, D. T. Ko, P. C. Austin, Y. He, R. Hopkins, J. Tarride, G. Blackhouse, C. Lazzam, E. A. Cohen, and R. Goeree. 2007. "Effectiveness and safety of drug-eluting stents in Ontario." The *New England Journal of Medicine* 357(14): 1393–1402.

Weitzen, S., K. L. Lapane, A. Y. Toledano, A. L. Hume, and V. Mor. 2005. "Weakness of goodness-of-fit tests for evaluating propensity score models: the case of the omitted confounder." *Pharmacoepidemiolgy and Drug Safety* 14(4): 227–238.

Chapter 4

Doubly Robust Estimation of Treatment Effects

Michele Jonsson Funk
Daniel Westreich
Chris Weisen
Marie Davidian

Abstract

Estimation of the effect of a treatment or exposure with a causal interpretation from studies where exposure is not randomized may be biased if confounding is not taken into appropriate account. Adjustment for confounding is often carried out through regression modeling of the relationships among treatment, confounders, and outcome. Doubly robust (DR) estimation produces a consistent effect estimator as long as one of two component regression models is correctly specified and assuming that there are no unmeasured confounders, giving the analyst two chances to correctly specify at least one of the regression models. In this chapter, we provide a brief introduction to DR estimators; present sample code using a SAS macro; illustrate the use of the macro with results from analyses of simulated data; and discuss issues including interpretation of estimates, assumptions, and limitations of this approach.

4.1 Introduction

Correct specification of the regression model is one of the most fundamental assumptions in statistical analysis. In an observational data analysis, it is common to estimate the causal effect of treatment using a regression model for the relationship between outcome, treatment, and confounders. Even when all relevant confounders have been measured, an unbiased estimator for the causal treatment effect can be obtained only if the model itself reflects the true relationship among treatment, confounders, and outcome. This is the case for a typical analysis in which the outcome is modeled as a function of exposure and covariates as well as propensity score-based methods, in which the exposure is modeled as a function of covariates. Outside of simulation studies, we can never know whether or not the model we have constructed accurately depicts those relationships. Thus, correct specification of the regression model is an unverifiable assumption. The DR estimator does not eliminate the need for such an assumption but does give the analyst two chances to satisfy it.

4.1.1 Conceptual Overview

Doubly robust (DR) estimation builds on the propensity score approach of Rosenbaum and Rubin (1983) and the inverse probability of weighting (IPW) approach of Robins and colleagues (Robins, 1998; Robins, 1999a; Robins, 1999b; Robins et al., 2000). DR estimation combines inverse probability weighting by a propensity score with regression modeling of the relationship between covariates and outcome for each treatment. It combines it in such a way that, as long as *either* the propensity score model *or* the outcome regression models are correctly specified, the effect of the exposure on the outcome will be correctly estimated, assuming that there are no unmeasured confounders (Robins et al., 1994; Robins, 2000; van der Laan and Robins, 2003; Bang and Robins, 2005). Specifically, one builds and fits a (binary) regression model for the probability that a particular patient received a given treatment as a function of that individual's covariates (the propensity score). Maximum likelihood regression is conducted separately within the exposed and unexposed populations to predict the mean response (outcome) as a function of confounders and risk factors. (These two sets of models are visually represented in Figure 4.1.) Finally, each individual observation is given a weight equal to the inverse of the probability of the treatment he/she received based on baseline covariates (as in IPW analysis) to create two pseudopopulations of subjects that represent the expected response in the entire population under those two treatment conditions. Results from simulations confirm that the estimator is consistent when an important confounder is omitted entirely from one of the two models (Lunceford and Davidian, 2004; Bang and Robins, 2005) and, in more realistic scenarios, when one of the component models is misspecified by categorizing a continuous variable when the true relation with the outcome is a function of the continuous form (Jonsson Funk and Westreich, 2008).

Figure 4.1 Component Models of the DR Estimator

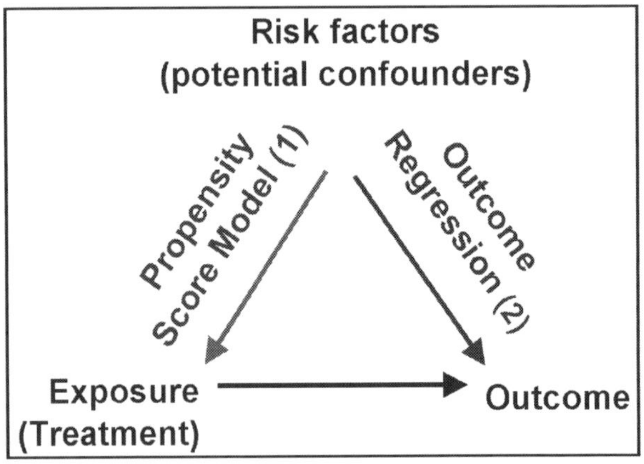

The DR estimator is an alternative to the usual approach of estimating the causal treatment effect based on a regression model for the relationships among the outcome and covariates and treatment (or using standard propensity scoring adjustment methods). If the outcome regression model is correctly specified, then the estimator for the causal effect will be at least as precise asymptotically as the DR estimator. However, if the outcome regression is misspecified, the resulting causal effect estimator need not be consistent for the true casual effect. The DR estimator is consistent if either the propensity score or treatment-specific outcome regression models are correct; thus, one trades a possible loss of precision in using the DR estimator for this additional protection.

The DR effect estimates have a marginal, rather than a conditional (on covariates), interpretation and are directly comparable to the effect estimates that one would obtain from a randomized trial in which a population is randomly assigned to receive treatment. Because the estimates from a standard outcome regression model have a conditional interpretation, the two estimates might not agree simply because they are averaging the effect in two different target populations. In particular, this could arise in the presence of effect measure modification (Kurth et al., 2006) or due to the non-collapsibility of the effect estimate (Stürmer et al., 2006; Petersen et al., 2006).

4.1.2 Statistical Expression and Assumptions

We use the following notation: Y is the observed response or outcome, Z is a binary treatment (exposure) variable taking values 0 or 1, and X represents a vector of baseline covariates. Y_1 and Y_0 are the counterfactual responses under treatment and no treatment, respectively (Hernán, 2004). All of these variables are further subscripted by i for subjects i=1, ..., n. In this example, the causal effect of interest is the difference in means if everyone in the population received treatment versus everyone not receiving treatment, or $\Delta=E(Y_1)-E(Y_0)$. In the following equation, $e(X,\beta)$ is a postulated model for the true propensity score (from logistic regression), and $m_0(X,\alpha_0)$ and $m_1(X,\alpha_1)$ are postulated regression models for the true relationship between the vector of covariates (confounders plus other prognostic factors) and the outcome within each stratum of treatment. With these definitions, the estimator of the causal effect is:

$$\hat{\Delta}_{DR} = n^{-1}\sum_{i=1}^{n}\Bigg[\underbrace{\frac{Z_iY_i}{e(X_i,\hat{\beta})}}_{\text{IPTW Estimator}} - \underbrace{\frac{\{Z_i - e(X_i,\hat{\beta})\}}{e(X_i,\hat{\beta})}m_1(X_i,\hat{\alpha}_1)}_{\text{"Augmentation"}}\Bigg] - n^{-1}\sum_{i=1}^{n}\Bigg[\underbrace{\frac{(1-Z_i)Y_i}{1-e(X_i,\hat{\beta})}}_{\text{IPTW Estimator}} - \underbrace{\frac{\{Z_i - e(X_i,\hat{\beta})\}}{1-e(X_i,\hat{\beta})}m_0(X_i,\hat{\alpha}_0)}_{\text{"Augmentation"}}\Bigg]$$

$$= \hat{\mu}_{1,DR} - \hat{\mu}_{0,DR}$$

The standard error for the DR estimator is estimated using the delta method (Casella and Berger, 2002). The sampling variance for the DR estimator is calculated as:

$$SE_{\hat{\Delta}_{DR}} = \sqrt{n^{-2}\sum_{i=1}^{n}\hat{I}_i^2}$$

where $\hat{I}_i$ is defined as follows:

$$\hat{I}_i = \left[\frac{Z_iY_i}{e(X_i,\hat{\beta})} - \frac{\{Z_i - e(X_i,\hat{\beta})\}}{e(X_i,\hat{\beta})}m_1(X_i,\hat{\alpha}_1)\right] - \left[\frac{(1-Z_i)Y_i}{1-e(X_i,\hat{\beta})} + \frac{\{Z_i - e(X_i,\hat{\beta})\}}{1-e(X_i,\hat{\beta})}m_0(X_i,\hat{\alpha}_0)\right] - \hat{\Delta}_{DR}$$

The DR estimator is consistent for the true value of Δ if the following assumptions are satisfied: 1) no unmeasured confounding (also called the *assumption of exchangeability*); 2) correct specification of at least one of the two component models; 3) positivity (the true propensity score is bounded away from 0 and 1 so that there is always a positive probability of receiving both treatments under any combination of covariates); and 4) stable unit treatment value (SUTVA) (Rubin, 1980), comprising consistency and no interference (Cox, 1958). The delta method standard error is appropriate when the sample size is sufficiently large and when both the propensity score model and the outcome regression models have been correctly specified. For reporting estimates from an analysis of data where the true propensity score and outcome regression models are not known and may have been misspecified, standard errors should be obtained using the bootstrap.

4.2 Implementation with the DR Macro

While several estimators have been found to have the doubly robust property (Robins et al., 2007), we will describe the augmented IPW estimator identified by Robins and colleagues (1994) that was subsequently recognized to be doubly robust (Scharfstein et al., 1999). This DR estimator has been implemented in a macro developed at the University of North Carolina at Chapel Hill for use with Base SAS (validated with SAS 9.1.3). The DR macro can be downloaded from the Resources section of http://harryguess.unc.edu/sas.htm along with the sample data. This chapter reflects the features of the macro as of version 1.0. Please review the readme file (ReadMe.pdf) for important information regarding setup and installation as well as updated details of features prior to use.

4.2.1 Getting Started

The DR macro runs two sets of models: one for the probability of receiving a dichotomous treatment or exposure (the propensity score) and another to predict either the probability of the outcome (for a dichotomous outcome) or its mean value (for a continuous outcome) within strata of the exposure (treatment-specific outcome regression models). We describe the general syntax for each model statement, the use of optional commands, and the resulting output in the following sections.

4.2.2 Specifying the Weight Model

The general weight (or propensity score) model is specified in the first MODEL statement using the form:

```
wtmodel exposure = <covariates> / method=dr dist=bin <other options>
```

We model the main exposure or treatment on the left side of the equal sign as a function of the covariates on the right side. `Method=dr` indicates that the DR estimation method should be used, while `dist=bin` indicates that this is a binary exposure. Therefore, logistic regression will be used to model the relationship between the covariates and the exposure.

The weight model should be specified with the same care and rigor that you would use in the specification of any other IPW or propensity score model based on substantive knowledge. Brookhart and colleagues (2006) have found that the propensity score (exposure) model should include all confounders as well as those covariates that are risk factors for the outcome.

`Z`
: is the Z score based on the delta method standard error.

`ProbZ`
: is the two-tailed probability that `deltadr=0` based on the Z score. Like the estimated standard error and Z score, this *p* value should be reported only when the weight and outcome regression models are known to be correctly specified.

Program 4.5 shows the related SAS code.

Program 4.5 Excerpt of SAS Code from DR Macro v1.0 for Calculation of DR Estimate of the Mean Difference Due to Exposure and Estimated Standard Error

```
/* combine M0 and M1 */
      data _modres01_(keep=&expvar &resvar __ps __m0 __m1 __exp01 __res01);
        merge _ps_ _modres0_ _modres1_;
        %if ("&desc"="") %then %do;
            __ps=1-__ps;
              __m0=1-__m0;
              __m1=1-__m1;
        %end;
      run;

/* create DR0 and DR1 and their difference DR1_DR0 statistics */
      data _dr01_;
        set _modres01_;
        dr0=((1-__exp01)*__res01+(__exp01-__ps)*__m0)/(1-__ps);
        dr1=(__exp01*__res01-(__exp01-__ps)*__m1)/__ps;
        dr1_dr0=dr1-dr0;
    run;

/* obtain mean, variance and n of difference DR1_DR0 */
/* and the means of DR0 and DR1 */
      proc means noprint data=_dr01_ vardef=n;
        var dr1_dr0 dr0 dr1;
        output out=_mdr01_(drop=_type_) mean=deltadr dr0 dr1 var=i2 vdr0 vdr1
n=__n;
      run;

/* get the SE of the difference */
/* and the two variance components */
      data _mdr01_;
        merge _mdr01_;
        SEdeltadr=sqrt(i2/__n);
        vdr0=vdr0/__n;
        vdr1=vdr1/__n;
      run;
```

In the case of a dichotomous outcome, a separate table with parameter estimates is displayed in the output. The following parameters, with their standard errors, Z scores and *p* values, are displayed. Program 4.6 shows the relevant SAS code.

`LogRiskRatio`
: The natural log of the risk ratio. Exponentiating this value returns the risk ratio.

`LogOddsRatio`
: The natural log of the odds ratio. Exponentiating this value returns the odds ratio.

Program 4.6 Excerpt of SAS Code from DR Macro v1.0 for Calculation of DR Estimates of the Mean Difference, Log Relative Risk, Log Odds Ratio, and Estimated Standard Errors

```
/* if the distribution of the response is binary */
/* get the ratio and the standard error of the ratio */
   %if (&mdist=BINOMIAL or &mdist=B or &mdist=BIN) %then %do;

      /* obtain the 2 variances and the covariance */
      ods listing close;
      proc corr cov data=_dr01_ vardef=n;
       var dr0 dr1;
        ods output cov=_cov_;
      run;
      ods listing;
      data _cov_;
        set _cov_;
        if _n_=1 then do;
          v0=dr0;
            v01=dr1;
        end;
        else do;
          v1=dr1;
         keep v0 v1 v01;
         output;
        end;
        retain v0 v01;
      run;

/* risk ratio, odds ratio and standard errors */

/* combine the covariance information with the means information */
/* get the variance estimates of some functions of the means */
      data _mdr01_;
        merge _mdr01_ _cov_;
/* derivatives */
/* log odds */
        alo=(1/(dr1*(1-dr1)));
        blo=(-1/(dr0*(1-dr0)));
/* mean difference */
        am=1;
        bm=-1;
/* log risk ratio */
        alrr=1/dr1;
        blrr=-1/dr0;
/* log odds ratio and log risk ratio */
         LogOddsRatio=log((dr1*(1-dr0))/((1-dr1)*dr0));
         LogRiskRatio=log(dr1/dr0);
/* special for DESCENDING */
         %if "&desc"="" %then %do;
           LogOddsRatio=-1*logoddsratio;
           LogRiskRatio=-1*logriskratio;
         %end;
/* standard error estimates */
    SELogOddsRatio=sqrt((alo*alo*v1+blo*blo*v0+2*alo*blo*v01)/__n);
        SEMeanDifference=sqrt((am*am*v1+bm*bm*v0+2*am*bm*v01)/__n);

SELogRiskRatio=sqrt((alrr*alrr*v1+blrr*blrr*v0+2*alrr*blrr*v01)/__n);
         drop alo blo am bm alrr blrr v0 v1 v01;
      run;
  %end;
```

4.3 Sample Analysis

4.3.1 Introduction to Sample Data

The examples presented here are based on a simulated observational cohort with 10,000 individuals. The main exposure is statin initiation at baseline (statin, p[statin=1]=0.51). The main outcomes are rmi1a (mean=-10.7, sd=4.7), which represents the change in lipid levels between the baseline and a follow-up visit, and mi1 (p[mi1=1]=0.19), which represents the occurrence of an acute myocardial infarction during the follow-up period for the cohort. The data set is structured as one record or observation per person with the individuals represented in rows. Because these data are simulated, we know the true causal effect of the exposure on the outcomes as well as the true relationships between the covariates and the exposure and between the covariates and the outcomes. In both cases, the true effect of statin use on the outcomes is null. While the true mean response for the continuous outcome in each treatment group is negative (representing a decrease in lipid levels at follow-up relative to the baseline), these are simulated data and the methods described here apply equally to an outcome with a mean positive value. The association between the exposure and the outcomes is confounded by seven variables, four continuous (Age, BMI, Chol, and Exer) and three dichotomous (Hs, Smk, and Hxcvd). In addition, there is one variable that is a risk factor only for the outcome (Female) and two variables that are risk factors only for the exposure (Black and Income).

To run these example analyses, download the simulated study data set from http://harryguess.unc.edu/sas.htm and create a libname for SampleData that points to the appropriate directory on your computer.

4.3.2 DR Analysis of a Continuous Outcome

This example represents an analysis of simulated data where the exposure of interest is statin use (statin) and the outcome of interest is a continuous cardiovascular disease score (rmi1a). The true effect of statin use on the outcome is null. Both the weight (propensity score) model and the regression model are specified correctly in this analysis (see Program 4.7):

Program 4.7 Call to DR Macro v1.0 for Analysis of rmi1a Outcome

```
title 'Continuous Example';
%dr(%str(options data=sampledata.study descending;
       wtmodel statin=hs smk hxcvd black bmi age income chol exer
         / method=dr dist=bin showcurves common_support=.99;
model rmi1a=hs female smk hxcvd bmi bmi2 age age2 chol exer /dist=n;)
);
```

The first component of the output is the usual SAS output from a logistic regression model (Program 4.1). From this, we can confirm the total number of observations and that the probability modeled is `statin=1`. These results also allow the analyst to identify covariates that are strongly associated with exposure and assess the fit of the model.

Output Node from rmi1a Analysis: Logistic Weight Model

```
                         The LOGISTIC Procedure

                            Response Profile

                    Ordered                          Total
                      Value        statin        Frequency

                          1        Yes                5073
                          2        No                 4927

                  Probability modeled is statin='Yes'.
...more results...

                Analysis of Maximum Likelihood Estimates

                                          Standard          Wald
          Parameter    DF    Estimate        Error    Chi-Square    Pr > ChiSq

          Intercept     1     -8.0728       0.2589      972.0943        <.0001
          hs            1      0.3587       0.0457       61.7075        <.0001
          smk           1     -0.4534       0.0529       73.4696        <.0001
          hxcvd         1      0.9101       0.0563      260.9287        <.0001
          black         1     -0.6783       0.0489      192.5989        <.0001
          bmi           1      0.0567      0.00460      152.1308        <.0001
          age           1      0.0590      0.00328      323.4639        <.0001
          income        1    6.171E-6     1.141E-6       29.2467        <.0001
          chol          1      0.0181     0.000599      916.7678        <.0001
          exer          1     0.00789     0.000917       74.0638        <.0001

...more results...
          Association of Predicted Probabilities and Observed Responses

                  Percent Concordant          77.8    Somers' D    0.557
                  Percent Discordant          22.1    Gamma        0.558
                  Percent Tied                 0.2    Tau-a        0.279
                  Pairs                   24994671    c            0.779
```

The next node in the results pane presents the mean, standard deviation, and minimum and maximum predicted probabilities (or propensity scores) stratified by exposure group. This allows the analyst to check the assumption of positivity. This assumption states that for each combination of characteristics, there must be a non-zero probability of being exposed and unexposed (Cole and Hernán, 2008). In the event that positivity is violated, consider whether this is a case of structural nonpositivity, in which it is not possible for individuals with a particular combination of characteristics to receive one of the exposures. Instances of structural nonpositivity suggest that these observations should not be included in the analysis. There may also be cases of random nonpositivity, particularly when some covariates are continuous. The regression models smooth over these instances of nonpositivity, but it is helpful to investigate the sensitivity of the findings to violation of the positivity assumption.

Output Node from rmi1a Analysis: Descriptive Statistics for Exposure Probability

```
        Descriptive Statistics For Exposure Probability
                        by Exposure Group

                                 Standard
statin          Mean            Deviation         Minimum        Maximum

 No           0.38962          0.21121          0.014905       0.96883
 Yes          0.62159          0.21006          0.037478       0.98576
```

The SHOWCURVES option produces a histogram that compares the distributions of the propensity score for the two levels of exposure with a nonparametric smoothed curve overlaid (see Figure 4.2, produced by Program 4.2). This allows the analyst to visually assess the degree to which there are unexposed individuals who can serve as counterfactuals for those who were exposed and vice versa.

Output Node from rmi1a Analysis: Propensity Score Curves Stratified by Exposure

Figure 4.2 Estimated Propensity Score Distributions Stratified by Exposure with Nonparametric Smoothed Curve

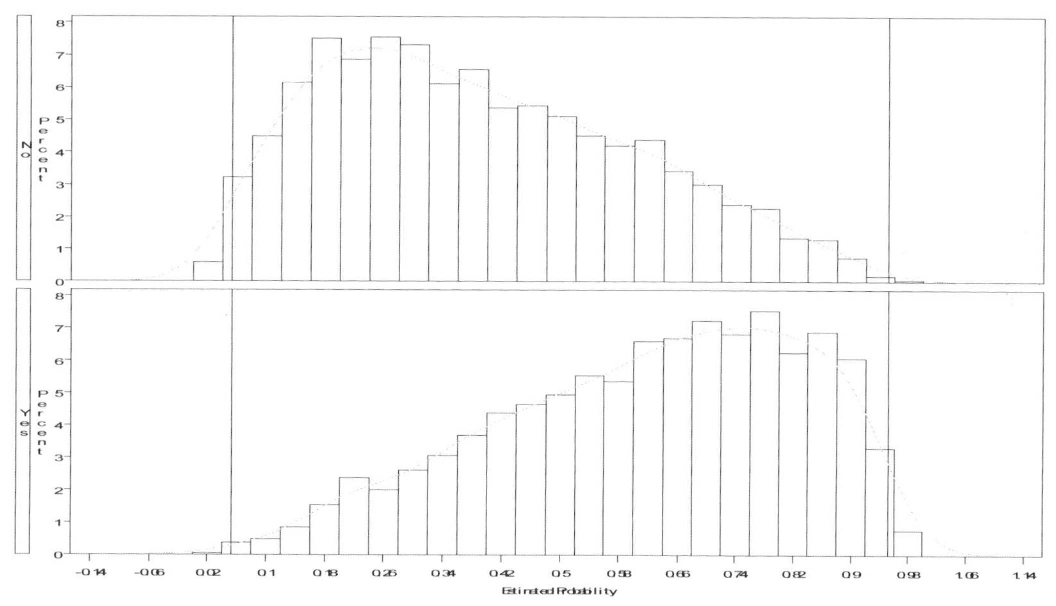

The COMMON_SUPPORT option directs the outcome regression model to trim off observations that lie at the extreme ends of the propensity score distribution in order to support sensitivity analyses.[1] Using `common_support=0.99`, the regression models are limited to those observations with a propensity score between the 0.5th percentile and the 99.5th percentile. The vertical dashed lines in Figure 4.2 indicate the boundaries for this portion of the data.

[1] We have used it in this example only to demonstrate its application. There is no indication that it is needed in these data based on the good overlap across the full range of the propensity score distributions.

The following two nodes present the results of linear regression within the unexposed (`statin=0`) and exposed (`statin=1`, not shown) groups, respectively (Program 4.3). The number of observations used may be less than the total number of observations in the data set (the number of observations read). In this example, there are 9,858 total observations rather than 10,000 because of the use of the COMMON_SUPPORT option, of which 4,857 (out of the original 4,927) were in the unexposed group and, therefore, contribute to the outcome regression among the unexposed (shown here). In addition, observations without complete data for all covariates are excluded in a case-wise deletion manner.

Output Nodes from rmi1a Analysis: Observation Information for Exposure=0 and GLM Outcome Model for Exposure=0

```
          Statin=0
                                  The GLM Procedure

                        Number of Observations Read          9858
                        Number of Observations Used          4857

<some results omitted here save space>

                                                  Standard
Parameter           Estimate              Error    t Value    Pr > |t|

Intercept       -35.24558550         0.63717979     -55.31      <.0001
hs               -0.96761996         0.02874527     -33.66      <.0001
female            1.50190505         0.02936782      51.14      <.0001
smk               2.02010820         0.03152377      64.08      <.0001
hxcvd             2.01384495         0.03986875      50.51      <.0001
bmi               0.12632269         0.02201941       5.74      <.0001
bmi2              0.00951336         0.00041793      22.76      <.0001
age               0.07753889         0.02195693       3.53      0.0004
age2              0.00121005         0.00020904       5.79      <.0001
chol              0.05018018         0.00036380     137.93      <.0001
exer             -0.02076545         0.00058327     -35.60      <.0001
```

Finally, under the node labeled `Print: DR Estimate`, we find the results of interest (Program 4.5). Again, the number of observations under `Used Obs` may be less than the total number of observations in the event of missing data for some observations for some covariates and/or use of the COMMON_SUPPORT option in the MACRO statement. Under `Modeled Mean for Statin=0`, we find the estimated mean response if all subjects in this cohort had been *unexposed* (`statin=0`) and, likewise under `Modeled Mean for Statin=1`, the estimated mean response if all subjects in this cohort had been *exposed* (`statin=1`). The doubly robust estimate (deltadr) of the average treatment effect (also known as the mean difference due to treatment) when we have specified both models correctly is a difference of 0.00 with a standard error of 0.02, a *p* value of 0.87, and a 95% confidence interval of -0.04 to 0.05 (calculated using the estimated standard error for the delta DR).

Output Node from rmi1a Analysis: DR Estimate

DR Estimates

Total Obs	Used Obs	Modeled Mean for STATIN=0	Modeled Mean for STATIN=1	deltadr	SEdeltadr	Z	Probz
10000	9858	-10.6783	-10.6744	.003914308	0.023986	0.16319	0.87037

Results from a standard linear outcome regression model including treatment and all covariates can be obtained, for comparison, using the following SAS code:

Program 4.8 Standard Linear Regression Model

```
proc reg data=sampledata.study;
model rmi1a=statin hs female smk hxcvd bmi bmi2 age age2 chol exer;
run;
```

Results from this model are shown here. The mean difference due to statin use conditional on all other covariates in a single linear regression model is -0.01, similar to the DR estimate. The standard error of the DR estimate (0.024) is slightly greater than that from the single linear regression model (0.022), as we would expect. Recall that the DR estimate used a sample in which some observations at the extreme were trimmed, so these are not strictly comparable estimates.

Output from Program 4.8—Standard Linear Regression Model

Parameter Estimates

Variable	DF	Parameter Estimate	Standard Error	t Value	Pr > |t|
Intercept	1	-34.70314	0.43740	-79.34	<.0001
statin	1	-0.01064	0.02229	-0.48	0.6333
hs	1	-0.96683	0.01994	-48.48	<.0001
female	1	1.51607	0.02032	74.60	<.0001
smk	1	2.02120	0.02303	87.76	<.0001
hxcvd	1	2.00006	0.02412	82.93	<.0001
bmi	1	0.10456	0.01507	6.94	<.0001
bmi2	1	0.00989	0.00027799	35.57	<.0001
age	1	0.06559	0.01463	4.48	<.0001
age2	1	0.00133	0.00013566	9.77	<.0001
chol	1	0.05039	0.00024814	203.06	<.0001
exer	1	-0.02034	0.00039787	-51.13	<.0001

4.3.3 DR Analysis of a Dichotomous Outcome

The second example represents an analysis of simulated data where the exposure of interest is statin use (`statin`) and the outcome of interest is a dichotomous variable indicating whether the subject experienced a myocardial infarction within the follow-up period (`mi1`). Both the weight (propensity score) model and the regression model are specified correctly:

Program 4.9 Call to DR Macro v1.0 for Analysis of mi1 Outcome

```
title 'Dichotomous Example';
%dr(%str(options data=sampledata.study descending;
      wtmodel statin=hs smk hxcvd black bmi age income chol exer
         / method=dr dist=bin showcurves;
model mi1=hs female smk hxcvd bmi bmi2 age age2 chol exer /dist=bin;
) );
```

As before, the first node in the results pane includes the complete output from the logistic regression model for the propensity score model. Because we specified the SHOWCURVES option, a graph of the two propensity score distributions is also produced. The results are identical because the same exposure and covariates were specified as in the previous example. There are two additional logistic regression nodes: the first for the model of the predicted response among the exposed and the second among the unexposed, respectively. The results of interest appear under the `Print: DR estimates` node (Program 4.6). These results include DR estimates of the risk (or probability) of the outcome had everyone in the population been untreated (dr0) or treated (dr1), the risk difference (delta DR), the log risk ratio, and the log odds ratio. In addition, the standard errors, Z score, and p value for each parameter are provided.

Output Node from mi1 Analysis: DR Estimate

```
     Sample size and DR Estimates

                         Modeled       Modeled
Total       Used        Mean for      Mean for
 Obs        Obs         STATIN=0      STATIN=1

10000      10000        0.19032       0.19540



                            Parameter Estimates

Parameter              Estimate       StdError         Z           ProbZ

Delta DR               0.005081       0.005667      0.89660       0.36993
Log Risk Ratio         0.026347       0.029545      0.89174       0.37253
Log Odds Ratio         0.032641       0.036556      0.89292       0.37190
```

Due to the noncollapsibility of the odds ratio, it is not particularly meaningful to compare the DR estimate of the odds ratio to that from a typical logistic regression model. Instead, we compare the DR estimate of the risk ratio to the risk ratio estimated using the GENMOD procedure (Spiegelman and Hertzmark, 2005). (Poisson regression is used in this case because of problems with convergence of binomial regression.)

Program 4.10 Analysis of mi1 Using Poisson Regression Model

```
title 'Estimate of RR using Poisson Regression';
proc genmod data=sampledata.study descending;
    class i;
    model mi1=statin hs female smk hxcvd bmi bmi2 age age2 chol exer
/dist=poisson link=log;
    repeated subject=i/type=ind;
    estimate 'log RR statin' statin 1/exp;
run;
```

The estimate of logrRR (0.12) is further from the true null value than the DR estimator (0.03), and the standard error of the logRR from Poisson regression is less efficient (0.04 vs. 0.03).

Output from Program 4.10—Poisson Regression Model

```
                              Contrast Estimate Results

                             Standard                                               Chi-
Label               Estimate Error       Alpha  Confidence  Limits      Square     Pr > ChiSq

Log RR statin         0.1151 0.0402      0.05   0.0363      0.1939      8.20        0.0042
Exp(log RR statin)    1.1220 0.0451      0.05   1.0370      1.2140
```

In the examples provided, the true forms of the propensity score and outcome regression models are used, but one can also explore the robustness of this method by intentionally misspecifying one of the two models using these sample data.

4.4 Summary

Given that we rarely know the true relations among exposures, outcomes, and confounders, the DR estimator is a potentially valuable tool for obtaining more robust effect estimates in observational studies of the effects (intended and unintended) of drugs, devices, and other interventions. The SAS macro described here makes this method relatively straightforward to apply to real-world analyses. But given the relative novelty of this estimator, we suggest that researchers take an especially careful approach to this type of analysis, with particular consideration of the method's limitations, the SAS macro's implementation in particular, and a variety of issues that remain under active debate. Given that this is a relatively new approach, we suggest using this method along with a more traditional bias adjustment approach as a sensitivity analysis.

4.4.1 Limitations

While the DR estimator provides the analyst with two chances to specify a regression model correctly, it still requires assumptions common to most regression models for causal effect estimation. While some of these can be verified, the most critical assumption of no unmeasured confounders is unverifiable. One of the two models must be correctly specified for the estimator to remain consistent, which means that all confounders must have been measured in order to be included in at least one of the models. In the event that neither model is correct, the estimator is no longer consistent and is not necessarily closer to the true effect than that from a single misspecified outcome regression model (Jonsson Funk and Westreich, 2008; Kang and Schafer, 2008).

Because this method reweights observations, the results can be sensitive to observations that are given a very large weight, as is the case with IPW methods more generally (Robins et al., 2000; Cole and Hernán, 2008). This can arise when an individual has a particular combination of characteristics that is almost always associated with one of the two exposure conditions. For instance, if there are 100 individuals over the age of 80 but only one of them is unexposed, that single unexposed individual will be reweighted in the final calculation of the treatment effect to count as 100 observations, making his or her outcome potentially overinfluential. In this situation, the analyst should first seek to understand which combinations of characteristics define these unusual individuals. Next, the analyst needs to make a decision based on the research question and substantive knowledge regarding whether these individuals are properly part of the population of interest. If so, then further investigations of effect measure modification would be appropriate in combination with sensitivity analyses to assess the degree to which the estimated treatment effect is sensitive to omission of individuals where there is limited positivity.

4.4.2 Practical Considerations

While there are other DR estimators and means of computing these estimators, the SAS macro for DR estimation described here has specific advantages and limitations. One advantage is that it provides estimates of the absolute risks, risk difference, and risk ratio in addition to the usual odds ratio for analyses of dichotomous outcomes. The macro also includes some built-in diagnostics to aid the analyst in evaluating the appropriateness of the propensity score (weight) model.

In terms of limitations, the current version (v1.0) is designed only to handle binary exposures and binary or continuous outcomes. In the event that there are more than two exposure groups, the analyst would need to conduct pairwise comparisons to make use of the macro. Estimated standard errors are provided for reference but appropriate estimates of the standard error and confidence limits should be obtained by bootstrapping for purposes of reporting results from original research where either the propensity score or outcome regression models may be misspecified. With respect to missing data, if a given observation has a missing value for any covariate, the individual's data will not be utilized, as is the case with most SAS procedures. While methods such as multiple imputation can be used to more adequately address missing data, the analyst will need to do so outside of the macro. Although the code used by the analyst to run the macro was designed to look much like a typical SAS procedure to improve its usability, there are some SAS conventions that are not currently recognized. Specifically, variables for interaction terms and higher order terms must be created in a DATA step—not within the MODEL statements. The CLASS statement is also not recognized and, therefore, all categorical variables should be coded using indicator variables. Other common statements such as WHERE and BY are also not recognized. Development of the macro is ongoing, so the analyst should review the documentation provided with the current version on the Web site to be aware of any changes subsequent to this publication.

4.4.3 Areas of Onoing Investigation

Doubly robust estimation is a relatively new method. As such, many questions remain to be answered about its performance in applied analyses and its optimal use. Key questions under active discussion include detecting and handling effect modification, selecting covariates for the propensity score and outcome regression models, using diagnostics, and addressing violations of the assumption of positivity.

4.5 Conclusion

Doubly robust estimation methods—which provide the analyst with two chances to correctly specify the true relationships among exposures, covariates and outcomes—are potentially valuable tools for epidemiologic research. In this chapter, we have presented a basic introduction to the method, provided specific instruction on the use of DR estimation as implemented with a

SAS macro, illustrated the use of the macro with two sample analyses of a simulated observational cohort, and discussed several issues that the analyst should take into consideration when using this approach.

References

Bang, H., and J. M. Robins. 2005. "Doubly robust estimation in missing data and causal inference models." *Biometrics* 61(4): 962–973.

Brookhart, M. A., S. Schneeweiss, K. J. Rothman, R. J. Glynn, J. Avorn, and T. Stürmer. 2006. "Variable selection for propensity score models." *American Journal of Epidemiology* 163(12): 1149–1156.

Casella, G., and R. L. Berger. 2001. *Statistical Inference*. Australia: Duxbury Press.

Cole, S. R., and M. A. Hernán. 2008. "Constructing inverse probability weights for marginal structural models." *American Journal of Epidemiology* 168(6): 656–64.

Cox, D. R. 1958. *Planning of Experiments*. New York: John Wiley & Sons, Inc.

Greenland, S. 2008. "Invited commentary: variable selection versus shrinkage in the control of multiple confounders." *American Journal of Epidemiology* 167(5): 523–529; discussion 530–531.

Harrell, F. E. 2001. *Regression Modeling Strategies: With Applications to Linear Models, Logistic Regression, and Survival Analysis*. New York: Springer-Verlag.

Hernán, M. A. 2004. "A definition of causal effect for epidemiological research." *Journal of Epidemiology and Community Health* 58(4): 265–71.

Jonsson Funk, M. L., and D. Westreich. 2008. "Doubly robust estimation under realistic conditions of model misspecification." *Pharmacoepidemiology and Drug Safety* 17(S1): S106.

Kang, J. D.Y., and J. L. Schafer. 2007. "Demystifying double robustness: a comparison of alternative strategies for estimating a population mean from incomplete data (with discussion)." *Statistical Science* 22(4): 523–580.

Kurth, T., A. M. Walker, R. J. Glynn, K. A. Chan, J. M. Gaziano, K. Berger, and J. M. Robins. 2006. "Results of multivariable logistic regression, propensity matching, propensity adjustment, and propensity-based weighting under conditions of nonuniform effect." *American Journal of Epidemiology* 163(3): 262–270.

Lunceford, J. K., and M. Davidian. 2004. "Stratification and weighting via the propensity score in estimation of causal treatment effects: a comparative study." *Statistics in Medicine* 23(19): 2937–2960.

Petersen, M. L., Y. Wang, M. J. van der Laan, and D. R. Bangsberg. 2006. "Assessing the effectiveness of antiretroviral adherence interventions: Using marginal structural models to replicate the findings of randomized controlled trials." *Journal of Acquired Immune Deficiency Syndromes* 43: S96–S103.

Robins, J. M. 1997. "Marginal structural models." In *ASA Proceedings* in the *Section on Bayesian Statistical Science.* Alexandria, VA: American Statistical Association, 1–10.

Robins, J. M. 1998. "Correction for non-compliance in equivalence trials." *Statistics in Medicine* 17(3): 269–302; discussion 387–389.

Robins, J. M. 1999a. "Association, causation, and marginal structural models." *Synthese* 121: 151–179.

Robins, J. M. 1999b. "Marginal structural models versus structural nested models as tools for causal inference." In *Statistical Models in Epidemiology: The Environment and Clinical Trials*. Edited by M. E. Halloran and D. Berry. IMA 116: 95–134. New York: Springer-Verlag.

Robins, J. M. 1999c. "Robust estimation in sequentially ignorable missing data and causal inference models." In *ASA Proceedings* in the *Section on Bayesian Statistical Science* 6–10.

Robins, J. M., A. Rotnitzky, and L. P. Zhao. 1994. "Estimation of regression coefficients when some of the regressors are not always observed." *Journal of the American Statistical Association* 89: 846–866.

Robins, J. M., M. A. Hernán, and B. Brumback. 2000. "Marginal structural models and causal inference in epidemiology." *Epidemiology* 11(5): 550–60.

Robins, J. M., M. Sued, Q. Lei-Gomez, and A. Rotnitzky. 2007. "Comment: Performance of double-robust estimators when 'inverse probability' weights are highly variable." *Statistical Science* 22(4): 544–559.

Rosenbaum, P. R., and D. B. Rubin. 1983. "The central role of the propensity score in observational studies for causal effects." *Biometrika* 70: 41–55.

Rubin, D. B. 1980. Comments on "Randomization analysis of experimental data in the Fisher randomization test." *Journal of the American Statistical Association* 75: 591–593.

Scharfstein, D. O., A. Rotnitzky, and J. Robins. 1999. "Adjusting for nonignorable drop-out using semiparametric nonresponse models." *Journal of the American Statistical Association* 94: C/R)1121–1146.

Spiegelman, D., and E. Hertzmark. 2005. "Easy SAS calculations for risk or prevalence ratios and differences." *American Journal of Epidemiology* 162: 199–200.

Stefanski, L. A., and D. D. Boos. 2002. "The calculus of M-estimation." *The American Statistician* 56: 29–38.

Stürmer, T., K. J. Rothman, and R. J. Glynn. 2006. "Insights into different results from different causal contrasts in the presence of effect-measure modification." *Pharmacoepidemiology and Drug Safety* 15(10): 698–709.

van der Laan, M. J., and J. M. Robins. 2003. *Unified Methods for Censored and Longitudinal Data and Causality*. New York: Springer-Verlag.

Chapter 5

Propensity Scoring with Missing Values

Yongming Qu
Ilya Lipkovich

Abstract

Propensity scores have been used widely as a bias reduction method to estimate the treatment effect in nonrandomized studies. Because many covariates are generally included in the model for estimating propensity scores, the proportion of subjects with at least one missing covariate can be relatively large. In this chapter, we review existing methods for estimating propensity scores when missing values are present. The methods include a complete covariate (CC) method, an indicator variable (IND) method, various multiple imputation (MI) methods, a missingness pattern (MP) method, and a multiple imputation missingness pattern (MIMP) method. We provide SAS programs to implement all five methods for a data set from a clinical study in osteoporosis. We also provide a SAS macro for pooling small patterns of missing data to increase the stability and efficiency of MP and MIMP estimators. Because estimation may be sensitive to model misspecification for imputation and/or propensity score estimation as well as to the tuning parameters of associated algorithms, we also suggest various sensitivity analyses.

5.1 Introduction

Observational studies are becoming increasingly important because they allow us to observe treatment outcomes for large numbers of subjects in real-world treatment practice. Well-designed observational studies could provide valuable information to enhance information from randomized controlled trials (Concato, Shah, and Horwitz, 2000). The propensity score concepts introduced by Rosenbaum and Rubin (1983) are tools for estimating causal effects of alternative treatments in the presence of imbalance in baseline covariate (*X*) distributions between treatment groups due to lack of randomization.

Let T denote a binary treatment group indicator. Throughout this chapter, we restrict attention to only two treatment groups, with T=0 indicating the reference treatment group and T=1 indicating the investigational or active treatment group. The propensity score $\Pr(T=1 \mid X)$, which is the probability of a subject being assigned to the active treatment given X, is essentially a mapping of multiple covariates onto a single, scalar valued variable. Propensity scores are typically estimated using a multiple logistic regression model, as follows:

$$\log[\Pr(T=1 \mid X)/(1-\Pr(T=1 \mid X))] = (1, X^T)\beta .$$

It has been shown that using propensity scores results in substantial reduction of bias in estimating the treatment effect when treatment assignments are subject to selection bias (Rosenbaum and Rubin, 1983). Furthermore, the propensity score method provides advantages compared to simply incorporating all the covariates in the model for the treatment effect. For example, propensity score methods tend to be more robust than direct covariate adjustment with respect to model overparameterizations (including too many covariates) and situations with different covariance matrices within treated and untreated groups (D'Agostino, 1998, page 2286.)

Propensity score methods encourage use of many covariates because only predicted probabilities of alternative treatment choices end up being used, while the relative magnitudes, numerical signs, and p-values of fitted coefficients tend to be ignored. The generally larger number of missing values recorded in observational studies, compared to well-controlled trials, implies that a large proportion of subjects have at least one missing covariate value. The first simple approach is using only the observations without missing covariates. We call this method the *complete covariate* (CC) method. Clearly, simply ignoring patients with at least one missing covariate value is not a viable strategy. A simple and intuitive way for handling categorical missing values is to treat a missing value for each categorical variable as an additional category. For a continuous covariate with missing values, we can impute the missing values with the marginal mean and create a new dummy variable to indicate the missingness. We call this the *indicator variable* (IND) method. However, creating this new value ignores any observed correlations among original covariate values and, thus, is not an efficient approach.

A more sophisticated method is to fit separate regressions in estimation of the propensity score for each distinct missingness pattern (MP) (D'Agostino, 2001). Although this approach includes all nonmissing values for those subjects with the same MP, it increases the variability of estimated propensity scores because only a subset of subjects is included in the propensity score model. A much more complicated and computationally intensive approach is to jointly model the propensity score and the missingness, and then use the EM/ECM algorithm (Ibrahim et al., 1999) or Gibbs sampling (D'Agostino et al., 2000) to estimate parameters and propensity scores. Because there is currently no SAS procedure to perform such analyses, the computational complexity makes this alternative approach less attractive and practical.

As a different approach, propensity scores in the presence of missing covariates could also be estimated using multiple imputation (MI) concepts proposed by Rubin (1978, 1987). Recently, Crowe, Lipkovich, and Wang (2009) studied the performance of different multiple imputation strategies in propensity score-based estimation through a simulation study. The central idea of MIs is to randomly fill in any missing values multiple times with sampling from the posterior predictive distribution of the missing values given the observed values, thereby creating a sequence of complete data sets. One advantage to this method is that each data set in the imputed sequence can be analyzed using standard complete data methods. Another advantage is that MI procedures allow us to include ancillary variables that, although they do not directly affect propensity scores, may none the less contain useful information about missing values in important variables.

Recently, Qu and Lipkovich (2009) developed a new method called *multiple imputation missingness pattern* (MIMP), which utilizes not only a multiple imputation method but also the pattern of missing data in the estimation of propensity scores. In this approach, missing data are imputed using a multiple imputation procedure. Then, the propensity scores are estimated from a logistic regression model including the covariates (with missing values imputed) and a factor (a set of indicator variables) indicating the missingness pattern for each observation. A simulation study showed that MIMP performs as well as MI and better than MP when the missingness mechanism is either "missing completely at random" or "missing at random," and it performs better than MI when data are missing not at random (Qu and Lipkovich, 2009).

We will use a data example from a clinical trial in osteoporosis to show how to estimate propensity scores in the presence of missing data for some covariates using the CC, IND, MI, MP, and MIMP methods. There are many ways to use these estimated propensity scores to estimate treatment effects, including regression, stratification, inverse probability weighting, matching, and some combinations of these (see Chapters 2–4 for detailed discussions of these methods). Note that each of the approaches for estimating propensity scores discussed in this chapter can be used in combination with any method of using the propensity scores to estimate treatment effects. In this chapter, for illustration, we use the inverse probability weighting (IPW) approach to estimate the treatment difference. It has been shown that standardizing the weights before performing the IPW estimation provides a more stable estimator for the treatment difference. Therefore, we use the standardized IPW estimation throughout this chapter. Specifically, the estimated treatment effects is estimated as the difference in mean outcome between the two treatment groups, $\hat{\theta}_d = \hat{\theta}_1 - \hat{\theta}_0$, where

$$\hat{\theta}_0 = \left(\sum_{j=1}^{n} (1-T_j)/(1-\hat{p}_j) \right)^{-1} \sum_{j=1}^{n} (1-\hat{p}_j)^{-1} Y_j (1-T_j),$$

$$\hat{\theta}_1 = \left(\sum_{j=1}^{n} T_j / \hat{p}_j \right)^{-1} \sum_{j=1}^{n} \hat{p}_j^{-1} Y_j T_j$$

and individual propensity scores, $\hat{p}_j$, are estimated from the logistic regression model described previously (Lunceford and Davidian, 2004).

5.2 Data Example

In this section, we apply the five methods of handling missing data when estimating propensity scores to a set of data from an osteoporosis study: Multiple Outcomes of Raloxifene Evaluation (MORE) (Delmas et al., 2002). In this study, 7,705 women with osteoporosis were randomly assigned to one of the three treatment groups with an intended ratio of 1:1:1 for placebo, raloxifene 60 mg/day, or raloxifene 120 mg/day and were followed up for 4 years. After 3 years of follow-up, women were allowed to take other bone-active agents such as bisphosphonates. In this analysis, we compared the change in the femoral neck bone mineral density (BMD) during the fourth year (Y) between women not taking bisphosphonates (referred to in this analysis as the *untreated* group, T=0) and women taking bisphosphonates (the *treated* group, T=1) among the 1,643 women who were originally randomized to placebo. Our primary analytic method for evaluating treatment difference is an analysis of variance (ANOVA) model for the outcome (Y) against the assigned treatment group (T). However, because taking bisphosphonates was not a randomized factor, the response variable Y in treated and untreated groups may be confounded due to selection bias. Therefore, we use a weighted ANOVA model with weights taken as the standardization of the inverse of the estimated probability of treatment received. Because PROC MIXED in SAS automatically standardizes the weights before performing the analysis, there is no need to explicitly compute standardized weights in the SAS program. These propensities were estimated using a logistic regression model with 16 covariates (Table 5.1): age at baseline (i.e., prior to randomization), body mass index (BMI) at baseline, family history of breast cancer, 5-year breast cancer risk score (Costantino et al.,1998) at baseline, whether a woman had had a hysterectomy at baseline, lumbar spine BMD at baseline, femoral neck BMD at baseline, change in lumbar spine BMD during the first 3 years, change in femoral neck BMD during the first 3 years, previous hormone replacement therapy status, prevalent vertebral fracture at baseline, new nonvertebral fracture in the first 3 years, new vertebral fracture in the first 3 years, weighted adverse event score during the first 3 years calculated as (1 × #mild AE + 2 × #moderate AE + 3 × #severe AE + 4 × #serious AE), smoking status at baseline, and baseline semi-quantitative vertebral fracture status (0=no fracture, 1=mild fracture, 2=moderate fracture, and 3=severe fracture).

A total of 1,643 women (1,512 with T=0 and 131 with T=1) were included in this sub-analysis and 603 women (36.7%) had at least one missing covariate. Table 5.1 displays the variable names and the numbers of missing values for women originally treated with the placebo. There were 14 distinct patterns of the missing data. The largest pattern included 1,040 subjects with no missing covariates, and each of the three smallest patterns consisted of only one subject.

Table 5.1 Variables in the Example Data Set

Variable Name	Variable Description	# Missing Observations
AGE	Age at MORE baseline	0
BMIR	Body mass index (BMI) at MORE baseline	1
GAILMORE	5-year breast cancer risk score	562
LSC	Change in lumbar spine BMD during the first 3 years	6
LTOTBMR	Lumbar spine BMD at baseline	6
FNC	Change in femoral neck BMD during the first 3 years	0
NECKBMDR	Femoral neck BMD at baseline	0
AESCORE	Weighted adverse event score during the first 3 years	0
SQ	Baseline semi-quantitative vertebral fracture status (0=no fracture, 1=mild fracture, 2=moderate fracture, and 3=severe fracture)	9
FAMHXBCN	Family history of breast cancer (Y/N)	41
KHYSYN	Whether hysterectomized at MORE baseline (Y/N)	0
NVFX	New nonvertebral fracture in the first 3 years (Y/N)	0
PREVHRT	Previous hormone replacement therapy status (Y/N)	3
PREVVERT	Prevalent vertebral fracture at MORE baseline (Y/N)	8
SMOKE	Smoking status at MORE baseline (Y/N)	23
VFX	New vertebral fracture in the first 3 years (Y/N)	8
FNBMD_C	Change in the femoral neck BMD during the fourth year (Outcome variable)	0
BISMORE	Taking bisphosphonates versus not taking (treatment group), (Y/N)	0

5.3 Using SAS for IPW Estimation with Missing Values

SAS procedures (MEANS, GLM, and MIXED) automatically standardize the weights before performing the analysis. Therefore, although there is no explicit code for standardizing the weights (defined as the inverse of the propensity scores in the SAS programs), the standardized IPW estimation is actually performed for all methods of handling missing data.

5.3.1 Complete Covariates (CC) Analysis

The CC method simply omits observations with at least one missing covariate. Program 5.1 shows the SAS code to perform the CC analysis and Output from Program 5.1 shows the results.

Program 5.1 Complete Covariate (CC) Analysis

```
PROC FORMAT;
   VALUE FORMATYN 0 = 'NO'
                  1 = 'YES';
RUN;

*********************************************************************;
* COMPLETE COVARIATE (CC) ANALYSIS;
*********************************************************************;

PROC LOGISTIC DATA = ANALDATA NOPRINT;
    MODEL BISMORE = &VARLIST;
    OUTPUT OUT=PRED PREDICTED=P;
RUN;


DATA PRED;
   SET PRED;
   IF BISMORE = 0 THEN PROB = P;
   IF BISMORE = 1 THEN PROB = 1-P;
   W = 1/PROB;
RUN;

PROC SORT DATA=PRED;
   BY BISMORE;
RUN;

TITLE 'ANALYSIS RESULTS USING THE COMPLETE COVARIATE (CC) METHOD';
PROC MIXED DATA = PRED;
   CLASS BISMORE;
   MODEL FNBMD_C = BISMORE;
   WEIGHT W;
   FORMAT BISMORE FORMATYN.;
   LSMEANS BISMORE/DIFF=ALL;
RUN;
```

Output from Program 5.1

```
ANALYSIS RESULTS USING THE COMPLETE COVARIATE (CC) METHOD

The Mixed Procedure

                                 Least Squares Means
         Bisphosphonates
         use in the 4th                     Standard
Effect   yr of MORE          Estimate          Error        DF     t Value     Pr > |t|

BISMORE  No                  -0.00225     0.001224      1038       -1.84       0.0668
BISMORE  Yes                 0.006102     0.001180      1038        5.17       <.0001


                            Differences of Least Squares Means

        Bisphosphonates   Bisphosphonates
        use in the 4th    use in the 4th          Standard
Effect  yr of MORE        yr of MORE  Estimate    Error      DF   t Value   Pr > |t|

BISMORE No                Yes        -0.00835  0.001700  1038   -4.91     <.0001
```

5.3.2 Indicator Variable (IND) Analysis

The IND approach is a straightforward method for categorical data where the missing value is treated as a special category. For continuous variables, we generally impute the missing values with the marginal means and create a dummy variable to indicate missingness. Program 5.2 shows the SAS code to perform the IND analysis and Output from Program 5.2 shows the results.

Program 5.2 Indicator Variable (IND) Analysis

```
*********************************************************************;
* INDICATOR VARIABLE (IND) ANALYSIS;
*********************************************************************;
PROC MEANS DATA = ANALDATA NOPRINT;
   VAR AGE BMIR GAILMORE LSC LTOTBMDR FNC NECKBMDR AESCORE SQ;
   OUTPUT OUT = ANALDATA_MEAN MEAN=AGE_M BMIR_M GAILMORE_M LSC_M
LTOTBMDR_M FNC_M NECKBMDR_M AESCORE_M SQ_M;
   BY STUDY;
RUN;

DATA ANALDATA_2;
   MERGE ANALDATA ANALDATA_MEAN;
   BY STUDY;
RUN;

DATA ANALDATA_IV;
   SET ANALDATA_2;
   ARRAY X{9} AGE BMIR GAILMORE LSC LTOTBMDR FNC NECKBMDR AESCORE SQ;
   ARRAY M{9} M1-M9;
   ARRAY XM{9} AGE_M BMIR_M GAILMORE_M LSC_M LTOTBMDR_M FNC_M NECKBMDR_M
            AESCORE_M SQ_M;
   DO I = 1 TO 9;
      IF X{I} = . THEN DO;
           M{I} = 1;
             X{I} = XM{I};
         END;
         ELSE M{I} = 0;
   END;
```

```
    ARRAY XC{7} FAMHXBCN KHYSYN NVFX PREVHRT PREVVERT SMOKE VFX;
    DO I = 1 TO 7;
       IF XC{I} = . THEN XC{I} = -1;
    END;
RUN;


PROC LOGISTIC DATA = ANALDATA_IV NOPRINT;
     CLASS FAMHXBCN KHYSYN NVFX PREVHRT PREVVERT SMOKE VFX;
     MODEL BISMORE = &VARLIST M1-M9;
     OUTPUT OUT=PRED PREDICTED=P;
RUN;

DATA PRED;
    SET PRED;
    IF BISMORE = 0 THEN PROB = P;
    IF BISMORE = 1 THEN PROB = 1-P;
    W = 1/PROB;
RUN;

PROC SORT DATA=PRED;
    BY BISMORE;
RUN;

TITLE 'ANALYSIS RESULTS USING THE INDICATOR VARIABLE (IND) METHOD';
PROC MIXED DATA = PRED;
    CLASS BISMORE;
    MODEL FNBMD_C = BISMORE;
    WEIGHT W;
    LSMEANS BISMORE/DIFF=ALL;
    FORMAT BISMORE FORMATYN.;
RUN;
```

Output from Program 5.2

ANALYSIS RESULTS USING THE INDICATOR VARIABLE (IND) METHOD

The Mixed Procedure

Least Squares Means

Effect	Bisphosphonates use in the 4th yr of MORE	Estimate	Standard Error	DF	t Value	Pr > |t|
BISMORE	No	-0.00217	0.001031	1641	-2.11	0.0354
BISMORE	Yes	0.008131	0.000995	1641	8.17	<.0001

Differences of Least Squares Means

Effect	Bisphosphonates use in the 4th yr of MORE	Bisphosphonates use in the 4th yr of MORE	Estimate	Standard Error	DF	t Value	Pr > |t|
BISMORE	No	Yes	-0.01030	0.001433	1641	-7.19	<.0001

5.3.3 Multiple Imputation (MI) Analysis

Applying MI for categorical predictors may be challenging because most commercially available statistical software for MI works with continuous data under an assumption of normality. Unfortunately, there is no current procedure in SAS to perform multiple imputation easily for categorical covariates. As an alternative, we could create dummy variables for categorical variables and perform MI treating the dummy variables as continuous variables, which is readily justified for binary variables. For example, let X=1 indicate a subject who smoked regularly at baseline, and X=0 indicate a subject who did not. The imputed value for X could then be, say, 0.4, indicating a subject who has a 40% chance of smoking. This might provide better information about a patient than rounding the probability down to 0 (no smoking). In this chapter, we impute missing binary predictors with probabilities without rounding down or up.

Another difficulty in applying MI inference in the context of propensity-based estimation of treatment effects is that using combining rules (Rubin, 1987) may result in variance estimators that are not valid because the uncertainty in estimated weights has not been accounted for. Another reason why Rubin's variance estimator may not be appropriate is that one's imputation model (for baseline covariates) and analysis model (for treatment effects) are unlikely to be compatible. See Meng (1994), Wang and Robins (1998), and Robins and Wang (2000) for more information. One general recipe for improving the variance estimator is bootstrapping the entire estimation procedure. This can be easily done using the available SAS macro suite for bootstrapping and implementing various bootstrap-based confidence intervals (http://cuke.hort.ncsu.edu/cucurbit/wehner/software/pathsas/jackboot.txt). In Section 5.3.6, we outline how to use this macro.

Program 5.3 shows the SAS code to perform the MI analysis and Output from Program 5.3 shows the results. Program 5.3 shows how to calculate the point estimator when PROC MI is used to impute missing values. Essentially, it is the average of the estimates from samples generated by multiple imputations.

Program 5.3 The Multiple Imputation (MI) Analysis

```
*********************************************************************;
* ANALYSIS RESULTS USING THE MULTIPLE IMPUTATION (MI) METHOD;
*********************************************************************;
PROC MI DATA = ANALDATA ROUND=.001 NIMPUTE=5 SEED=6731205
OUT=IMPUTED_DATA NOPRINT;
   VAR &VARLIST FNBMD_C BISMORE;
RUN;


PROC LOGISTIC DATA = IMPUTED_DATA NOPRINT;
    MODEL BISMORE = &VARLIST;
   OUTPUT OUT=PRED PREDICTED=P;
   BY _IMPUTATION_;
RUN;


DATA PRED;
   SET PRED;
   IF BISMORE = 0 THEN PROB = P;
   IF BISMORE = 1 THEN PROB = 1-P;
   W = 1/PROB;
RUN;

PROC SORT DATA=PRED;
   BY _IMPUTATION_ BISMORE;
RUN;

ODS LISTING CLOSE;
ODS OUTPUT LSMEANS = LSM DIFFS=DIFFS;
```

```
PROC MIXED DATA = PRED;
   CLASS BISMORE;
   MODEL FNBMD_C = BISMORE;
   WEIGHT W;
   BY _IMPUTATION_;
   LSMEANS BISMORE/ DIFF=ALL;
RUN;
ODS LISTING;

TITLE 'ANALYSIS RESULTS USING THE MULTIPLE IMPUTATION (MI) METHOD';
TITLE2 'POINT ESTIMATES BY TREATMENT GROUP';
PROC MEANS DATA=LSM;
   CLASS BISMORE;
   VAR ESTIMATE;
   FORMAT BISMORE FORMATYN.;
RUN;

TITLE2 'POINT ESTIMATE FOR THE TREATMENT DIFFERENCE';
PROC MEANS DATA = DIFFS;
   VAR ESTIMATE;
RUN;
```

Output from Program 5.3

```
ANALYSIS RESULTS USING THE MULTIPLE IMPUTATION (MI) METHOD
POINT ESTIMATES BY TREATMENT GROUP

The MEANS Procedure

                         Analysis Variable : Estimate

Bisphosphonates
use in the 4th      N
yr of MORE        Obs    N          Mean         Std Dev          Minimum
Maximum
-------------------------------------------------------------------------------------
No                  5    5    -0.0021784     0.000011247       -0.0021881      -
0.0021606

Yes                 5    5     0.0083319     0.000191791        0.0081308
0.0086499
-------------------------------------------------------------------------------------
ANALYSIS RESULTS USING THE MULTIPLE IMPUTATION (MI) METHOD
POINT ESTIMATE FOR THE TREATMENT DIFFERENCE

The MEANS Procedure

                 Analysis Variable : Estimate

N          Mean          Std Dev          Minimum          Maximum
----------------------------------------------------------------------
5    -0.0105103     0.000189049       -0.0108240       -0.0103159
----------------------------------------------------------------------
```

The following SAS code produces the MI estimators of treatment effect with naïve estimates of standard error using PROC MIANALYZE. Specifically, it proceeds in three steps: first one creates multiple data sets without missing baseline values by imputation using a multivariate normal model (PROC MI), then one computes IPW estimates of treatment effects for each completed data set (PROC MIXED), and finally one computes a single MI estimator of treatment effect and associated approximate 95% confidence interval (CI) using Rubin's combining rules (PROC MIANALYZE).

Note that PROC MIANALYZE has different formats for input data sets PARMS and COVB for SAS versions 8 and 9. Our example assumes use of SAS 9. Remember also that the variance estimator from PROC MIANALYZE may not be valid for the reasons mentioned here. Program 5.4 shows the SAS code to summarize the estimates from the MI method using PROC MIANALYZE and Output from Program 5.4 shows the results.

Program 5.4 Summarize the Estimates from the MI Method Using PROC MIANALYZE

```
TITLE2 'ESTIMATE THE TREATMENT DIFFERENCE USING PROC MIANALYZE';
DATA FOR_MI_EST (KEEP = _IMPUTATION_ EFFECT ESTIMATE RENAME=(EFFECT=
                 PARAMETER));
   SET DIFFS;
   EFFECT = 'DIFF';
RUN;

DATA FOR_MI_COV (KEEP = _IMPUTATION_ ROWNAME BISMORE DIFF );
   SET DIFFS;
   DIFF = STDERR**2;
   ROWNAME = "DIFF";
RUN;

PROC MIANALYZE PARMS=FOR_MI_EST COVB=FOR_MI_COV;
   MODELEFFECTS DIFF;
   ODS OUTPUT PARAMETERESTIMATES=MI_EST
              VARIANCEINFO=MI_VAR;
RUN;
```

Output from Program 5.4

```
ANALYSIS RESULTS USING THE MULTIPLE IMPUTATION (MI) METHOD
ESTIMATE THE TREATMENT DIFFERENCE USING PROC MIANALYZE

The MIANALYZE Procedure

              Model Information

PARMS Data Set               WORK.FOR_MI_EST
COVB Data Set                WORK.FOR_MI_COV
Number of Imputations        5

              Multiple Imputation Variance Information

               -----------------Variance-----------------
Parameter          Between         Within           Total        DF

DIFF          3.5739427E-8    0.000002072     0.000002115    9729.1

          Multiple Imputation Variance Information

                  Relative        Fraction
                  Increase         Missing          Relative
Parameter      in Variance     Information        Efficiency

DIFF              0.020696        0.020478          0.995921

                  Multiple Imputation Parameter Estimates

Parameter          Estimate       Std Error    95% Confidence Limits          DF

DIFF              -0.010510        0.001454     -0.01336      -0.00766    9729.1

                       Multiple Imputation Parameter Estimates

                                                                t for H0:
Parameter           Minimum          Maximum          Theta0   Parameter=Theta0   Pr > |t|

DIFF              -0.010824        -0.010316               0             -7.23     <.0001
```

The two data sets passed to PROC MIANALYZE contain estimated treatment effects (data set FOR_MI_EST) and their associated variance-covariance matrices (squared estimated standard errors in data set FOR_MI_COV) for each imputation. The output of PROC MIANALYZE contains information on partitioning of the total variance associated with estimated treatment effect into between- and within-imputation pieces, multiple imputation parameter estimates, approximate 95% confidence intervals based on *t*-distributions, and total variance. Note that for a finite number of imputations (*M*), Rubin's variance estimator is inconsistent because it has a non-degenerate chi-squared limiting distribution. Therefore, a standard Wald-type inference based on the normal distribution is invalid and a *t*-distribution is used (Rubin, 1987). The impact of missing covariates on the final estimates of treatment effect can also be assessed by the fraction of missing information (about treatment effect), which is fairly low in this case (only 2%).

5.3.4 Missingness Pattern (MP) Analysis

The MP method essentially estimates propensity scores separately for each missingness pattern by including only variables without missing values within a missingness pattern. As a result, the independent variables included in the propensity score estimation models differ across missingness patterns. One challenge in implementing MP analysis is that usually there are some missingness patterns with a small number of observations, which renders estimation using the described model unstable. To address this problem, we developed an algorithm for pooling small missingness patterns according to their similarities to reach a prespecified minimum number of observations in each pattern (Qu and Lipkovich, 2009). After combining similar patterns, we impute all missing values within each pooled pattern with the marginal means (to avoid "holes") and estimate the propensity scores using a logistic regression model. In this example, we pooled missingness patterns with a minimum of 100 observations for each pooled cell. Program 5.5 provides a macro to create these pooled patterns.

Program 5.5 Macro to Pool Small Missingness Pattern

```
***************************************************************************;
* Input parameters:
*     indata = input data set;
*     outdata = output data set;
*     varlist = a list of variables to be included in the propensity score
estimation;
*     M_MP_MIN = minimum number of observations for each missing pattern.
*              Missing patterns with less than MIN_MP observations will be
pooled;
***************************************************************************;
%MACRO MP_ASSIGN(MSDATA = , OUTDATA =, VARLIST =, N_MP_MIN = 100);

     /* Determine how many variables to include in the propensity score
estimation */
     %LET N = 1;
       %LET VARINT = ;
     %DO %UNTIL(%QSCAN(&VARLIST., &N. , %STR( )) EQ %STR( ));
            %LET VAR = %QSCAN(&VARLIST. , &N. , %STR( ));
            %LET VARINT = &VARINT  &VAR.*MP;
          %LET N = %EVAL(&N. + 1);
     %END;
       %LET KO = %EVAL(&N-1);
       %LET M_MISSING = %EVAL(&N-1);
       %PUT &VARINT;
       %PUT &KO;
       %PUT &M_MISSING;
```

```
/* Create indicators for missing values and missingness patterns */
DATA MS;
   SET &MSDATA;
     ARRAY MS{&M_MISSING} M1-M&M_MISSING.;
     ARRAY X{&M_MISSING} &VARLIST;
     MV = 0;
     DO I = 1 TO &M_MISSING;
        IF X{I} = . THEN MS{I} = 1;
          ELSE MS{I} = 0;
        MV = 2*MV + MS{I};
     END;
     MV = MV + 1;
     DROP I;
RUN;

/* Only keep one record for each missingness pattern */
PROC SORT DATA = MS OUT = PATTERN NODUPKEY;
   BY MV;
RUN;

/* Calculate the number of observations in each missingness pattern */
PROC FREQ DATA = MS NOPRINT;
   TABLES MV / OUT = M_MP(KEEP = MV COUNT);
RUN;

DATA PATTERN;
   MERGE PATTERN M_MP;
     BY MV;
RUN;

PROC SORT DATA = PATTERN;
   BY DESCENDING COUNT;
RUN;

/* Assign missingness pattern to new index from the largest to the smallest */
DATA PATTERN;
   RETAIN M1-M&M_MISSING MV COUNT MV_S;
   SET PATTERN;
     KEEP M1-M&M_MISSING MV COUNT MV_S;
     MV_S = _N_;
RUN;

PROC IML;
   USE PATTERN;
      READ ALL INTO A;
   CLOSE PATTERN;
   MS = A[, 1:&M_MISSING];
   MV = A[, 1+&M_MISSING];
   N_MP = A[, 2+&M_MISSING];
   MV_S = A[, 3+&M_MISSING];

   M_MP = NROW(MS);
   M = NCOL(MS);

   /* Calculate the distance between missingness patterns */
   DISTANCE = J(M_MP, M_MP, 0);
   DO I = 1 TO M_MP;
      DO J = 1 TO I-1;
           D = 0;
           DO L = 1 TO M;
              D = D + ( (MS[I,L]-MS[J,L])*(MS[I,L]-MS[J,L]) );
             END;
```

```
            DISTANCE[I,J] = D;
            DISTANCE[J,I] = D;
      END;
END;

I = 0;
K_MV_POOL = 0;
MV_POOL = J(M_MP, 1, 0);

  /*Pooling small missingness patterns according to their similarities to
   reach a prespecified minimum number of observations (&N_MP_MIN) in each
   pattern */

DO WHILE( I < M_MP);
   I = I + 1;
   IF MV_POOL[I] = 0 THEN
     DO;
      K_MV_POOL = K_MV_POOL + 1;
          N_MP_POOL = N_MP[I];
      IF N_MP_POOL >= &N_MP_MIN THEN
        DO;
             MV_POOL[I] = K_MV_POOL;
        END;
        ELSE
        DO;
             IF I < M_MP THEN
               DO;
                 A = DISTANCE[(I+1):M_MP, I];
                     B = MV[(I+1):M_MP];
                     C = N_MP[(I+1):M_MP];
                     D = MV_S[(I+1):M_MP];
                     E = MV_POOL[(I+1):M_MP];
                     TT = A || B || C || D || E;
                     CALL SORT( TT, {1 3});
                     J = 0;
                     DO WHILE( (N_MP_POOL < &N_MP_MIN) & (I+J < M_MP) );
                   J = J+1;
                        IF (TT[J,5] = 0) THEN
                        DO;
                           N_MP_POOL = N_MP_POOL + TT[J,3];
                             TT[J,5] = K_MV_POOL;
                        END;
                     END;
               END;
               IF ( N_MP_POOL >= &N_MP_MIN ) THEN
               DO;
                  MV_POOL[I] = K_MV_POOL;
                  DO K = 1 TO J;
                     MV_POOL[TT[K,4]] = K_MV_POOL;
                  END;
               END;
               ELSE
               DO J = I TO M_MP;
                  SGN_TMP = 0;
                  K = 1;
                  DO WHILE(SGN_TMP = 0 & K <= M_MP);
                     DO L = 1 TO M_MP;
                          IF (DISTANCE[J,L] = K) & (MV_POOL[J]=0) &
                                                  (MV_POOL[L]>0) THEN
                          DO;
                               MV_POOL[J] = MV_POOL[L];
                                 SGN_TMP = 1;
                          END;
```

```
                                    END;
                                    K = K + 1;
                              END;
                        END;

               END;
         END;
      END;

      MV_FINAL = MV || MV_POOL;

      VARNAMES={'MV' 'MV_POOL'};
      CREATE MVPOOL FROM MV_FINAL[COLNAME=VARNAMES];
      APPEND FROM MV_FINAL;
QUIT;

PROC SORT DATA = MVPOOL;
   BY MV;
RUN;

PROC SORT DATA = MS;
   BY MV;
RUN;

/* The variable MVPOOL in the &OUTDATA set indicates the pooled missingness
pattern */

DATA &OUTDATA(RENAME=(MV=MP_ORIG MV_POOL=MP));
   MERGE MS MVPOOL;
   BY MV;
RUN;

%MEND MP_ASSIGN;
```

Program 5.6 shows the SAS code to perform the MP analysis after the macro %MP_ASSIGN is applied. Output from Program 5.6 shows the results.

Program 5.6 The Missingness Pattern (MP) Analysis

```
**********************************************************************;
* MISSINGNESS PATTERN (MP) METHOD;
**********************************************************************;

%MP_ASSIGN(MSDATA = ANALDATA, OUTDATA = ANALDATA2, VARLIST = &VARLIST,
N_MP_MIN = 100);

PROC MEANS DATA = ANALDATA2 NOPRINT;
   VAR &VARLIST;
   OUTPUT OUT = MN MEAN = XM1-XM16;
   BY STUDY;
RUN;

DATA TEMP;
   MERGE ANALDATA2 MN;
   BY STUDY;
RUN;

DATA TEMP;
   SET TEMP;
   ARRAY X{16} &VARLIST;
   ARRAY XM{16} XM1-XM16;
```

```
   DO I = 1 TO 16;
      IF X{I} = . THEN X{I} = XM{I};
   END;
   DROP I;
RUN;

PROC SORT DATA = TEMP;
   BY MP;
RUN;

PROC LOGISTIC DATA = TEMP NOPRINT;
   CLASS MP;
   MODEL BISMORE = &VARLIST;
   OUTPUT OUT=PRED PREDICTED=P;
   BY MP;
RUN;


DATA PRED;
   SET PRED;
   IF BISMORE = 0 THEN PROB = P;
   IF BISMORE = 1 THEN PROB = 1-P;
   W = 1/PROB;
RUN;

PROC SORT DATA=PRED;
   BY BISMORE;
RUN;

TITLE 'ANALYSIS RESULTS USING THE MISSINGNESS PATTERN (MP) METHOD';
PROC MIXED DATA = PRED;
   CLASS BISMORE;
   MODEL FNBMD_C = BISMORE;
   WEIGHT W;
   LSMEANS BISMORE/DIFF=ALL;
   FORMAT BISMORE FORMATYN.;
RUN;
```

Output from Program 5.6

ANALYSIS RESULTS USING THE MISSINGNESS PATTERN (MP) METHOD

The Mixed Procedure

Least Squares Means

Effect	Bisphosphonates use in the 4th yr of MORE	Estimate	Standard Error	DF	t Value	Pr > |t|
BISMORE	No	-0.00222	0.001021	1641	-2.18	0.0295
BISMORE	Yes	0.007187	0.000987	1641	7.28	<.0001

Differences of Least Squares Means

Effect	Bisphosphonates use in the 4th yr of MORE	Bisphosphonates use in the 4th yr of MORE	Estimate	Standard Error	DF	t Value	Pr > |t|
BISMORE	No	Yes	-0.00941	0.001420	1641	-6.63	<.0001

5.3.5 Multiple Imputation Missingness Pattern (MIMP) Analysis

The MIMP method essentially is a combination of MI and MP methods. First of all, missing values are multiply imputed. Then, for each imputed data set, propensity scores are estimated using the baseline covariates and the categorical variable for the missingness pattern. Similar to the MP method, we combine small missingness patterns to reach a minimum of 100 observations for each cell. Once we create data sets with indicators for pooled patterns (as shown in Section 5.3.4), we simply apply PROC MI to this data set (as shown in Section 5.3.3). Program 5.7 shows the SAS code to perform the MIMP analysis and Output from Program 5.7 shows the results.

Program 5.7 The Multiple Imputation Missingness Pattern (MIMP) Analysis

```
*************************************************************************;
* Multiple Imputation Missingness Pattern (MIMP) Method;
*************************************************************************;

PROC MI DATA = ANALDATA2 ROUND=.001 NIMPUTE=5 SEED=6731205 OUT=IMPUTED_DATA
NOPRINT;
   VAR &VARLIST FNBMD_C BISMORE;
RUN;


PROC LOGISTIC DATA = IMPUTED_DATA NOPRINT;
   CLASS MP;
    MODEL BISMORE = &VARLIST MP;
   OUTPUT OUT=PRED PREDICTED=P;
   BY _IMPUTATION_;
RUN;


DATA PRED;
   SET PRED;
   IF BISMORE = 0 THEN PROB = P;
   IF BISMORE = 1 THEN PROB = 1-P;
   W = 1/PROB;
RUN;

PROC SORT DATA=PRED;
   BY _IMPUTATION_ BISMORE;
RUN;


ODS OUTPUT LSMEANS = LSM DIFFS=DIFFS;
PROC MIXED DATA = PRED;
   CLASS BISMORE;
   MODEL FNBMD_C = BISMORE;
   WEIGHT W;
   BY _IMPUTATION_;
   LSMEANS BISMORE/ DIFF=ALL;
RUN;


TITLE 'ANALYSIS RESULTS USING THE MULTIPLE IMPUTATION MISSINGNESS PATTERN
(MIMP) METHOD';
TITLE2 'POINT ESTIMATES BY TREATMENT GROUP';
PROC MEANS DATA=LSM;
   CLASS BISMORE;
   VAR ESTIMATE;
   FORMAT BISMORE FORMATYN.;
RUN;
```

```
TITLE2 'POINT ESTIMATE FOR THE TREATMENT DIFFERENCE';
PROC MEANS DATA = DIFFS;
   VAR ESTIMATE;
RUN;
```

Output from Program 5.7

```
ANALYSIS RESULTS USING THE MULTIPLE IMPUTATION MISSINGNESS PATTERN (MIMP) METHOD
POINT ESTIMATES BY TREATMENT GROUP

The MEANS Procedure

                           Analysis Variable : Estimate

Bisphosphonates
use in the 4th       N
yr of MORE         Obs   N         Mean        Std Dev         Minimum         Maximum
----------------------------------------------------------------------------------------
No                   5   5   -0.0021775    0.000011208      -0.0021870      -0.0021596

Yes                  5   5    0.0083296    0.000190528       0.0081254       0.0086443
----------------------------------------------------------------------------------------


ANALYSIS RESULTS USING THE MULTIPLE IMPUTATION MISSINGNESS PATTERN (MIMP) METHOD
POINT ESTIMATE FOR THE TREATMENT DIFFERENCE

The MEANS Procedure

                  Analysis Variable : Estimate

N          Mean          Std Dev           Minimum           Maximum
--------------------------------------------------------------------
5    -0.0105070      0.000187855        -0.0108178        -0.0103096
--------------------------------------------------------------------
```

One can also use PROC MIANALYZE to get the point estimate for the treatment difference. However, the variance estimation from PROC MIANALYZE is not valid. This approach is shown in Program 5.8, and Output from Program 5.8 shows the results.

Program 5.8 Summarize the Estimates from the MIMP Method Using PROC MIANALYZE

```
TITLE2 'ESTIMATE THE TREATMENT DIFFERENCE USING PROC MIANALYZE';
DATA FOR_MIMP_EST (KEEP = _IMPUTATION_ EFFECT ESTIMATE RENAME=(EFFECT=
PARAMETER));
   SET DIFFS;
   EFFECT = 'DIFF';
RUN;

DATA FOR_MIMP_COV (KEEP = _IMPUTATION_ ROWNAME BISMORE DIFF );
   SET DIFFS;
   DIFF = STDERR**2;
   ROWNAME = "DIFF";
RUN;

PROC MIANALYZE PARMS=FOR_MIMP_EST COVB=FOR_MIMP_COV;
   MODELEFFECTS DIFF;
   ODS OUTPUT PARAMETERESTIMATES=MI_EST
              VARIANCEINFO=MI_VAR;
RUN;
```

Output from Program 5.8

```
ANALYSIS RESULTS USING THE MULTIPLE IMPUTATION MISSINGNESS PATTERN (MIMP) METHOD
ESTIMATE THE TREATMENT DIFFERENCE USING PROC MIANALYZE

The MIANALYZE Procedure

             Model Information

PARMS Data Set              WORK.FOR_MIMP_EST
COVB Data Set               WORK.FOR_MIMP_COV
Number of Imputations       5


            Multiple Imputation Variance Information

             -----------------Variance-----------------
Parameter          Between          Within             Total         DF

DIFF          3.5289507E-8     0.000002072       0.000002115    9972.9

       Multiple Imputation Variance Information

                  Relative          Fraction
                  Increase           Missing          Relative
Parameter      in Variance       Information        Efficiency

DIFF              0.020436          0.020224          0.995972


                  Multiple Imputation Parameter Estimates

Parameter         Estimate         Std Error    95% Confidence Limits          DF

DIFF             -0.010507          0.001454     -0.01336      -0.00766   9972.9

                       Multiple Imputation Parameter Estimates

                                                                    t for H0:
Parameter          Minimum           Maximum           Theta0   Parameter=Theta0    Pr > |t|

DIFF             -0.010818         -0.010310                0              -7.23      <.0001
```

5.3.6 Obtaining Bootstrap Confidence Intervals

Direct estimation of standard errors for the point estimators in all of these propensity score-based IPW methods is challenging because the additional variability in the estimated weights is difficult to account for. Therefore, we use bootstrap methods to estimate the standard error and the confidence interval for the point estimates. The SAS macros %BOOT and %BOOTCI (http://cuke.hort.ncsu.edu/cucurbit/wehner/software/pathsas/jackboot.txt) provide nonparametric estimates of standard errors and various bootstrap confidence intervals (including the popular bias-corrected accelerated [BCa] method; Efron, 1987) for the IPW treatment difference. First, we need to create a user-defined macro that has to be named %ANALYZE. This macro computes the point estimate of the IPW treatment difference that will be repeatedly called from the %BOOT and %BOOTCI macros. Next, the %BOOT and %BOOTCI macros are called to compute bootstrap estimates. Note that the %ANALYZE macro must have two parameters: *data* to identify the input data set and *out* to name the output data set. Program 5.9 is an illustration of the %ANALYZE macro and calls to the %BOOT and %BOOTCI macros.

Program 5.9 Estimation of the Variance and Confidence Interval Using the Bootstrap Method

```
/*************************************************************************************
      MIMP_ANALYSIS is a macro which calculates CC, MI, MP and MIMP estimates;
      Q_METH indicates the method
*************************************************************************************/

%INCLUDE 'BOOTS.SAS'; /* the file can be found in
http://cuke.hort.ncsu.edu/cucurbit/wehner/software/pathsas/jackboot.txt */

%MACRO ANALYZE(DATA=BMDPS, OUT= );
   %MIMP_ANALYSIS(INDATA = &DATA, VARLIST = &VARLIST, Y = FNBMD_C, G =
BISMORE, M_MP_MIN = 100);

   PROC SORT DATA = EST OUT = &OUT;
      BY Q_METH;
   RUN;
%MEND ANALYZE;
PROC PRINTTO LOG=NOLOG;
RUN;

TITLE 'BOOSTRAP: NORMAL ("STANDARD") CONFIDENCE INTERVAL WITH BIAS
CORRECTION';
TITLE2;
%BOOT(DATA=BMDPS, ALPHA=.05, SAMPLES=1000, RANDOM=123, ID=Q_METH);

TITLE 'BOOTSTRAP BCA';
%BOOTCI(BCA, ID=Q_METH);

PROC PRINTTO;
RUN;
```

Carpenter and Bithell (2000) used simulation to show that the BCa bootstrap method generally produces reliable results, even if the distribution of the test statistic is far from symmetric. In this example, we use BCa bootstrapping to estimate confidence intervals for the data set in Section 5.2 (see Table 5.2). The naive estimator (a direct unweighted estimator of treatment effect using a *t*-test) appears to overestimate the treatment difference. The CC method had the widest confidence interval and the MP method had wider confidence intervals than the MI and MIMP methods, whereas the last two methods produced similar results. It should be noted that for this example, the 95% confidence intervals produced by the CC and MP methods contained 0 while those for the MI and MIMP methods did not.

Table 5.2 The Mean (95% CI) of the Change in Femoral Neck BMD (g/cm^2) During the Fourth Year of MORE Study for Women Assigned to Placebo (n = 1,643)*.

Method	Untreated (n=1512)	Treated (n=131)	Treated vs. Untreated
NAIVE	-0.002(-0.004,-0.001)	0.011(0.006, 0.017)	0.013(0.007, 0.019)
CC	-0.002(-0.004,-0.001)	0.006(-0.002, 0.020)	0.008(0.000, 0.022)
MP	-0.002(-0.004,-0.001)	0.007(-0.003, 0.016)	0.009(-0.001, 0.018)
MI	-0.002(-0.003,-0.001)	0.009(0.002, 0.017)	0.011(0.004, 0.019)
MIMP	-0.002(-0.003,-0.001)	0.009(0.002, 0.017)	0.011(0.004, 0.019)

*Results are from Qu and Lipkovich (2009). The estimates for MI and MIMP were slightly different from the SAS output presented previously due to the choice of different seeds in PROC MI.

5.4 Sensitivity Analyses

Estimation of treatment effects using propensity scores may be sensitive to the misspecification of imputation and propensity score models, as well as to the tuning parameters of the associated algorithms. To address this issue, we discuss several strategies for performing sensitivity analysis in the context of propensity-based analyses with missing data.

5.4.1 Varying Analytic Methods

Examples of alternative analytic methods were illustrated in Section 5.3. Within each method, one can also vary parameters. For example, one can vary the minimum pattern size to test how sensitive the results are to the selection of the minimum size of the pooled pattern in MP and MIMP. We also recommend, as illustrated here, computing propensity-stratified estimates of treatment effects in addition to IPW estimates.

The SAS code here constructs five strata (subgroups, bins) based upon fitted values of propensity for treatment and computes the corresponding stratified estimators of treatment effects. This can be done in various ways. For example, one can compute treatment effects within each stratum and combine them by weighting inversely to the square of estimated standard errors. In general, this approach is not recommended because it always down-weights results from the strata with highly different observed treatment fractions and up-weighs results from the strata with nearly equal observed treatment fractions. Here we follow a stratified regression (SR) approach described in D'Agostino (1998) and Lunceford and Davidian (2004) that combines stratification on propensity scores and regression and computes the overall estimator of treatment effect as an average of regression-adjusted estimators within each strata. Specifically, for stratum s, a regression-based estimator of treatment effect is computed as follows:

$$\hat{\theta}_d^{(s)} = n_s^{-1} \sum_{j \in Q_s} \{ m_j^{(s)}(1, X_j, \hat{\alpha}^{(s)}) - m_j^{(s)}(0, X_j, \hat{\alpha}^{(s)}) \},$$

where Q_s is the set of indices of subjects with estimated propensity scores falling within stratum s; n_s is the size of stratum s; $m_j^{(s)}(1, \boldsymbol{X}_j, \hat{\boldsymbol{\alpha}}^{(s)})$ denotes the predicted outcome for subject j using regression of the form $m(T, \boldsymbol{X}, \boldsymbol{\alpha}) = E(Y \mid T, \boldsymbol{X})$ fitted to the data within stratum s, with predictors T and $\boldsymbol{X}$, and $\hat{\boldsymbol{\alpha}}^{(s)}$ representing the vector of estimated parameters. When a linear regression model is used, as in the following example, the estimated treatment effect within stratum is simply the estimated regression coefficients for treatment, $\hat{\alpha}_T^{(s)}$.

In this example, shown in Program 5.10, the estimated propensity scores are divided into K=5 strata and the overall SR estimator of treatment effect is computed as an average of strata-specific estimators based on linear regression within each stratum, $\hat{\theta}_d^{SR} = K^{-1} \sum_{s=1}^{K} \hat{\theta}_d^{(s)}$. The estimate of standard error can be obtained using bootstrapping, as explained in Section 5.3.6.

This alternative stratified estimator may be more robust compared to the IPW estimator when the estimated propensity for the treatment actually received is close to 0 for a few patients, resulting in these few subjects having undue impact on the overall estimated treatment difference. Program 5.10 shows the SAS code to perform the SR method and Output from Program 5.10 shows the results. The SR estimate for the treatment effect is 0.0099.

Program 5.10 Illustration of the Sensitivity Analysis Using Propensity Score Stratified Regression Estimator

```
/* THIS STEP CAN BE REPLACED WITH ANY METHOD FOR OBTAINING PROPENSITY SCORES */
PROC LOGISTIC DATA = ANALDATA DESC NOPRINT;
    MODEL BISMORE = &VARLIST;
    OUTPUT OUT=PRED PREDICTED=P;
RUN;

/* DEFINE THE QUINTILES WITH PROC RANK (GROUP=5) */
PROC RANK DATA = PRED OUT=PRED GROUPS=5;
   VAR P;
   RANKS PS_STRATA;
RUN;

PROC SORT DATA=PRED; BY PS_STRATA; RUN;

ODS LISTING CLOSE;
ODS OUTPUT SOLUTIONF=SF;
PROC MIXED DATA = PRED (WHERE=(PS_STRATA NE .));
   BY PS_STRATA;
   MODEL FNBMD_C = BISMORE &VARLIST/SOLUTION;
RUN;
ODS LISTING;


TITLE 'ESTIMATING TREATMENT EFFECT BY ADJUSTING FOR BASELINE COVARIATES WITHIN
EACH STRATA';
PROC MEANS DATA = SF N MEAN;
   CLASS PS_STRATA;
   TYPES PS_STRATA ();
   VAR ESTIMATE;
   where effect = 'BISMORE';
RUN;
```

Output from Program 5.10

```
ESTIMATING TREATMENT EFFECT BY ADJUSTING FOR BASELINE COVARIATES WITHIN EACH STRATA

The MEANS Procedure

Analysis Variable : Estimate

  N
Obs      N             Mean
-------------------------
  5      5        0.0099243
-------------------------

      Analysis Variable : Estimate

    Rank for        N
  Variable P      Obs       N              Mean
-----------------------------------------
           0        1       1        0.0144995

           1        1       1        0.0102909

           2        1       1        0.0023628

           3        1       1        0.0143711

           4        1       1        0.0080970
-----------------------------------------
```

5.4.2 Using Different Imputation Strategies

For methods involving multiple imputation, try several imputation models using different sets of predictors for imputation. It has been suggested (Meng, 1994; Schafer, 1997) that it is better to include as many variables as possible in one's imputation model, because omitting an important covariate results in an incorrect analysis while keeping an irrelevant predictor may only lower efficiency. Also, a recent simulation study comparing performance of different imputation strategies for propensity-based estimation (Crowe, Lipkovich, and Wang, 2009) showed that including treatment (*T*) and treatment outcome (*Y*) in imputation models improves estimation of the treatment effect. While it may appear counterintuitive to incorporate future outcomes in the imputation model for baseline covariates, it makes the imputation model more compatible with the analysis model (ANOVA for *Y* and *T*, in our case) and, therefore, helps reduce bias in estimating the treatment effect (Meng, 1994). Note that, in our examples of multiple imputation in Sections 5.3.3 and 5.3.5, we include both treatment and outcome variables in addition to baseline covariates in the VAR statement of PROC MI.

It is useful to evaluate the impact of missingness by examining the fraction of missing information (FMI), which is part of the output from PROC MIANALYZE. While the FMI may be substantial when estimating some of the coefficients of the propensity score model, the overall impact of missing covariates may be fairly low when estimating treatment effects (which, after all, is the ultimate goal of one's analysis). This is the case because variables that have the largest FMI may contribute little to the probability of treatment assignment. In our example, the FMI for estimating the treatment difference was only about 2% (see the output in Section 5.3.3); for some variables included in the logistic model, it was fairly large, such as for FAMHXBCN (30%) and GAILMORE (31%). However, these variables were not significant predictors of treatment assignment, given other covariates, and, therefore, their missing values did not contribute much to the uncertainty associated with estimating treatment effects. On the other hand, the FMI for the most significant predictor of treatment assignment, LTOTBMDR, FNC, and NECKBMDR was estimated as <0.1%, 0.1%, and 0.1%, respectively. Program 5.11 shows the SAS code of PROC MIANALYZE for logistic regression coefficients. Output from Program 5.11 shows the results.

Program 5.11 Calculation of the Fraction Missing Information

```
/**** ASSESING FRACTION MISSING INFORMATION FOR COEFFICIENTS IN PS  MODEL
*****/
PROC MI DATA = ANALDATA ROUND=.001 NIMPUTE=5 SEED=6731205 OUT=IMPUTED_DATA
NOPRINT;
   VAR &VARLIST FNBMD_C BISMORE;
RUN;

ODS LISTING;
ODS OUTPUT PARAMETERESTIMATES = _EST
           COVB= COV;
PROC LOGISTIC DATA = IMPUTED DATA;
   MODEL BISMORE = &VARLIST/COVB;
   OUTPUT OUT=PRED PREDICTED=P;
BY  IMPUTATION_;
RUN;
TITLE 'ANALYSIS RESULTS USING THE MULTIPLE IMPUTATION (MI) METHOD';
DATA  EST;
  SET  EST;
  RENAME VARIABLE=PARAMETER;
  KEEP _IMPUTATION_ VARIABLE ESTIMATE;
RUN;
```

```
PROC MIANALYZE PARMS=_EST COVB=_COV;
  MODELEFFECTS INTERCEPT &VARLIST;
  ODS OUTPUT PARAMETERESTIMATES=MI_EST
             VARIANCEINFO=MI_VAR;
RUN;
```

Output from Program 5.11

Multiple Imputation Variance Information

Parameter	Relative Increase in Variance	Fraction Missing Information	Relative Efficiency
intercept	0.003791	0.003784	0.999244
AGE	0.041368	0.040481	0.991969
BMIR	0.003756	0.003749	0.999251
FAMHXBCN	0.380552	0.301688	0.943096
GAILMORE	0.395063	0.310298	0.941567
KHYSYN	0.000864	0.000863	0.999827
LSC	0.008437	0.008401	0.998323
LTOTBMDR	0.000264	0.000264	0.999947
FNC	0.001002	0.001001	0.999800
NECKBMDR	0.001434	0.001433	0.999713
NVFX	0.001993	0.001991	0.999602
PREVHRT	0.003607	0.003601	0.999280
PREVVERT	0.008648	0.008610	0.998281
AESCORE	0.007936	0.007904	0.998422
SMOKE	0.073996	0.071100	0.985979
SQ	0.010930	0.010870	0.997831
VFX	0.002259	0.002256	0.999549

Multiple Imputation Parameter Estimates

Parameter	Estimate	Std Error	95% Confidence Limits		DF
intercept	-3.910976	1.415616	-6.68554	-1.13641	280408
AGE	0.032916	0.016281	0.00099	0.06484	2534.8
BMIR	0.011069	0.027360	-0.04256	0.06469	285733
FAMHXBCN	-0.131857	0.410049	-0.95444	0.69073	52.643
GAILMORE	-0.130776	0.168963	-0.47017	0.20862	49.879
KHYSYN	-0.042621	0.230992	-0.49536	0.41011	5.37E6
LSC	5.866674	1.922807	2.09796	9.63539	57142
LTOTBMDR	2.713227	0.893752	0.96150	4.46495	5.73E7
FNC	9.155874	2.772187	3.72249	14.58926	3.99E6
NECKBMDR	4.221311	1.430553	1.41748	7.02515	1.95E6
NVFX	-0.255861	0.294621	-0.83331	0.32159	1.01E6
PREVHRT	-0.245808	0.210377	-0.65814	0.16652	309625
PREVVERT	-0.338755	0.372863	-1.06957	0.39206	54417
AESCORE	-0.015502	0.007301	-0.02981	-0.00119	64523
SMOKE	0.562806	0.311964	-0.04951	1.17512	842.65
SQ	-0.134405	0.184790	-0.49660	0.22779	34218
VFX	-0.600087	0.282802	-1.15437	-0.04581	787654

5.4.3 Handling Extreme Weights

One major drawback for the IPW estimator is that it can produce unstable estimators if there are extreme large or small weights when the propensity scores are close to 0 or 1. One immediate remedy is to set boundaries for the weights. For example, for propensity scores $< \delta$, we set them to be δ; for propensity scores $> 1 - \delta$, we set propensity scores to be $1 - \delta$, where δ is an empirical small number. In our experience, we used $\delta = 0.001$ in some simulations, and it yields great results. For the data example presented in Section 5.3, there were no very small or large weights, so we did not use this empirical technique. Program 5.12 shows how to set boundaries for weights to produce stable estimators.

Program 5.12 Setting Boundaries for the Weights Derived from Propensity Scores

```
%LET DELTA = 0.001;
DATA PRED;
    SET PRED;
    IF . < P < &DELTA. THEN P = 0.001;
    IF P > 1-&DELTA. THEN P = 1-&DELTA.;
RUN;
```

5.5 Discussion

We have presented several methods of estimating propensity scores in the presence of missing values for some covariates. The CC method simply includes only subjects without any missing covariates. The IND method creates dummy variables to indicate the missingness. The MP method estimates the propensity scores within each missingness pattern. For some missingness patterns with a small number of observations, we proposed a method to pool small missingness patterns according to their similarities. The MI method estimates propensity scores with missing values imputed by multiple imputations. The MIMP method essentially combines the MI and MP methods by first imputing missing values with multiple imputations and then including information on the missingness pattern as a covariate in estimating propensity scores.

These approaches to estimating propensity scores can be combined with any propensity score-based method to estimate the treatment difference in the presence of treatment selection bias. In this chapter, all the analytic methods presented were based on the assumption of two treatment groups and used standardized inverse-probability weighted ANOVA with estimated propensities from a logistic regression. When more than two treatment arms are present, propensities are vectors of probabilities that sum to 1. The IPW approach is thus easily extended, with probabilities estimated using a multinomial logistic model (e.g., in SAS using PROC LOGISTIC with GLOGIT in its MODEL statement). Sometimes multiple treatment groups can be naturally ordered (e.g., when representing increasing levels of exposure/dose), and propensity scores can be estimated using ordinal logistic regression as shown in Leon and Hedeker (2005).

If the proportion of subjects with at least one missing value is low (e.g., < 10%), intuitively all approaches handling missing values will produce similar results. Therefore, one can choose the most convenient method such as the complete covariate analysis.

References

Carpenter, J. and J. Bithell. 2000. “Bootstrap confidence intervals: when, which, what? A practical guide for medical statisticians.” *Statistics in Medicine* 19: 1141–1164.

Concato, J., N. Shah, and R. I. Horwitz. 2000. “Randomized, controlled trials, observational studies, and the hierarchy of research designs.” The *New England Journal of Medicine* 342: 1887–1892.

Costantino. J., M. Gail, S. Pee, et al. 1999. “Validation studies for models projecting the risk of invasive and total breast cancer incidence.” *Journal of the National Cancer Institute* 91: 1541–1548.

Crowe, B., I. Lipkovich, and O. Wang. 2009. “Comparison of several imputation methods for missing baseline data in propensity scores analysis of binary outcome.” *Pharmaceutical Statistics*. In Press. DOI: 10.1002/pst.389.

D'Agostino, R. B. 1998. "Tutorial in biostatistics: propensity score methods for bias reduction in the comparison of a treatment to a non-randomized control group." *Statistics in Medicine* 17(19): 2265–2281.

D'Agostino, Jr., R. B., and D. B. Rubin. 2000. "Estimating and using propensity scores with partially missing data." *Journal of the American Statistical Association* 95: 749–759.

D'Agostino, R., W. Lang, M. Walkup, and T. Morgon. 2001. "Examining the impact of missing dData on propensity score estimation in determining the Effectiveness of self-monitoring of blood glucose (SMBG)." *Health Services & Outcomes Research Methodology* 2: 291–315.

Delmas, P. D., K. E. Ensrud, J. D. Adachi, et al. 2002. "Efficacy of raloxifene on vertebral fracture risk reduction in postmenopausal women with osteoporosis: four-year results from a randomized clinical trial." *The Journal of Clinical Endocrinology & Metabolism* 87(8): 3609–3617.

Efron, B. 1987. "Better bootstrap confidence intervals." *Journal of the American Statistical Association* 82: 171–185.

Horvitz, D. G., and D. J. Thompson. 1952. "A generalization of sampling without replacement from a finite universe." *Journal of the American Statistical Association* 47(260): 663–685.

Ibrahim, J., S. Lipitz, and M. Chen. 1999. "Missing covariates in generalized linear models when the missing data mechanism is non-ignorable." *Journal of the Royal Statistical Society, Series B* (Statistical Methodology) 61: 173–190.

Leon, A. C., and D. Hedeker. 2005. "A mixed-effects quintile-stratified propensity adjustment for effectiveness analyses of ordered categorical doses." *Statistics in Medicine* 24: 647–658.

Little, R. J., and D. B. Rubin. 2002. *Statistical Analysis with Missing Data*. 2d ed. New York: Wiley-Interscience.

Lunceford, J. K., and M. Davidian. 2004. "Stratification and weighting via the propensity score in estimation of causal treatment effects: a comparative study." *Statistics in Medicine* 23: 2937–2960.

Meng, X. L. 1994. "Multiple-imputation inferences with uncongenial sources of input." *Statistical Science* 9: 538–573; discussion 558–573.

Qu, Y., and I. Lipkovich. 2009. "Propensity score estimation with missing values using a multiple imputation missingness pattern (MIMP) approach." *Statistics in Medicine*. 28:1402–1414.

Robins, J. M., A. Rotnitzky, and L. P. Zhao. 1994. "Estimation of regression coefficients when some regressors are not always observed." *Journal of the American Statistical Association* 89: 846–866.

Robins, J. M., and N. Wang. 2000. "Inference for imputation estimators." *Biometrika* 87: 113–124.

Rosenbaum, P. R. 1987. Model-based direct adjustment." *Journal of the American Statistical Association* 82: 387–394.

Rosenbaum, P. R., and D. B. Rubin. 1983. "The central role of the propensity score in observational studies for causal effects." *Biometrika* 70: 41–55.

Rosenbaum, P. R., and D. B. Rubin. 1984. "Reducing bias in observation studies using subclassification on the propensity score." *Journal of the American Statistical Association* 79: 516–524.

Rubin, D. B. 1978. "Multiple imputations in sample surveys: a phenomenological Bayesian approach to nonresponse." In the ASA Proceedings in the Section on *Survey Research Methods* 20–28. Alexandria, VA: American Statistical Association.

Rubin, D. B. 1987. *Multiple Imputation for Nonresponse in Surveys*. New York: John Wiley & Sons, Inc.

Schafer, J. L. 1997. *Analysis of Incomplete Multivariate Data*. London: Chapman and Hall/CRC.

Wang, N., and J. M. Robins. 1998. "Large-sample theory for parametric multiple imputation procedures." *Biometrika* 85: 935–948.

Xie, J., and C. Liu. 2005. "Adjusted Kaplan-Meier estimator and log-rank test with inverse probability of treatment weighting for survival data." *Statistics in Medicine* 24: 3089–3110.

Chapter 6

Instrumental Variable Method for Addressing Selection Bias

R. Scott Leslie
Hassan Ghomrawi

Abstract

Observational data can provide powerful answers to research questions when properly addressing selection bias due to non-randomization. The medical literature has relied mostly on conventional regression and propensity score methods, which rely on observed variables, to adjust for selection bias. Such methods might deliver biased estimates due to unmeasured confounding. In this chapter, we introduce the instrumental variable method, an econometric method, to adjust for selection bias and illustrate its use in evaluating treatment effects on medication compliance. If properly applied, this method might be more useful in addressing selection bias.

6.1 Introduction

A key strength of observational studies is their ability to estimate the effect of treatments and interventions in real-world conditions. However, the lack of random group assignment may impose a serious threat to the results of observational studies (D'Agostino and Kwan, 1995).

Non-randomized groups usually differ on observed and unobserved characteristics, which in turn result in differential selection into treatment groups. This non-random sampling selection is one form of selection bias that distorts the effect of treatment on outcomes. In other words, it is unclear whether the observed treatment effect is due to the treatment itself or to the differential selection into treatment groups due to non-randomization.

This selection bias problem has been shown to have a substantial impact on the treatment effect in some studies, while in other studies adjusting for selection bias has resulted in minor changes in the treatment effect (Wang, 2005; Foster, 2000; McClellan, 2000; Grimes, 2002; Glesby, 1996). Therefore, several studies caution that overestimating the selection bias may lead to further biased estimates (Hernán, 2006; Stukel, 2007). In this chapter, we provide an overview of instrumental variable (IV) methodology and demonstrate an example of applying this approach to adjust for selection bias using administrative claims data. The IV approach is an econometric method that is less prevalent in the medical literature than methods of matching, stratification, conventional regression, and propensity scoring, but it may have advantages over these methods if used appropriately.

6.2 Overview of Instrumental Variable Method to Control for Selection Bias

Observational studies that lack randomization of subjects into treatment groups must address selection bias to properly estimate the effect of treatment while addressing potential confounds. Instrumental variable (IV) analysis is a common tool in economics and social sciences to adjust for selection bias but less used in health care research. Where conventional selection adjustment methods use only observed variables, the IV method, on the other hand, acknowledges that a set of observed variables may not capture residual confounding due to unobserved factors (Angrist et al., 1996). By implementing the IV method, researchers find variables, called *instruments* or *instrumental variables*, which are highly correlated with the treatment selection but not directly correlated with the outcome variable. When incorporated into the analysis, the IV creates additional variance that is unaccounted for from the observables to obtain an unbiased estimate of the effect of treatment on the outcome. In 2000, the *Health Services Research* journal published a special supplemental issue devoted to IV analysis (McClellan and Newhouse, 2000). This issue contains explanations of the methodology and provides examples of its use in health outcomes research.

Figure 6.1 illustrates how an instrumental variable works. Observable risk factors or confounders (*X*) (such as age, gender, and co-morbid conditions) may affect both the outcome (*Y*) and treatment (*T*). The presence of this association makes treatment allocation dependent on observables and not truly an independent variable. That is, treatment is correlated with the error term in the model. Thus, estimating the effect of treatment (*T*) on outcome (*Y*) without any adjustment creates difficulty in deciphering cause and effect between treatment and outcome. Traditional regression methods can account for observables but won't capture bias from unobservables. The goal of IV analyses is to find an instrument or instruments that are correlated with treatment selection but are not *directly* correlated with the outcome variable. These IVs are then used in estimating a treatment effect that is independent from the observables (*X*). The objective is to mimic randomization of subjects into treatment groups to be able to attribute changes in outcome due to treatment rather than observables.

Figure 6.1 Schematic Representation of IV Methodology

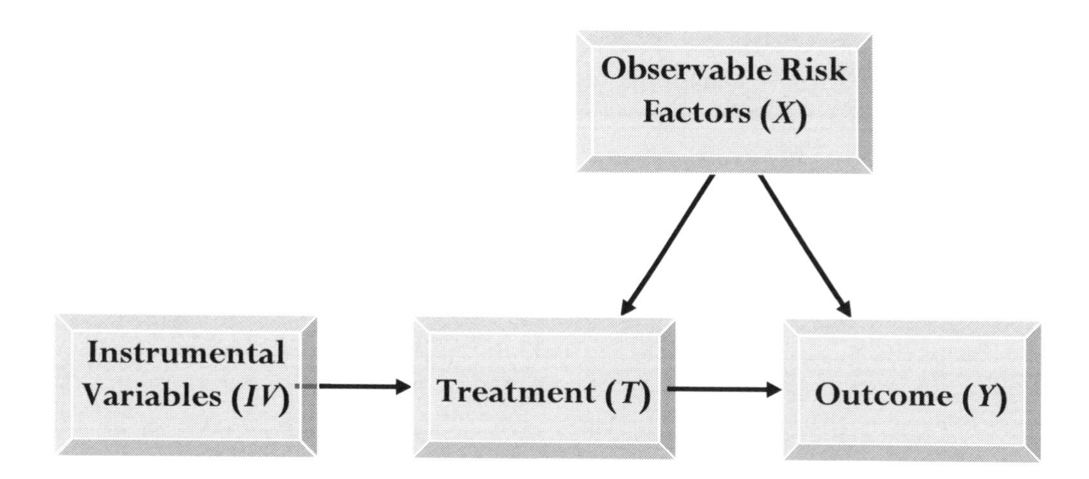

While the intuition of IV methodology is appealing, the difficulty in finding a valid instrument may be the reason for its relatively limited use. For the IV method to overcome unmeasured confounding, several assumptions must be addressed (Angrist, 1996; Landrum, 2001; Greenland, 2000). Most noteworthy assumptions include the independence assumption, exclusion restriction, and non-zero causal effect of the instrument on treatment. The independence assumption states the lack of relation between the instrument and the observed risk factors. The exclusion restriction requires that the IV have no effect on the outcome other than through treatment or that the IV affect the outcome exclusively through treatment. The non-zero causal effect of the instrument on treatment assumes that the instrument is associated with treatment or a predictor of treatment.

In order to estimate a treatment effect that is adjusted for selection bias using the instrumental variable approach, two equations need to be estimated. The first equation estimates the effect of the IV and observables (X) on treatment (T). The second equation estimates the effect of observables (X) and treatment (T) on outcome (Y). The maximum likelihood ratio method is usually used in conducting this two-stage regression estimation of treatment on outcome. Using the Heckman two-stage estimation to calculate the inverse Mills ratio is another way to accomplish the IV approach (Heckman, 1978).

The remaining sections of this chapter discuss an example of using the instrumental variable methodology to evaluate the effect of drug choice on medication adherence in a population of diabetic patients. Determining differences between treatments is important because increased adherence to medications may indicate better diabetes disease management, which consequently may slow disease progression. These data are often used when deciding on a preferred treatment for larger populations. We conducted our instrumental variable analysis using the Qualitative and Limited Dependent Model (QLIM) procedure in SAS/ETS.

6.3 Description of Case Study

A large pharmacy claims database was used to identify newly started patients using one of two oral antidiabetic medications in a 7-month time period (*N*=19,433). The purpose of the study was to compare compliance rates over a 180-day period between the two treatments. Compliance was measured as the proportion of days a medication was covered or supplied to the patient after treatment initiation (Benner, 2002). Patients new to therapy, or *new starts*, were chosen for review because this sample gives a more accurate estimate of initial compliance with the medication. New starts are also less confounded by previous medication use and more exposed to selection of treatment through the prescriber. We suspected the presence of selection bias because evidence shows the two drug treatments differ in patient tolerance, adverse events, and side effects, which possibly influence treatment selection as well as compliance with each drug (Lago et al., 2007; Lincoff et al., 2007). Additionally, selection of treatment is influenced by recent findings, changes in clinical guidelines, and policy changes (Schneeweiss, 2002). Knowing that traditional regression techniques may fall short in estimating the treatment net effect on the outcome, we chose the IV approach to minimize bias attributed to unmeasured data.

The TABULATE procedure code in Program 6.1 was used to create a table displaying patient characteristics by drug treatment for the new starts sample. Additionally, PROC TTEST and PROC FREQ were used to test for differences and associations between groups. Descriptors include demographic variables (age, gender), type of health plan insurance, and medication use in a 6-month period prior to treatment initiation (baseline period). Age was the age of the patient at date of treatment initiation (index date). Type of insurance was categorized by health maintenance organization (HMO) or other. Prior medication use was measured for sulfonylureas, antihypertensives, lipid lowering agents as well as asthma and antidepressant medications. Refill patterns of medications for chronic diseases, or maintenance medications, were used to estimate patient compliance behavior with the following prescribed dosings.

Program 6.1 Displaying Patient Characteristics by Drug Treatment Using PROC TABULATE

```
proc format;
  picture pct 0-100=009.0% (mult=1000);
run;

proc tabulate data=newstarts;
  class tx;
  var age age_18to44 age_45to54 age_55to64 age_65plus b_hmo b_medicaid
      b_medicare b_self pre_sulf _0106 _0109 _0112 _0113 _0149 female
      maintrefillratio pre_stc_class_cnt_subset pre_drug_cnt_subset;
  table N='Member Count'*f=comma8.
       (age='Age')*(mean std='SD')*f=4.1
       (age_18to44='Age Group 18-44' age_45to54='Age Group 45-54'
          age_55to64='Age Group 55-64' age_65plus='Age Group >=65'
          female='Female')*(mean='')*f=pct.
       (b_hmo='HMO Enrollee')*(mean='')*f=pct.
       (pre_drug_cnt_subset='# of Drugs Utilized')*(mean std='SD')*f=4.1
       (maintrefillratio='Maintenance Medication Refill %')*(mean='')*f=pct.
       (pre_sulf='Sulfonylurea' _0106='Hypertension' _0109='Lipid
          Irregularity' _0112='Pain Management' _0113='Antidepressant'
          _0149='Asthma')*(mean='')*f=pct.
       , tx='Treatment' /box='Unadjusted Demographic and Baseline
          Characteristics';
run;
```

```
proc ttest data=newstarts;
  var age pre_drug_cnt_subset maintrefillratio;
  class tx;

proc freq data=newstarts;
  tables tx*(female b_hmo pre_sulf _0106 _0109 _0112 _0113 _0149)/chisq;
run;
```

Output from Program 6.1

Unadjusted Demographic and Baseline Characteristics		Treatment	
		Drug A	Drug B
Member Count		611	815
Age	Mean	55.5	56.0
	SD	11.8	12.6
Age Group 18-44		16.3%	16.3%
Age Group 45-54		30.9%	28.3%
Age Group 55-64		32.8%	34.1%
Age Group >=65		19.8%	21.2%
Female		44.6%	46.3%
HMO Enrollee *		65.3%	74.8%
# of Drugs Utilized	Mean	3.1	3.3
	SD	3.1	3.8
Maintenance Medication Refill % *		36.3%	41.3%
Sulfonylurea		27.6%	31.5%
Hypertension		56.6%	57.7%
Lipid Irregularity		34.5%	38.7%
Pain Management *		21.1%	26.1%
Antidepressant		14.5%	13.6%
Asthma *		7.2%	10.6%

* $p < .05$

Output from Program 6.1 describes the two treatment groups. Those observables that differed significantly in the two groups of patients include type of insurance (proportion of patients enrolled in an HMO), previous refill rate for maintenance medication, asthma medication use, and pain medication use. Differences in observables between groups led us to believe differences existed in unobservables between the two groups.

To compare methods to control for selection bias, our analytic plan proceeds as follows. We use three methods in estimating the difference in outcome between Drug A and Drug B. First, a simple *t*-test crudely compares the mean compliance rates for drugs A and B using PROC TTEST. Second, we use conventional ordinary least squares regression to compare drug effectiveness on compliance for Drugs A and B, adjusting for measured covariates. Third, we estimate compliance rates for the two treatments, adjusting for selection bias using the IV method.

Our compliance outcome was measured as the proportion of days the medication was supplied over the 180-day period; hence, the maximum allowable value was 1. Mean compliance for Drug A and Drug B was 0.4774 and 0.5122, respectively. The unadjusted comparison of mean compliance values using PROC TTEST (Program 6.2) indicates the difference is approaching statistical significance ($p = 0.0609$) at the 0.05 level of significance. This unadjusted 3% difference in compliance between treatments indicates better compliance to prescribed dosings, which may translate into better diabetes disease management. Such evidence can influence formulary management decisions on the preferred treatment for large populations. Displaying distributions of the outcome for the two treatment groups can be done using the CLASS statement in PROC UNIVARIATE, as shown in Program 6.2.

Program 6.2 Computation of *t*-test Comparison of Mean Compliance Values and Generation of Histograms

```
proc ttest data=newstarts;
  var pdc;
  class tx;

proc univariate data=newstarts noprint plot;
  var pdc;
  class tx;
  histogram pdc / ctext=purple cfill=blue
    kernel (k=normal color=green w=3 l=1)
    normal (color = red w=3 l= 2)
    ncols=1 nrows=2;
  inset n='N' (comma6.0) mean='Mean' (6.2) median='Median' (6.2)
    mode='Mode'(6.2)
    normal kernel(type)/ position=NW;
run;
```

Output from Program 6.2

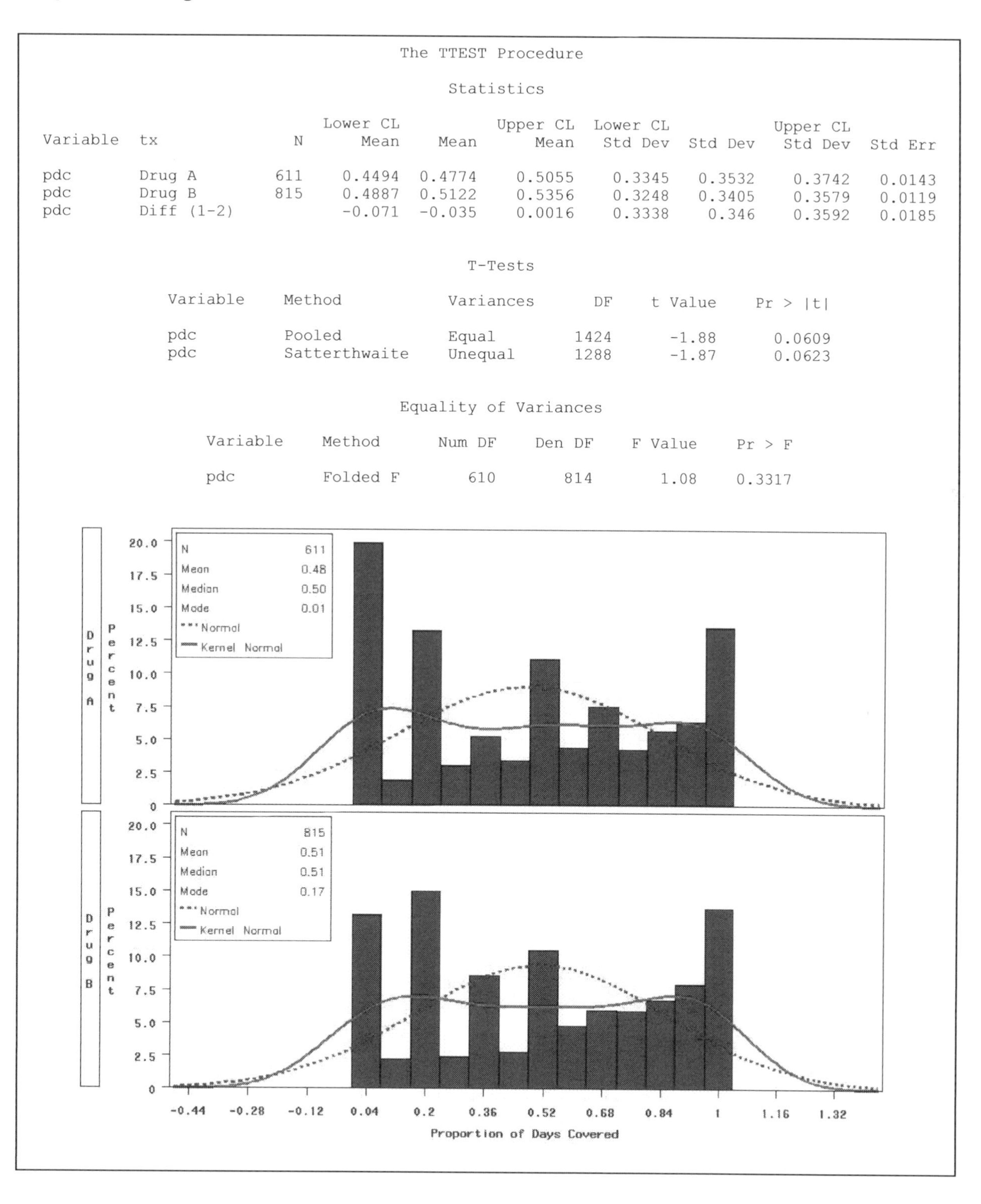

The TTEST Procedure

Statistics

Variable	tx	N	Lower CL Mean	Mean	Upper CL Mean	Lower CL Std Dev	Std Dev	Upper CL Std Dev	Std Err
pdc	Drug A	611	0.4494	0.4774	0.5055	0.3345	0.3532	0.3742	0.0143
pdc	Drug B	815	0.4887	0.5122	0.5356	0.3248	0.3405	0.3579	0.0119
pdc	Diff (1-2)		-0.071	-0.035	0.0016	0.3338	0.346	0.3592	0.0185

T-Tests

Variable	Method	Variances	DF	t Value	Pr > |t|
pdc	Pooled	Equal	1424	-1.88	0.0609
pdc	Satterthwaite	Unequal	1288	-1.87	0.0623

Equality of Variances

Variable	Method	Num DF	Den DF	F Value	Pr > F
pdc	Folded F	610	814	1.08	0.3317

6.4 Traditional Ordinary Least Squares Regression Method Applied to Case Study

Using ordinary least squares regression methods to adjust for observed risk factors, we obtained adjusted estimates of compliance for the two treatment groups. The GLM procedure can conduct an analysis of variance to calculate least squares means while using the Tukey-Kramer (Kramer, 1956) adjustment for multiple comparisons (Program 6.3). Tests of univariate associations with the outcome were used to select the independent variables in this model.

Program 6.3 Creating Adjusted Outcome Values Using PROC GLM

```
proc glm data=newstarts;
  class tx age_18to44 female b_hmo pre_sulf _0112;
  model pdc = tx age_18to44 female b_hmo maintrefillratio _0112
    /solution;
  lsmeans tx/OM ADJUST=TUKEY PDIFF CL;
quit;
```

Output from Program 6.3

```
                      The GLM Procedure
                      Least Squares Means
          Adjustment for Multiple Comparisons: Tukey-Kramer

                                                 H0:LSMean1=
                                                   LSMean2
                 tx          pdc LSMEAN             Pr > |t|

                 Drug A      0.47863394              0.0747
                 Drug B      0.51124635


          tx          pdc LSMEAN       95% Confidence Limits

          Drug A        0.478634        0.451623       0.505645
          Drug B        0.511246        0.487889       0.534604


                   Least Squares Means for Effect tx

                      Difference          Simultaneous 95%
                         Between        Confidence Limits for
          i    j           Means         LSMean(i)-LSMean(j)

          1    2       -0.032612        -0.068480       0.003255
```

Adjusted compliance means for Drug A and Drug B are 0.4786 and 0.5112, respectively. The difference between means using the Tukey-Kramer adjustment shows no statistically significant difference in mean compliance values. Comparing these adjusted mean values to unadjusted mean values (Section 6.3) shows little change when adjusting for these observables.

6.5 Instrumental Variable Method Applied to Case Study

Suspecting that selection bias is not resolved with standard ordinary least squares methods, we employed the IV method. Among the few studies that apply the IV approach when comparing the treatment effectiveness of drugs, Brookhart and colleagues (2006, 2007) used physician prescribing preference as an instrumental variable when assessing drug treatment effectiveness on morbidity and mortality outcomes. The authors used these preference-based instruments in two separate studies to assess the risk of gastrointestinal toxicity associated with nonsteroidal anti-inflammatory drug treatment and the mortality in elderly patients using types of antipsychotic medications. Replicating their instruments, we used the last prescription written by the prescriber for the drug class (Drug A or Drug B) as the instrument for our study. Brookhart and colleagues hypothesized that a physician's immediate history of prescribing as measured by the last written prescription estimates the prescriber's preference for one treatment or another. That choice, according to the hypothesis, therefore, affects the choice of treatment for the prescriber's next patient. We believed that in our study this measure would act as a valid instrument because it influences the treatment choice but is uncorrelated with the outcome for the next patient. To construct our IV, prescribers of the initial prescription for each of the 1,426 study patients were identified. Prescription claims for these prescribers for the two drugs were extracted in a period preceding this initial prescription to calculate the prescriber's preference. Prescribers were classified as a Drug A prescriber or a Drug B prescriber based on their most recent prescription in the drug class. Some prescribers were not identified correctly. Some prescribers had no history of prescribing either drug; therefore, patients with these physicians were excluded from the analysis. A total of 1,226 prescribers were classified.

As stated earlier, the validity of an instrumental variable relies on many assumptions. Administrative data can't confirm these assumptions, but they can be used to look into the credibility of the assumptions. To test the validity of our method, we first looked at the distribution of the IV to show that prescribers' preference to prescribe these two drugs varied. Preference for Drug A or Drug B for the 1,226 identified prescribers was 47% and 53%, respectively. To address the non-zero causal effect of IV treatment assumption, we evaluated associations between the instrument and treatment selection by using PROC FREQ to estimate how well our instrument predicted treatment or the extent of prescriber preference in predicting the treatment choice of the prescriber's next patient (Program 6.4). Results showed a strong, positive relationship between our IV and treatment selection. Prescribers with a preference for Drug A were more than three times more likely to prescribe Drug A for the identified patient in our sample (OR = 3.44, CI = 2.766 – 4.293).

To address the independence assumption, we checked relationships between our IV and observables factors. Potential violations of the independent assumption could include differing patient profiles by prescriber group (that is, Drug A prescribers treating patients who are much different than patients seen by Drug B prescribers). A stratification of patient demographic and baseline characteristics by prescriber preference using the TABULATE, TTEST, and FREQ procedures can compare observables by the instrument. More complicated models can address time variant clustering relationships (Brookhart, 2007). Smaller differences between groups indicate treatment choice by the prescriber for the previous patient is unrelated to the observables of the current patient. Those differences that persist suggest possible violations of this assumption; however, those covariates can be addressed later in the two-stage least squares regression.

prescriber that may affect outcome (Brookhart, 2006). Prescriber preference might affect compliance through other services provided by the prescriber or because of differing skill level among providers. However, review of the literature shows patients' long-term adherence to medications is mostly due to the self-efficacy of the patient or the patient's beliefs and behavior (Bodenheimer et al., 2002; Jerant et al., 2005) rather than instruction by the prescriber (Haynes, 2002). The degree of physician skill on our compliance outcome is difficult to measure so we use this research to defend the possibility of violating the exclusion restriction.

Program 6.4 Code Used in Validating IV Assumptions

```
proc freq data=newstarts;
  tables iv*tx/chisq measures;
run;

proc format;
  picture pct 0-100=009.0% (mult=1000);
run;

proc tabulate data=newstarts;
  class tx iv;
  var age age_18to44 age_45to54 age_55to64 age_65plus b_hmo b_medicaid
      b_medicare b_self pre_sulf _0106 _0109 _0112 _0113 _0149 female
      maintrefillratio pre_stc_class_cnt_subset pre_drug_cnt_subset;
  table N='Member Count'*f=comma8.
      (age='Age')*(mean std='SD')*f=4.1
      (age_18to44='Age Group 18-44' age_45to54='Age Group 45-54'
        age_55to64='Age Group 55-64' age_65plus='Age Group >=65'
        female='Female')*(mean='')*f=pct.
      (b_hmo='HMO Enrollee')*(mean='')*f=pct.
      (pre_drug_cnt_subset='# of Drugs Utilized')*(mean std='SD')*f=4.1
      (maintrefillratio='Maintenance Medication Refill
        %')*(mean='')*f=pct.
      (pre_sulf='Sulfonylurea' _0106='Hypertension' _0109='Lipid
        Irregularity' _0112='Pain Management' _0113='Antidepressant'
        _0149='Asthma')*(mean='')*f=pct.
     , iv='IV (Prescriber Preference)' /box='Unadjusted Demographic and
        Baseline Characteristics';
run;
```

Output from Program 6.4

Table of iv by tx			
iv	tx		
Frequency Percent Row Pct Col Pct	Drug A	Drug B	Total
Drug A	390 27.35 58.56 63.83	276 19.35 41.44 33.87	666 46.70
Drug B	221 15.50 29.08 36.17	539 37.80 70.92 66.13	760 53.30
Total	611 42.85	815 57.15	1426 100.00

Statistic	DF	Value	Prob
Chi-Square	1	125.9656	<.0001
Likelihood Ratio Chi-Square	1	127.5668	<.0001
Continuity Adj. Chi-Square	1	124.7647	<.0001
Mantel-Haenszel Chi-Square	1	125.8773	<.0001
Phi Coefficient		0.2972	
Contingency Coefficient		0.2849	
Cramer's V		0.2972	

Estimates of the Relative Risk (Row1/Row2)			
Type of Study	Value	95% Confidence Limits	
Case-Control (Odds Ratio)	3.4463	2.7665	4.2931
Cohort (Col1 Risk)	2.0138	1.7717	2.2890
Cohort (Col2 Risk)	0.5843	0.5281	0.6465

Unadjusted Demographic and Baseline Characteristics		IV (Prescriber Preference)	
		Drug A	Drug B
Member Count		666	760
Age*	Mean	54.7	56.7
	SD	11.7	12.6
Age Group 18-44		18.3%	14.6%
Age Group 45-54		28.5%	30.2%
Age Group 55-64		35.8%	31.5%
Age Group >=65		17.2%	23.5%
Female		45.1%	46.0%
HMO Enrollee*		66.0%	74.8%
# of Drugs Utilized	Mean	2.8	3.5
	SD	3.0	3.9
Maintenance Medication Refill %		35.1%	42.8%
Sulfonylurea*		26.7%	32.6%
Hypertension*		53.0%	61.0%
Lipid Irregularity*		33.0%	40.3%
Pain Management		22.0%	25.6%
Antidepressant		13.5%	14.4%
Asthma		8.5%	9.7%

* $p < .05$.

This output reinforces our choice of instrument for estimating treatment effectiveness in the presence of unmeasured confounding. Next, we applied the two-stage IV method to our study example. First, we used our instrument variable and other observables to predict the treatment (see Figure 6.2).

Figure 6.2 Schematic Representation of First Stage of IV Analysis

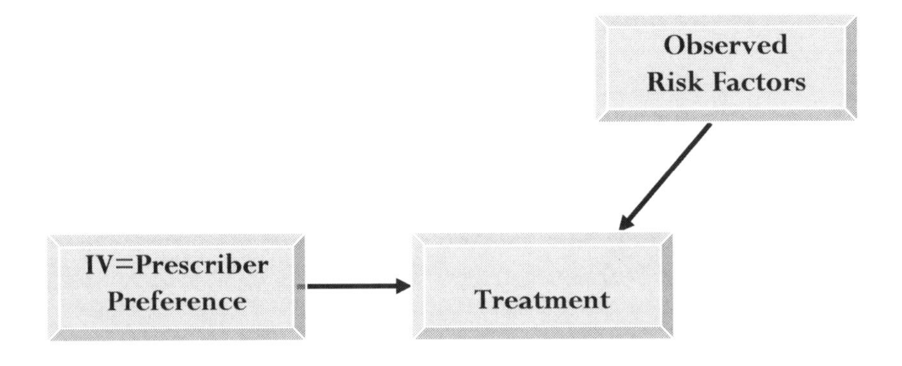

In the second stage of the process, an outcome equation approximates the compliance outcome by using the predicted treatment (from the first model) and other observables (see Figure 6.3). This two-stage approach has the advantage of incorporating the predicted treatment into the outcome model because it represents the portion of treatment selection related to prescriber preference.

Figure 6.3 Schematic Representation of Second Stage of IV Analysis

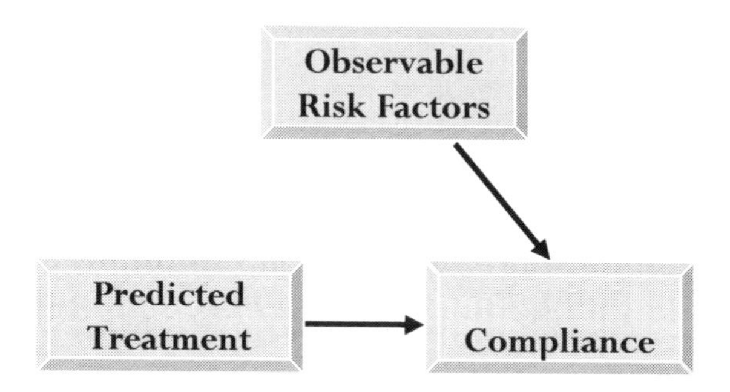

6.6 Using PROC QLIM to Conduct IV Analysis

The two-stage IV process described here can be done in one step using the Qualitative and Limited Dependent Model (QLIM) procedure in SAS/ETS. We chose the QLIM procedure because of its capability to analyze models that involve simultaneous relationships. This fits our example because we are simultaneously estimating treatment selection and compliance. The QLIM procedure let us submit two model statements in one procedure, allowing us to simultaneously estimate an unbiased effect of treatment on the outcome.

Proper modeling in PROC QLIM requires a subject-level data set (for example, one observation per patient). A quick look at the data set using PROC PRINT shows noteworthy variables of the data set (Program 6.5).

Program 6.5 Creating IV-Adjusted Outcome Value Using PROC QLIM

```
proc print data=newstarts (obs=10);
  var tx druga iv pdc age female b_hmo copay_idxdrug
      pre_drug_cnt_subset
      pre_sulf _0106 _0109 _0112 _0113 _0149 maintrefillratio;
run;

proc qlim data = newstarts ;
  class iv;
  model druga = iv age female copay_idxdrug pre_drug_cnt_subset
       maintrefillratio pre_sulf _0106 _0109 _0112 _0113 _0149 /discrete;
  model pdc = age female copay_idxdrug pre_drug_cnt_subset
       maintrefillratio pre_sulf _0106 _0109 _0112 _0113 _0149
       /select(druga=0);
  output out=drugb predicted;
run;
```

where

druga = treatment selection indicator

tx = treatment classification variable

iv = instrumental variable (prescriber preference)

pdc = outcome (compliance as proportion of days of medication covered)

age = age of patient at date of treatment initiation (index date)

female = indicator variable

b_hmo = HMO enrollee

copay_idxdrug = patient co-payment for initial prescription

Remaining variables describe utilization in the pre-treatment baseline period:

pre_drug_cnt = number of distinct medications utilized

pre_sulf = use of sulfonylurea

_0106 = use of antihypertensive

_0109 = use of asthma medication

_0112 = use of pain medication

_0113 = use of lipotropic

_0149 = use of antidepressant

maintrefillratio = refill percentage for maintenance medications

The first MODEL statement is a selection equation that uses the probit model (indicated by using the DISCRETE option) and creates the predicted probability of each subject receiving Drug B based on our IV and other observables. The second MODEL statement is the outcome equation, which uses linear regression to model the compliance outcome while controlling for covariates. This assesses the effect of the treatment while controlling for the probability produced from the first equation plus other believed confounders. Some believe that including independent variables other than the treatment group in this step is redundant because they are included in the first MODEL statement. We believe that adding variables to the model provides additional information on predictors of the outcome. The selection model can include covariates believed to be predictive of treatment where the outcome model can include covariates prognostic of outcome. The OUTPUT statement creates a data set named DrugB. With the addition of the PREDICTED option, the newly created data set includes all variables from the input data set plus two new variables named P_druga and P_pdc, which contain predicted values of the treatment and compliance values, respectively. The predicted compliance outcome values are generated for all subjects in the sample, assuming that all patients have been prescribed Drug B.

Output from Program 6.5

Obs	tx	druga	iv	pdc	age	female	b_hmo	copay_id xdrug	pre_drug _cnt_ subset	pre_ sulf	_0106	_0109	_0112	_0113	_0149	Maintrefill ratio
1	Drug A	1	Drug B	0.00556	55	0	0	23.000	11	1	1	1	0	1	0	0.45946
2	Drug B	0	Drug B	0.16667	76	1	0	20.000	0	0	0	0	0	0	0	0.00000
3	Drug A	1	Drug A	0.07222	44	1	0	0.000	10	1	0	0	1	0	0	0.00000
4	Drug B	0	Drug B	0.91111	74	1	0	15.333	4	1	1	0	0	0	0	0.50000
5	Drug B	0	Drug B	0.16667	77	0	0	7.000	1	1	1	0	0	0	0	1.00000
6	Drug A	1	Drug A	0.61667	74	0	0	109.362	5	1	0	0	0	0	0	0.00000
7	Drug B	0	Drug A	0.16667	59	1	0	0.000	5	1	1	1	1	0	0	0.00000
8	Drug A	1	Drug B	0.28333	51	1	0	0.000	4	0	1	1	1	0	1	0.22222
9	Drug B	0	Drug A	0.27778	43	1	0	0.000	17	1	1	1	1	1	1	0.29167
10	Drug A	1	Drug A	0.16667	69	0	0	0.000	2	0	0	0	0	0	0	1.00000

Parameter Estimates

Parameter		Estimate	Standard Error	t Value	Approx Pr > |t|
pdc.Intercept		0.468902	0.064961	7.22	<.0001
pdc.age		0.001444	0.000929	1.55	0.1201
pdc.female		-0.068086	0.022960	-2.97	0.0030
pdc.copay_idxdrug		-0.001525	0.000305	-4.99	<.0001
pdc.pre_drug_cnt_subset		-0.001683	0.004240	-0.40	0.6915
pdc.maintrefillratio		0.168015	0.036034	4.66	<.0001
pdc.pre_sulf		-0.042180	0.025716	-1.64	0.1010
pdc._0106		-0.001649	0.025733	-0.06	0.9489
pdc._0109		0.047814	0.025504	1.87	0.0608
pdc._0112		-0.045605	0.028238	-1.61	0.1063
pdc._0113		-0.008500	0.034562	-0.25	0.8057
pdc._0149		-0.006435	0.038786	-0.17	0.8682
_Sigma.pdc		0.297051	0.009963	29.82	<.0001
druga.Intercept		-0.420098	0.186430	-2.25	0.0242
druga.iv	Drug A	0.740991	0.074652	9.93	<.0001
druga.iv	Drug B	0	.	.	.
druga.age		-0.000008433	0.003272	-0.00	0.9979
druga.female		-0.112074	0.076919	-1.46	0.1451
druga.copay_idxdrug		0.000094205	0.001086	0.09	0.9308
druga.pre_drug_cnt_subset		0.004108	0.014939	0.28	0.7833
druga.maintrefillratio		-0.206794	0.118055	-1.75	0.0798
druga.pre_sulf		-0.100354	0.087456	-1.15	0.2512
druga._0106		0.108600	0.088306	1.23	0.2188
druga._0109		-0.078342	0.087028	-0.90	0.3680
druga._0112		-0.211746	0.098552	-2.15	0.0317

Parameter Estimates					
Parameter		Estimate	Standard Error	t Value	Approx Pr > |t|
druga._0113		0.105211	0.117267	0.90	0.3696
druga._0149		-0.179984	0.139948	-1.29	0.1984
_Rho		-0.235728	0.162230	-1.45	0.1462

Output from the QLIM procedure in Program 6.5 includes a table of parameter estimates for both MODEL statements (first for the outcome equation and second for the treatment selection equation), indicating direction and magnitude of the effect of each independent variable. Of most importance are the treatment selection/IV parameter (drugb.iv in our example), which indicates the effect of the IV on treatment selection, and the _rho parameter estimate, which indicates correlation between the error terms in the two equations. A significant rho parameter estimate indicates the presence of treatment selection bias in the outcome equation. The drugb parameter estimate indicates a strong effect of the IV on treatment selection (*p* <. 0001), and the _rho parameter estimate indicates the effect of treatment selection bias on the outcome. In this case, the estimate is -0.235728 (*p*=0.1462).

A second submission of this code was done to estimate compliance values if all patients received Drug A. By changing the SELECT option in the first MODEL statement to `druga=1` we generated predicted compliance values if all patients used Drug A. Comparing these predicted compliance values to the first scenario—wherein all patients were assumed to have used Drug B—gave us comparative effectiveness on compliance. Mean estimated compliance if all members were on Drug A was 0.5353. Mean estimated compliance if all patients were on Drug B was 0.5276. After running code for both scenarios, the two newly generated data sets were sorted and merged by subject. Using this final patient-level data set, containing predicted compliance values for each scenario, we can compare means using a paired *t*-test via PROC TTEST to test for an estimated treatment difference.

6.7 Comparison to Traditional Regression Adjustment Method

Table 6.1 compares results from the IV approach to an unadjusted result and, more notably, to a traditional regression adjustment method (adjusted OLS model) that adjusts for observables. The mean unadjusted compliance for Drug A and Drug B was 47.7% and 51.2%, respectively. Calculating adjusted compliance values using PROC GLM show the mean values change slightly, although the model controls for the various factors. Calculated values from the QLIM procedure show the effect of selection bias. Mean compliance values increase to 0.5390 and 0.55327 for Drug A and Drug B, respectively. Although our example shows minimal change in compliance when using the IV approach, many studies show considerable differences between methods (Brookhart, 2006; Landrum, 2001).

Table 6.1 Mean Compliance by Treatment: IV Model vs. Adjusted Model

Model	Treatment	Compliance Outcome	95% Confidence Limits	
Unadjusted Model				
	Drug A	0.477	0.449	0.504
	Drug B	0.512	0.488	0.535
	Estimated Treatment Difference	-0.034	-0.071	0.001
Regression Adjusted Model				
	Drug A	0.478	0.451	0.505
	Drug B	0.511	0.487	0.534
	Estimated Treatment Difference	-0.032	-0.068	0.003
IV Adjusted Model				
	Drug A	0.535	0.530	0.540
	Drug B	0.527	0.522	0.533
	Estimated Treatment Difference	0.007	0.003	0.011

6.8 Discussion

Where traditional regression adjustment techniques use observable measures to control for confounding, IV methods rely on instrumental variables to account for measured as well as unmeasured factors. This added element of the IV approach is valuable when compared with conventional methods to adjust for risk factors such as propensity scoring. The rather large assumption with propensity scoring is that all factors that affect group assignment and outcome are used in modeling. The abundance of unmeasured factors should not be overlooked by researchers. Among patient attitudes and other influencing factors, selection of treatment or group assignment is also prompted by changing guidelines and policies (Schneeweiss, 2002). Implementation of IV methods can be especially helpful when analyzing data sets not generated for the purpose of the research question. That is, studies relying on existing databases contain limited information. Those studies that can prospectively gather data on hypothesized confounders may depend less on unobservables.

Challenges to IV methods include the difficulty of identifying a proper instrument and of validating the instrument when found. Exercise caution when using an instrument because it could do more harm than good (Murray, 2006). Validation of instruments by subject matter experts is helpful to counter arguments of invalid instruments. The relationship between IV and treatment is based on hypothesis. It is empirically hard to test. Murray (2006) points to using a conditional likelihood ratio test when an instrument is weakly correlated with treatment. Another trade-off when using the two-stage least squares estimator is the presence of larger standard errors as compared with ordinary least squares.

In the demonstrated example, available data allowed us to address some but not all assumptions stated by Angrist (1996) and Landrum (2001). The stable unit treatment value assumption states that there is no relationship between the treatment statuses of other patients. We assumed that the prescriber's preference affects the treatment of the next patient. It is unlikely that one patient's treatment influences another patient's choice of treatment. It was also challenging to address the monotonicity of our instrument. It holds naturally that if a patient received Drug A from a Drug B prescriber, the patient would have also received Drug A from a Drug A prescriber. The difficulty in addressing the many assumptions for IV validity provides evidence of the difficulty in finding a strong instrument. In many examples, consistency of results using a combination of methods may suggest limited selection bias and/or not capturing the bias with observed and unknown data elements.

Limitations to study design that are present for both methods include the possibility that actual compliance may differ from observed compliance. Also, there may well be additional predictors of treatment selection and adherence that are not captured, including patient attitudes, socioeconomic status, education level, and number of other medications used.

One can conduct the IV method with SAS procedures other than SAS/ETS using the same two-step process described in our example. The LOGISTIC and GENMOD procedures can both estimate predicted probabilities for a response value. Using PROC LOGISTIC for the first treatment selection model would create the predicted treatment based on the IV. With these predicted treatment values, we could conduct the second step, the outcome model, using PROC GLM to assess treatment on the outcome while controlling for the predicted treatment values plus other observables that may affect the outcome. In other case studies, PROC REG or PROC LOGISTIC can be used depending on the nature of the outcome. We are not, however, aware of developed and validated SAS code that could be readily used.

6.9 Conclusion

Although observational studies can yield unique findings on treatment effectiveness on outcomes in routine care settings, the non-randomized nature of observational studies calls for addressing potential selection bias. Using conventional regression techniques that account for observables may resolve some bias, but it may also be biased when covariates are correlated with the error term in the model. Accounting for unobservables is necessary to maximize bias control; however, no method can totally eliminate selection bias when you are using observational data.

In this study, we demonstrate that controlling for observables alone shows little adjustment from crude, unadjusted mean values in compliance between two drug treatments. When using an IV approach that contains additional variance that is unaccounted for from the observables, we created a less biased estimate of the treatment effect on our compliance outcome. The result was a change in mean compliance values, with the conclusion that there was no difference in compliance between treatments.

We showed only one approach to conducting IV methods. Variations to IV approach depend on the type of treatment and the type of outcome, such as multiple treatments and nonlinear outcome measures.

Although IV methodology is less known and less widely used in observational and clinical studies, it can be used in conjunction with traditional risk adjustment techniques, such as propensity scoring and multivariable regression, to reduce selection bias. If applied correctly, IV can adjust for unobservables and add value to comparative effectiveness studies.

Acknowledgments

The authors would like to thank M. Alan Brookhart, Bradley Martin, and reviewers for their guidance, review, and comments.

References

Angrist, J. D., G. W. Imbens, D. B. Rubin, and J. M. Robins. 1996. "Identification of Causal Effects Using Instrumental Variables." *Journal of the American Statistical Association* 91: 444–455.

Benner, J. S., R. J. Glynn, H. Mogun, P. J. Neumann, et al. 2002. "Long-term Persistence in Use of Statin Therapy in Elderly Patients." The *Journal of the American Medical Association* 288: 455–456.

Bodenheimer, T., K. Lorig, H. Holman, and K. Grumbach. 2002. "Patient Self-Management of Chronic Disease in Primary Care." The *Journal of the American Medical Association* 288(19): 2469–2475.

Brookhart, M. A., et al. 2006. "Evaluating Short-Term Drug Effects Using a Physician-Specific Prescribing Preference as an Instrumental Variable." *Epidemiology* 17(3): 268–275.

Brookhart, M. A., et al. 2007. "Evaluating Validity of an Instrumental Variable Study of Neuroleptics: Can Between-Physician Differences in Prescribing Patterns Be Used to Estimate Treatment Effects?" *Medical Care* 45: 10: 116–122.

Brookhart, M. A., and S. Schneeweiss. 2007. "Preference-Based Instrumental Variable Methods for the Estimation of Treatment Effects: Assessing Validity and Interpreting Results." *The International Journal of Biostatistics* 3: Article 14.

D'Agostino, Sr., R. B., and H. Kwan. 1995. "Measuring Effectiveness: What to Expect Without a Randomized Control Group." *Medical Care* 33 (4 supplements): AS95–AS105.

Foster, E.M. 2000. "Is More Better Than Less? An Analysis of Children's Mental Health Services." *Health Services Research* 35(5 Pt 2): 1135–1158.

Glesby, M.J., and D. R. Hoover. 1996. "Survivor Treatment Selection Bias in Observational Studies: Examples From the AIDS Literature." *Annals of Internal Medicine* 124: 999–1005.

Greenland, S. 2000. "An Introduction to Instrumental Variables for Epidemiologists." *International Journal of Epidemiology* 29: 722–729.

Grimes, D.A., and K. F. Schulz. 2002. "Bias and Causal Associations in Observational Research." The *Lancet.* 359: 248–252.

Haynes, R. B., H. P. McDonald, and A. X. Garg. 2002. "Helping Patients Follow Prescribed Treatment: Clinical Applications." The *Journal of the American Medical Association* 288 (22): 2880–2883.

Heckman, J. J. 1978. "Dummy Endogenous Variables in a Simultaneous Equation System." *Econometrica* 46: 931–959.

Hernán, M. A., and J. M. Robins. 2006. "Instruments for Causal Inference: an Epidemiologist's Dream?" *Epidemiology* 17, 4: 360–372.

Jerant, A. F., M. M. Von Friederichs-Fitzwater, and M. Moore. 2005. "Patients' Perceived Barriers to Active Self-Management of Chronic Conditions." *Patient Education & Counseling* 57(3): 300–307.

Kramer, C. Y. 1956. "Extension of Multiple Range Tests to Group Means with Unequal Numbers of Replications." *Biometrics* 12(3): 307–310.

Lago, R. M., P. P. Singh, and R. W. Nesto. 2007. "Congestive Heart Failure and Cardiovascular Death in Patients with Prediabetes and Type 2 Diabetes Given Thiazolidinediones: A Meta-Analysis of Randomised Clinical Trials." The *Lancet.* 370(9593): 1129–1136.

Landrum, M. B., and J. Z. Ayanian. 2001. "Causal Effect of Ambulatory Specialty Care on Mortality Following Myocardial Infarction: A Comparison of Propensity Score and Instrumental Variable Analyses." *Health Services and Outcomes Research Methodology* 2: 221–245.

Lincoff, A. M., K. Wolski, S. J. Nicholls, and S. E. Nissen. 2007. "Pioglitazone and Risk of Cardiovascular Events in Patients With Type 2 Diabetes Mellitus: A Meta-Analysis of Randomized Trials." The *Journal of the American Medical Association* 298(10): 1180–1188.

McClellan, M., B. J. McNeil, and J. P. Newhouse. 1994. "Does More Intensive Treatment of Acute Myocardial Infarction in the Elderly Reduce Mortality? Analysis Using Instrumental Variables." The *Journal of the American Medical Association* 272(11): 859–866.

McClellan, M. B., and J. P. Newhouse. 2000. "Overview of the Special Supplement Issue." *Health Services Research* 35: 5 (Part 2): 1061–1069.

Murray, M. P. 2006. "Avoiding Invalid Instruments and Coping with Weak Instruments." *Journal of Economic Perspectives* 20(4): 111–132.

Schneeweiss, S., et al. 2002. "Quasi-Experimental Longitudinal Designs to Evaluate Drug Benefit Policy Changes with Low Policy Compliance." *Journal of Clinical Epidemiology* 55(8): 833–841.

Stukel, T. A., E. S. Fisher, D. E. Wennberg, and D. A. Alter. 2007. "Analysis of Observational Studies in the Presence of Treatment Selection Bias: Effects of Invasive Cardiac Management on AMI Survival Using Propensity Score and Instrumental Variable Methods." The *New England Journal of Medicine* 297: 278–285.

Wang, P. S., S. Schneeweiss, and J. Avorn. 2005. "Risk of Death in Elderly Users of Conventional vs. Atypical Antipsychotic Medications." The *Journal of the American Medical Association* 353: 2335–2341.

Chapter 7

Local Control Approach Using JMP

Robert L. Obenchain

Abstract

The local control approach to adjustment for treatment selection bias and confounding in observational studies is illustrated here using JMP because local control is best implemented and applied in highly visual ways. The local control approach is also unique because it hierarchically clusters patients in baseline covariate *x*-space; applies simple nested analysis of variance (ANOVA) models (treatment within cluster); and ends up being highly flexible, non-parametric, and robust. Although the local control approach is classical rather than Bayesian, its primary output is a full distribution of local treatment differences (LTDs) that contains all potential information relevant to patient differential responses to treatment. All concepts are illustrated using freely distributable data on 10,000 patients that were generated to be like those from a published cardiovascular registry containing 996 patients.

7.1 Introduction

The key roles played by blocking and randomization in the statistical design of experiments are universally recognized. This chapter emphasizes that relatively simple variations on these same concepts can lead to powerful and robust analyzes of observational studies. Because adequate blocking and randomization usually is not (or cannot be) incorporated into the data collection phase of observational research, the two variations (local control and resampling) that we discuss here are both applied *post hoc*.

Since the work of Cochran (1965, 1968), many methods for analysis of observational data have stressed formation of subclasses, subgroups, or clusters of patients leading to treatment comparisons that summarize locally defined outcome averages and/or differences. Traditionally, local control is just another name for blocking. Here, the local control approach is characterized as being a dynamic process in which the number and size of patient clusters (subgroups) is not pre-specified. Rather, built-in sensitivity analyses are used first to identify and then to focus on only the most relevant patient comparisons. This strategy ends up reducing treatment selection bias and revealing the full distribution of local treatment differences (LTDs) (that is, it identifies any patterns of patient differential response).

At least since the work of Fisher (1925), *randomization* has consistently been placed at the top of the hierarchy of research principles. See Concato and colleagues (2000). After all, randomization of patients to treatment is essential in all situations where nothing is known about the patients except their treatment choice(s) and observed outcomes. Without randomization in this situation, there would be no reason to believe (or at least hope) that the treated and untreated groups were comparable before treatment and definitely no way to identify meaningful patient subgroups and demonstrate that they are comparable in any way!

7.1.1 Fundamental Problems with Randomization in Human Studies

The main, practical problem with randomization of patients to treatment is that, due to ethical or pragmatic considerations, humans with acute conditions can be randomized at most one, single time. In other words, crossover designs are not possible. In theory, a single randomization can make a real difference. However, to get anywhere, one must then also be willing to make an almost endless litany of unverifiable assumptions about causal effects and counterfactual outcomes. See Holland (1986) on Rubin's causal model.

By the way, rather than using old-fashioned, complete randomization (where balance is merely expected on long-range averages), it is now widely recognized that the only way to come anywhere close to assuring relatively good balance in a study featuring only one treatment randomization per patient is to use separate, dynamic randomizations within each block of patients who are most comparable at baseline (McEntegart, 2003). Still, patients do not like to be randomized and blinded to the treatment they receive. As a result, the treatment arms of most studies typically tend, due to differential patient dropout over time, toward becoming unbalanced on baseline x-characteristics of the patients who end up being evaluable.

For me, the bottom line is simply that randomization unquestionably yields powerful and robust inferences only when each experimental subject can be exposed (like animals in cages, plots in a field, or Fisher's lady tasting tea) to a sequence of blinded challenges, ideally of variable length.

Example: Consider the following experiment on a collection (finite, nonrandom sample) of ancient coins of different designs and grades (amounts of circulation). Suppose each coin is to be treated by either being flipped in the usual way or else spun on edge on a hard flat surface, resulting in an observed outcome designated as either heads or tails. See Gelman and Nolan (2002) and Diaconis and colleagues (2007), especially Figure 7. How much information could randomization to treatment (flip vs. spin) add to this experiment under the stifling restriction that each coin is both treated and tested only one time? Due to such severe limitations on randomization in this experiment, nothing particularly interesting can be inferred about either the fairness of the coins or the effects of the treatments!

Situations where very little is known about the patients actually entering a study are rare. In fact, researchers frequently have such a good idea of which patient baseline characteristics are predictive of outcomes (and/or treatment choices) that they would not consider performing a serious (prospective or retrospective) study without first confirming that these key patient characteristics will be observed in each patient.

Here, we propose using a form of resampling (without replacement) in Section 7.3.3 to verify that an observed LTD distribution is salient. To avoid any possibility of bad luck in a single randomization of all patients to an exhaustive set of distinct subgroups, we certainly recommend accumulating results across multiple, independent resamples (default: 25 replications).

7.1.2 Fundamental Local Control Concepts

When performing a local control (LC) analysis, the more one knows about the most relevant pre-treatment characteristics of the patients, the better. This information is used to form blocks retrospectively. Blocks are potentially meaningful patient subgroups, which one might call empirically defined strata or subclasses (Cochran, 1965, 1968) or clusters. Because human subjects are notoriously heterogeneous in terms of their (baseline) x-characteristics, there really is little reason for optimism about reproducibility of findings when one cannot at least make treatment comparisons within subgroups of patients who really are very much alike.

Most importantly, a key feature of the LC approach is that one can indeed verify that the local subgroups one has formed reveal statistically meaningful differences, which are called *salient treatment differences* here. The basic LC terminology needed to establish the concept of salient differences is as follows.

Within any subgroup that contains both treated and untreated patients, the local treatment difference (LTD) is defined as the mean outcome for treated patient(s) minus the mean outcome for untreated patient(s). Because LTDs are calculated from mean outcomes, the local numbers of patients treated or untreated do not need to be balanced (that is, occur in a 1:1 ratio) for the LTD to be an unbiased estimate of the unknown, true local difference.

Any subgroup containing only treated patient(s) or only untreated patient(s) is said to be uninformative. The LTD for this subgroup is not estimable and is represented in JMP and SAS by the missing value symbol, a period.

When all N available patients are divided into K mutually exclusive and exhaustive subgroups (or clusters) of patient(s), each containing one or more patients ($K \leq N$), the corresponding LTD distribution consists of K values for the LTDs within the distinct subgroups, some of which may be missing values. The sufficient statistic for a given LTD distribution is assumed to be its empirical cumulative distribution function (CDF), where the height of the step at each observed, non-missing LDT value is (total number of patients in that subgroup) / (total number of patients within all informative subgroups). Because these steps can be of different heights, the CDF is described here as *patient weighted*. Because observed LTDs are heteroskedastic (due to variation in within-subgroup treatment fractions and to local heteroskedasticity in outcomes as well as to variation in subgroup sizes), several alternative weightings for CDFs could also be considered.

A useful rule of thumb is that $K \leq (N/11)$, so that the overall average number of patients per subgroup is at least 11. While smaller subgroups tend to be more local, they also tend to become uninformative about their LTD, thereby wastefully discarding information and increasing overall uncertainty.

In the LC approach, the CDF for an observed LTD distribution resulting from K subgroups of well-matched patients is compared with the CDF for the corresponding artificial LTD distribution, defined as follows. An *artificial LTD distribution* results from randomly assigning the N observed patient outcomes to K subgroups of the same size and with the same fractions of treated and untreated patients as the K observed subgroups. The precision of the overall, artificial LTD CDF is typically deliberately increased by merging several complete replications (typically 25) of independent, random assignments of N patients to K clusters. In particular, note that patient ***x***-characteristics are deliberately ignored when forming artificial LTD distributions; specifically, only the observed patient-level ***y***-outcomes and their observed ***t***-treatment assignments are used to estimate an LTD distribution. The artificial replicates can then be merged (averaged) or maximum and minimum values can be calculated at individual *y*-values.

When the CDF for an observed LTD distribution is truly different (in a possibly subtle way) from its corresponding artificial CDF, the observed LTD distribution is said to be *salient*. After all, like the overall comparison of all treated patients with all untreated patients in the full data set, treatment comparisons based upon randomly defined subgroups are biased whenever differential treatment selection or other confounding (***x***-characteristic imbalance) information is present. In sharp contrast, the observed LTDs formed within subgroups of truly comparable patients are unbiased.

When the empirical distributions of biased and unbiased estimates are not distinguishable from each other, the unbiased estimates are certainly not clearly superior to the biased estimates! Once the CDFs for the observed and artificial LTD distributions are seen to be truly different, the logical explanation is that the observed LTD distribution has been (at least partially) adjusted for treatment selection bias and confounding.

Similarly, the mean LTD value across the subgroups that constitute a salient LTD distribution is the corresponding adjusted main effect of treatment. Finally, the empirical CDF for a salient LTD distribution is assumed here to constitute an adjusted sufficient statistic for addressing questions about patient differential response to treatment as function(s) of their ***x***-characteristics.

7.1.3 Statistical Methods Most Useful in Local Control

The LC concepts discussed and illustrated in this chapter rely heavily on cluster analysis methodology (see, for example, Kaufman and Rousseeuw [1990]) applied to the observed baseline *x*-characteristics of patients. Clustering is a form of unsupervised learning (Barlow, 1989); no information from the ultimate outcome variables (*y*) or treatment assignment indicators (*t*) is used to guide (supervise) formation of patient clusters. While the bad news is that patient clustering is an extremely difficult (NP* hard) computational task, the good news is that several

* Non-deterministic polynomial-time.

versatile and relatively fast (approximate) algorithms have been developed recently. For example, see Fraley and Raftery (2002) or Wegman and Luo (2002).

In the early phases of an LC analysis, the only statistical modeling and estimation tools needed are those of a simple nested ANOVA model with effects for clusters, for treatment within cluster, and for error in Table 7.1.

Table 7.1 Nested ANOVA Table with Effects for Treatment within Cluster

Source	Degrees of Freedom	Interpretation
Clusters (Subgroups)	K = Number of Clusters	Cluster Means are Local Average Treatment Effects (LATEs) when *X*s are Instrumental Variables (IVs)
Treatment within Cluster	I = Number of Informative Clusters $\leq K$	Local Treatment Differences (LTDs) are of interest when *X* Variables either are or are not IVs.
Error	Number of Patients − K − I	Outcome Uncertainty and/or Model Lack of Fit

In Sections 7.3.2 and 7.3.3, we will see that the LC focuses on new ways to analyze, visualize, and interpret nested treatment effects and their uncertainty.

While the LC approach to adjustment for selection bias and confounding clearly makes very good sense intuitively, it may be comforting to some readers to note that the basic strategy and tactics of LC are also fully compatible with the propensity scoring (PS) principles of Rosenbaum and Rubin (1983, 1984) as well as with the clustering-based instrumental variable (IV) approach of McClellan, McNeil, and Newhouse (1994). The appendix to this chapter discusses the common foundational aspects shared by both the PS and LC approaches.

7.1.4 Contents of the Remaining Sections of Chapter 7

Section 7.2 introduces the LSIM10K numerical example that will be used to illustrate LC analyses. Section 7.3 outlines the four basic phases of a local control analysis and then illustrates that LC can lead to deeper and more detailed insights than the traditional approaches described in Section 7.2. Finally, Section 7.4 provides some conclusions about LC as well as a brief, general discussion of the advantages and disadvantages of LC methodology relative to

- covariate adjustment using global multivariable models
- inverse probability weighting
- propensity score matching or subgrouping
- instrumental variable approaches

7.2 Some Traditional Analyses of Hypothetical Patient Registry Data

7.2.1 Introduction to the LSIM10K Data Set

We have tried to gain access to any of a number of relatively large and rich data sets that have recently been described and analyzed in high profile, published observational studies, typically using some form of covariate adjustment for treatment selection bias as well as confounding among predictors of outcome. Unfortunately, the owners of these data sets often refuse to share them publicly.

We ultimately decided to simulate a data set with a relatively large number of patients (10,325), yielding data that can be distributed on the CD that accompanies this publication. This simulated patient registry-like data will also be used to illustrate a wide assortment of alternative methodologies, like the traditional, global analyses outlined in Sections 7.2.2 through 7.2.4.

To make the simulated data at least somewhat realistic, the Linder Center data described and analyzed in Kereiakes and colleagues (2000) served as our simulation starting point. This study collected 6-month follow-up data on 996 patients who underwent an initial percutaneous coronary intervention (PCI or angioplasty) in 1997 and were treated with usual care alone or usual care plus a relatively expensive blood thinner (IIB/IIIA cascade blocker). We decided to simulate the same two-outcome *y*-variables (measures of treatment effectiveness and cost) and use the same basic variable correlations and patient clustering patterns observed among seven patient baseline *x*-characteristics (listed here) in the original data set. These patient characteristics apparently help quantify differences in disease severity and/or patient frailty between treatment groups. In any case, they proved to be predictive of outcome and/or treatment selection.

The LSIM10K.SAS7BDAT data set contains the values of 10 simulated variables for 10,325 hypothetical patients. To simplify analyses, the data contain no missing values. The 10 variables are defined as follows:

mort6mo
: This binary, numeric variable characterizes 6-month mortality. It contains either 0, to indicate that the patient survived for 6 months, or 1, to indicate that the patient did not survive for 6 months.

cardcost
: This variable contains the cumulative, cardiac-related charges, expressed in 1998 dollars, incurred within 6 months of the patient's initial PCI. Reported costs are truncated by death for patients with `mort6mo=1`.

trtm
: This binary, numeric variable identifies treatment selection. It contains either 0, to indicate usual care alone, or 1, to indicate usual care augmented with a hypothetical blood thinner.

stent
: This binary, numeric variable identifies coronary stent deployment. A value of 0 means that no stent was deployed, while a value of 1 means that a stent was deployed.

height
: This numeric variable records the patient's height rounded to the nearest centimeter. These integer values range from 133 to 197.

female
: This binary, numeric variable equals 0 for male patients or 1 for female patients.

diabetic
: This binary, numeric variable equals 0 for patients with no diagnosis of diabetes mellitus or 1 for patients with a diagnosis of diabetes mellitus.

acutemi
: This binary, numeric variable equals 0 for patients who had not recently suffered an acute myocardial infarction or 1 for patients who had suffered an acute myocardial infarction within the previous 7 days.

ejfrac
: This numeric variable records the patient's left ejection fraction rounded to the nearest full percentage point. These integer values range from 18 to 77 percent.

ves1proc
: This numeric variable records the number of vessels involved in the patient's initial PCI. These integer values, ranging from 0 to 5, may be best viewed as six ordinal values. Here, we treat ves1proc as either a factor with 6 levels (5 degrees of freedom) or as continuous (1 degree of freedom when entering a model linearly).

7.2.2 Analyses of Mortality Rates and Costs Using Covariate Adjustment

The observed 6-month mortality rate among 4,679 treated patients in the LSIM10K data is 1.218%, while that among 5,646 untreated patients is 3.719%, which corresponds to a mortality risk ratio of more than 3:1 in favor of treatment. Equivalently, the risk percentage difference (treated minus untreated) of –2.501% is highly significant (*t*-statistic = –8.38, two-tailed *p*-value = 0.0000+).

A simple model appropriate for covariate adjustment (also called multivariable modeling) of 6-month mortality using the LSIM10K data would be logistic regression of the binary mortality indicator, mort6mo, on the binary trtm indicator plus all seven baseline patient characteristics (say, with height and ejfract entering linearly and model degrees of freedom = 12, not counting the intercept). The area under the receiver operating characteristic (ROC) curve is 0.7107 for this model, and it suffers no significant lack of fit. On the other hand, the R-squared statistic for this simple model is 0.0653, which is quite poor (low).

Most importantly, the implied predictions of 6-month mortality from this logistic model average 0.01218 for treated patients and 0.03720 for untreated patients, which are essentially the same as those previously observed, unadjusted results (differing only in the fifth decimal place). In other words, covariate adjustment essentially accomplishes nothing on average when outcomes are discrete.

When outcome measures are continuous, such as the 6-month cardiac-related cost variable (cardcost), covariance adjustment methods can be more interesting. For example, the mean costs in the LSIM10K data are $15,188 when untreated and $15,443 when treated; the *t*-statistic for the unadjusted difference in mean cost between treatment groups (+$255) is *t* = 1.24, with a *p*-value of 0.892. Using the simple linear covariate adjustment multivariable model with 12 degrees of freedom (R-squared = 0.0364), with right-hand-side structure identical to the logit model described previously, the least squares mean costs are \$12,176 when untreated and \$12,305 when treated. The t-statistic for the adjusted difference in mean cost (+\$129) is $t = 0.62$, with a p-value of 0.538. Thus, covariate adjustment methods clearly can accomplish something when outcomes are continuous. However, smooth, global models offer little hope for making realistic adjustments for treatment selection bias and confounding. Typically, they provide only relatively poor fits to large data sets covering numerous, heterogeneous patient subpopulations.

A highly touted variation on these sorts of covariate adjustment modeling is known as *inverse probability weighting* (IPW). This approach typically uses simple logistic or linear regression models like the ones considered here, but each observed patient outcome is then weighted inversely proportional to the conditional probability that he/she would receive the observed choice of treatment given his/her baseline x-characteristics. These estimated conditional probabilities are called *fitted propensity scores* and the appropriate calculations and graphical displays are illustrated next, in Section 7.2.3. We will then use the propensity score estimates from Section 7.2.3 to illustrate the IPW approach in Section 7.2.4.

7.2.3 Analyses of Mortality Rates Using Estimated Propensity Score Deciles

The conditional probability that a patient will choose a specified treatment given his/her baseline x-characteristics is that patient's true propensity score. The conditional probability of that patient choosing some other treatment is thus (1–PS). Propensity score estimates are typically generated by fitting a logit (or probit) model to binary indicators, trtm = 0 or 1, of observed choices for given patient baseline x–characteristics. Because all attention will ultimately be focused only on the resulting propensity score estimates (rather than on any p-values or other characteristics of the model), no penalties are assumed to result from overfitting. Thus, researchers typically fit nonparsimonious global models; here, we fit a full factorial-to-degree-two logit model in all seven available covariates. This model uses up 46 degrees of freedom, not counting the intercept.

The area under the ROC curve is 0.6993 for this model, and it suffers no significant lack of fit. On the other hand, the R-squared statistic for this model is 0.0867, which is again quite poor (low).

An essential feature of satisfactory propensity score estimates is that they behave, at least approximately, like unknown, true propensity scores. Specifically, conditioning upon (rounded) propensity score estimates should yield pairs of x-covariate distributions (treated vs. untreated) that are not significantly different. After all, conditioning upon true propensity scores would make all such pairs of subdistributions identical; see equation A.2 in the appendix. In other words, if patients are sorted by estimated propensity scores and divided into 10 ordered deciles (in the current context, 10 subgroups of size 1,032 or 1,033 patients each), then the pairs of within propensity score decile subdistributions (treated vs. untreated) for every x-covariate should be approximately the same. For example, Figure 7.1 shows (in the left panel) the relatively dissimilar marginal distributions of ejfract within the two treatment arms, which is due to treatment selection bias and confounding. On the other hand (in the right panel), we see the 10 pairs of relatively well-matched subdistributions of ejfract by treatment choice, which is due to subgrouping using estimated propensity score deciles. Again, in the left panel, note that the lower tail of the marginal ejfract distribution (that is, patients with the most severe impairment in circulation) tends to be dominated by treated patients. Meanwhile, within the 10th estimated propensity score decile (last pair of box plots in the right panel), note that the corresponding pair of conditional distributions for ejfract appears nearly identical.

Figure 7.1 Marginal and Within Propensity Score Decile Distributions of ejfract by Treatment

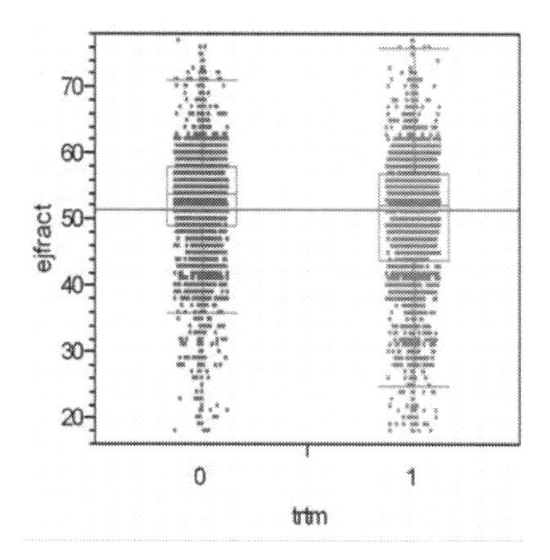

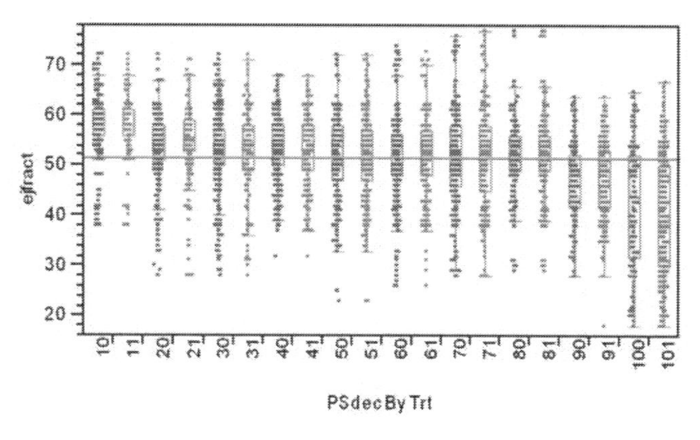

What may not be particularly clear from Figure 7.1 is that the treatment ratio is more than 3:1 (791 treated to 241 untreated) within the 10th estimated propensity score decile. In fact, the within propensity score decile treatment ratios are not very close to 1:1 here except in deciles 5, 6, and 7. See Figure 7.3. As a result, it is best to think of the objective of subgrouping via estimated propensity score deciles as being formation of valid blocks of patients. Within each block, the x-covariate distributions for treated and untreated patients need to be almost the same, yet the treatment fractions within each block may be quite different across blocks (deciles).

As well as examining these sorts of plots for each continuous x-covariate, researchers need to compare the corresponding $2 \times L$ contingency tables for each discrete x-covariate (factor) with L levels. In other words, researchers need to verify that the patient deciles implied by their propensity score estimates do indeed constitute 10 valid blocks of patients. This propensity score modeling/validation process can be somewhat tedious and time-consuming, at least when mismatches in x-covariate distributions don't go away! Again, propensity score estimates are clearly inadequate and unrealistic when they cannot be verified to at least approximately behave like unknown, true propensity scores.

An even more elementary requirement of estimated propensity scores is that they do indeed predict the observed local fractions of patients actually treated, as demonstrated by the least squares regression fit in Figure 7.2. As a direct result, the observed numbers of treated and untreated patients are expected to vary by propensity score decile to reveal the familiar X-shaped pattern of Figure 7.3.

Figure 7.2 Estimated Within Decile Propensity Score Means vs. Observed Fractions of Patients Treated

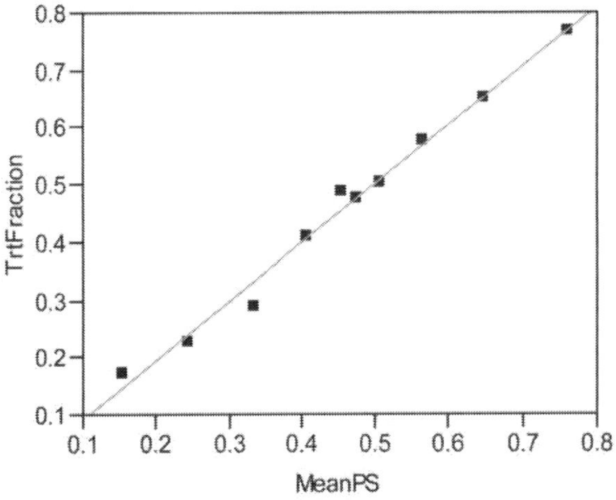

Local Fraction Treated = –0.0101 + 1.0223 * Mean Estimated Propensity Score within Decile

Figure 7.3 Numbers of Treated and Untreated Patients by Propensity Score Decile

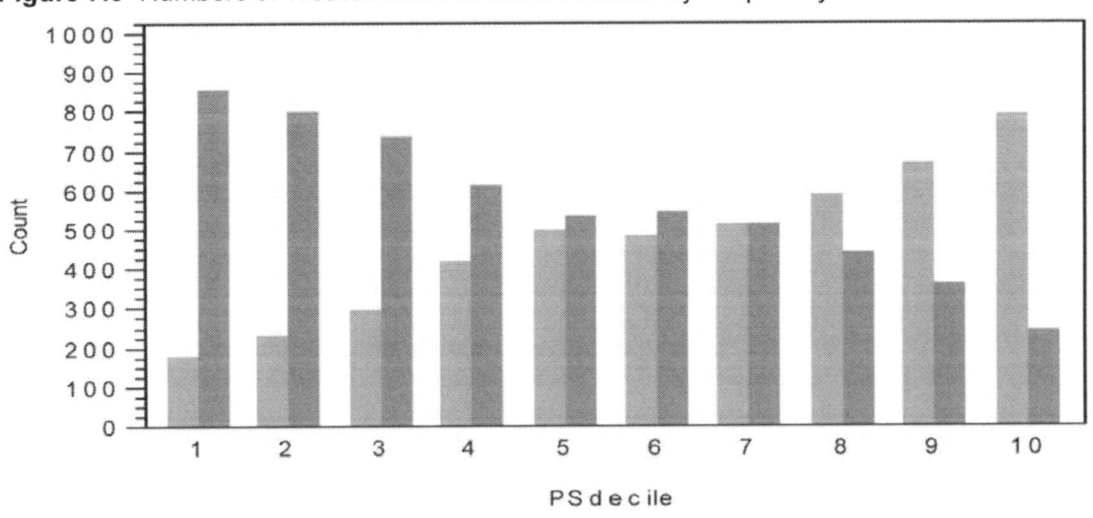

Another fundamental concept that differentiates the propensity score (and local control) approaches from covariate adjustment (CA) and IPW modeling is that it can be best to simply ignore the data from certain patients. For example, if all the patients with the lowest propensity score estimates in the first decile of Figure 7.3 were untreated, then the data from these patients should be set aside. Similarly, if all the patients with the highest propensity score estimates in the 10th decile of Figure 7.3 were treated, then their data should also be set aside. A more technical explanation for these sorts of patient exclusions is discussed next.

The distributions of propensity score estimates are portrayed in Figure 7.4 using histograms with 40 cells each. Only those patients within the common support of these two distributions are considered sufficiently comparable to be included in propensity score analyses. For the LSIM10K data, these two distributions luckily have essentially the same range, from 0.025 to 0.925. For pairs (treated vs. untreated) of distributions of propensity score estimates with different ranges, data from all patients falling outside of the maximum range supported by both distributions should be set aside. The propensity score deciles should then be formed using only the patients falling within this maximum supported range.

Figure 7.4 Detailed Histograms of Estimated Propensity Scores

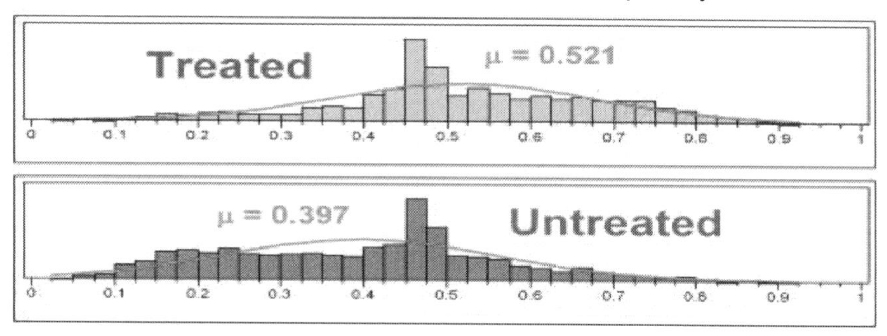

The remaining steps in a propensity score decile analysis are

1. compute the LTDs within each decile and their variances
2. compute the LTD main effect = the average of within decile LTDs across deciles and its variance
3. compute the *t*-statistic and *p*-value for the test of significance of the LTD main effect

For the LSIM10K data, $t = -2.95$ and $p = 0.026$. Note in Figure 7.5 that the hypothetical treatment in the LSIM10K data tends to deliver its greatest, incremental mortality benefit to the patients in the ninth and 10th propensity score deciles (that is, those who are most likely to choose/receive it). In summary, compared with the covariate adjustment approach that used a global ("wrong") model, the propensity score deciles approach yields a much larger (less biased) estimate for the main effect of treatment with somewhat lower (more realistic) precision.

Figure 7.5 LTDs for 6-Month Mortality (Treated minus Untreated) by Propensity Score Decile

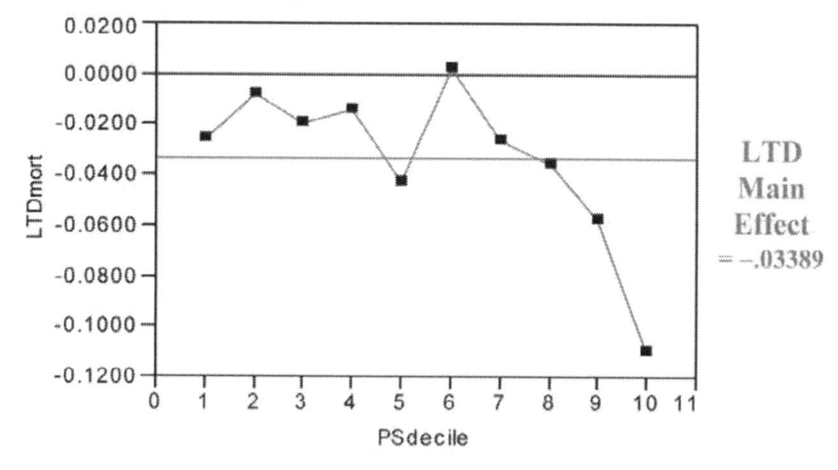

7.2.4 Analyses of Mortality Rates and Costs Using Inverse Probability Weighting

The model appropriate for inverse probability weighting of 6-month mortality on the LSIM10K data would be a (weighted) logistic regression with the binary trtm indicator and all seven baseline patient characteristics as dependent variables (again, with height and ejfract entering linearly and model degrees of freedom = 12, not counting the intercept). Here, the IPW is proportional to 1/PS for treated patients or 1/(1–PS) for untreated patients. To give results comparable to those from the unweighted analyses of Section 7.2.2, the estimated weights need to be rescaled to sum to 10,325, which is the total number of patients in the LSIM10K data. Without this rescaling, the weights here would sum to 20,796, which would yield a false increase in implied precision equivalent to assuming that the data are available for more than twice as many patients as actually are available!

The rescaled weights that sum to 10,325 range from 0.519 to 11.38 and are summarized in Figure 7.6. The mean weight for untreated patients is then 0.9114 (that is, less than one for the larger sample of 5,646 patients) while that for treated patients is 1.1050 (that is, more than one for the smaller sample of 4,679 patients).

Figure 7.6 IPWs for Treated or Untreated Patients Derived from Propensity Score Estimates

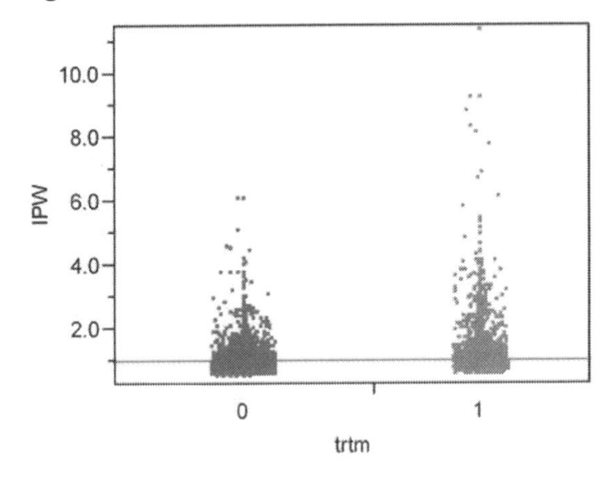

The area under the ROC curve for the resulting IPW prediction of 6-month mortality increases to 0.7550, again with no significant lack of fit. On the other hand, the R-squared statistic for this simple model is still only 0.1041, which is poor. The IPW predictions of 6-month risk of mortality average 0.01278 for treated patients and 0.03994 for untreated patients. The IPW adjusted main effect difference in mortality is thus 0.02716, which differs from the observed, unadjusted difference in the third decimal place. In other words, the IPW variation on covariate adjustment also accomplishes very little on average for a binary outcome.

Figure 7.7 compares predictions of the risk of 6-month mortality from simple logistic regression models, including the least squares regression of covariance adjustment risks (the unweighted logit) on IPW risks. The correlation between these risk predictions is 0.9177, so the fitted slope is 0.8421.

Using an IPW linear covariance adjustment model (with R-square = 0.0312), the IPW least squares mean costs are $13,761 when untreated and $13,647 when treated, and the *t*-statistic for the adjusted difference in mean cost (–$114) is $t = -0.56$, with a *p*-value of 0.573. Thus, while IPW methods do change the numerical sign of the estimated cost difference (treated minus untreated), this difference remains insignificant statistically. The fact remains that smooth, global models offer little hope for making realistic adjustments for treatment selection bias and confounding.

Figure 7.7 IPW versus Unweighted Predictions of 6-Month Risk of Mortality

Treated or Untreated

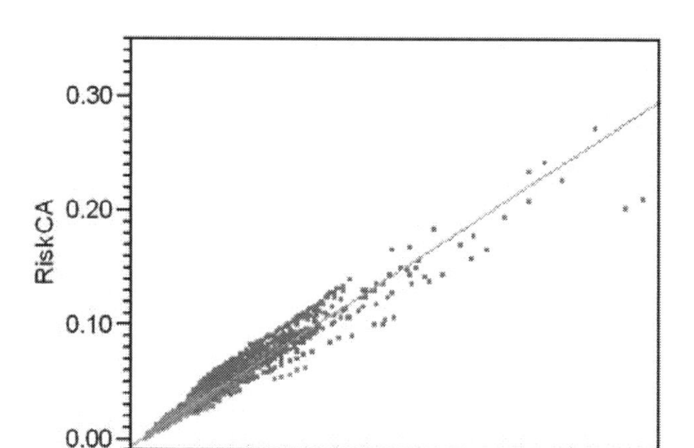

RiskCA = 0.00259 + 0.8421*RiskIPW

7.3 The Four Phases of a Local Control Analysis

7.3.1 Introduction to the Four Tactical Phases of a Local Control Analysis

Start by examining Table 7.2, which gives a brief title and description for each of the four phases of local control analysis. Sections 7.3.2 through 7.3.5 then provide more detailed motivations for each phase as well as illustrations of the use of JMP scripts on the LSIM10K.SAS7BDAT data set plus detailed interpretations for the resulting graphical and tabular outputs.

7.3.2 Phase One: Revealing Bias in Global Estimates by Making Local Comparisons

The local control approach is a highly graphical and computationally feasible way to bypass validation of propensity score estimates (as discussed in Section 7.2.3) and still end up with an even better (more robust) view of treatment effects that has been fully adjusted for treatment selection bias, local imbalance in treatment fractions, and confounding.

The primary concept behind the local control approach is that, within all data sets, comparisons between treated and untreated patients who are most similar should be more relevant than the same sorts of comparisons between dissimilar patients. Unfortunately, the *x*-covariate(s) most relevant to determining patient similarity may not be known or may be unobserved (missing from the data set).

Table 7.2 The Four Tactical Phases of Local Control Analysis

Phase One LC Tactics: Revealing Bias in Global Estimates by Making Treatment Comparisons More and More Local	The first phase of LC analysis needs to be highly interactive so that the researcher can literally see not only the direction and magnitude of potential bias introduced by treatment selection (channeling) and confounding but also the extent to which this bias can be reduced by simply increasing the number (and thereby decreasing the size) of relevant, local patient clusters. The primary objective in phase one is to identify the most revealing Local Treatment Difference (LTD) distribution (that is, an ideal number of clusters) when using available patient ***x***-characteristics to define clusters and also weighting them equally. Systematic exploration of alternative clustering strategies and tactics are best postponed until phase three.
Phase Two LC Tactics: Determining Whether an Observed LTD Distribution is Salient (Statistically Meaningful)	As pointed out in the second paragraph of Section 7.1.2, a key feature of the LC approach is that a researcher can indeed verify whether an observed set of patient ***x***-space clusters yields a meaningful LTD distribution. The artificial distribution resulting from random assignment of treated or untreated patients to the same number of clusters with the same within-cluster treatment fractions deliberately ignores all observed patient ***x***-characteristics. If the observed and artificial LTD distributions are not different, the observed LTD distribution is, for all practical purposes, meaningless. The key principle here is that, like the overall comparison(s) between treated and untreated groups within the full data set, comparisons within artificial subgroups are also biased whenever ***x***-imbalance and/or confounding are present. Differences between an observed LTD distribution and its artificial LTD distribution thus provide strong evidence of removal of bias and/or adjustment for confounding. Again, treatment comparisons made strictly within clusters of patients with highly comparable characteristics (other than treatment choice) are relatively unbiased. The LC approach emphasizes these most relevant comparisons and de-emphasizes all less local (less relevant) comparisons.

Table 7.2 (*continued*)

Phase Three LC Tactics: Performing Systematic Sensitivity Analyses	In the third (and most important) phase of LC analysis, a researcher explores the implications of using alternative ways to form clusters (for example, using different subsets of the available ***x***-covariates, different patient similarity or dissimilarity metrics, alternative clustering algorithms and [again] various numbers of clusters). Because this third phase is tedious and repetitive, it is best performed by invoking algorithms using some form of batch mode processing. The primary objective in phase three is to identify, say, the three most interesting LTD distributions that are typical (representative) of all the salient LTD distributions that have been identified. For example, which distribution is typical of the salient distributions most favorable to treatment? Which distribution is most representative of the LTD distributions least favorable to treatment? And, which LTD distribution is most typical of all salient distributions?
Phase Four LC Tactics: Identifying Baseline Patient Characteristics Predictive of Differential Treatment Response	Because results from the first three phases of LC analyses can make the differential patient response question moot, the LC approach rightfully postpones all causal and/or predictive types of analyses until last. Once the LTD for a cluster has been estimated, an extremely helpful LC tactic is to replace the observed outcomes for all patients in that cluster (whether treated or untreated) with this LTD value. As we will see, this simple tactic can be a big help in evaluating fitted models and making them more relevant and easy to interpret. Traditional covariate adjustment (CA) methods using global, parametric models (possibly combined with inverse probability weighting, IPW) are disadvantaged in the sense that they essentially have to start here at what is really the final, least well-defined, and potentially most frustrating phase of LC analysis. The researcher may well find that differential response is really rather difficult to predict.

In any case, the logical way to start learning about the potential value of concentrating upon local (within-subgroup) treatment comparisons is to simply jump in by using whatever patient baseline *x*-characteristics one does have to literally see, using the JMP scripts illustrated here, how far they can take you.

A convenient way to launch my JMP Script Language (*.JSL) files for automating local control analyses is to select Edit → Customize → Menus and Tool Bars in JMP to modify the list of **Analyze** options on the JMP main menu. Figure 7.8 illustrates that I have chosen the fifth and sixth positions on my JMP **Analyze** menu to display icons and titles for my local control and artificial LTD distribution scripts.

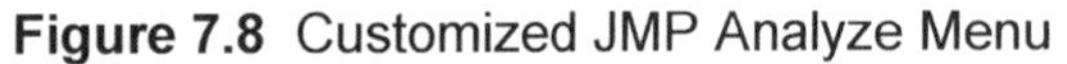

Figure 7.8 Customized JMP Analyze Menu

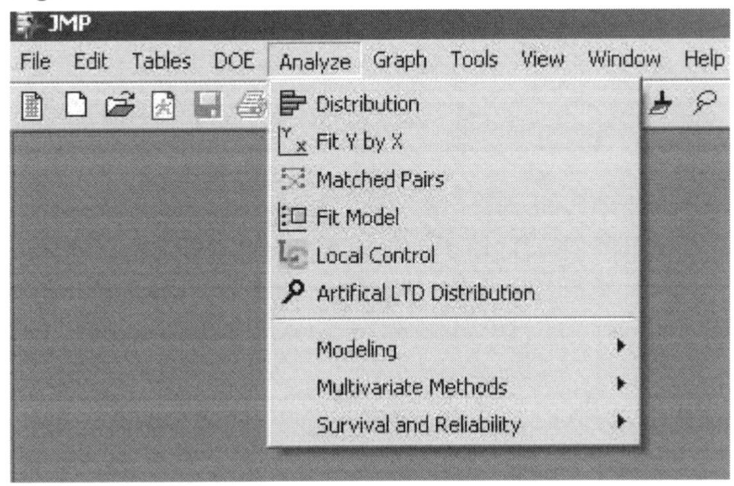

If no data set is currently open in JMP when the **Local Control** menu option is selected, JMP first displays the dialog box for opening a *.JMP or *.SAS7BDAT data set, as is illustrated in Figure 7.9. To follow along with the computations illustrated here, open the LSIM10K data set.

JMP then displays the customized Select Columns dialog box, as shown in Figure 7.10. Note that the figure shows that the first two columns (mort6mo and cardcost) were first highlighted (using left mouse shift-clicks) in the left-hand variable list and then transferred to the right-hand side by clicking on the **y, Outcomes** selection box. Similarly, the third column (trtm) was selected as the **t, Treatment Factor**, while columns four to ten (stent, height, …, ves1proc) were selected as the seven **x, Predictors** of outcome and/or treatment choice.

Figure 7.9 Open Data File Dialog Box with the LSIM10K Data Set Highlighted

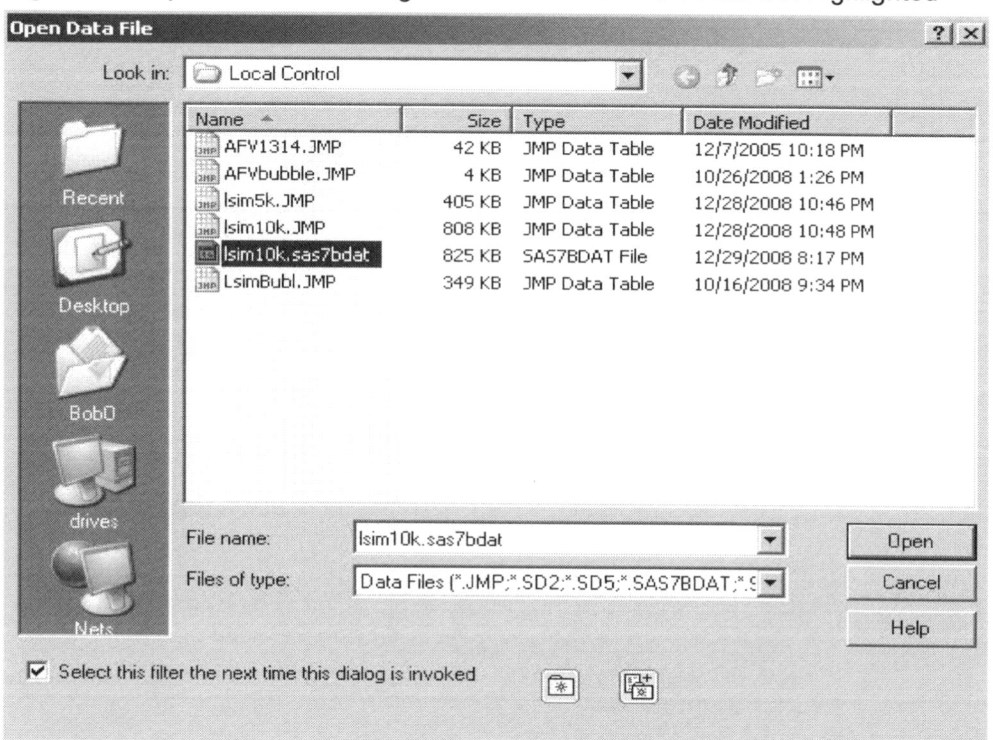

Figure 7.10 JMP Select Columns Dialog Box for Local Control

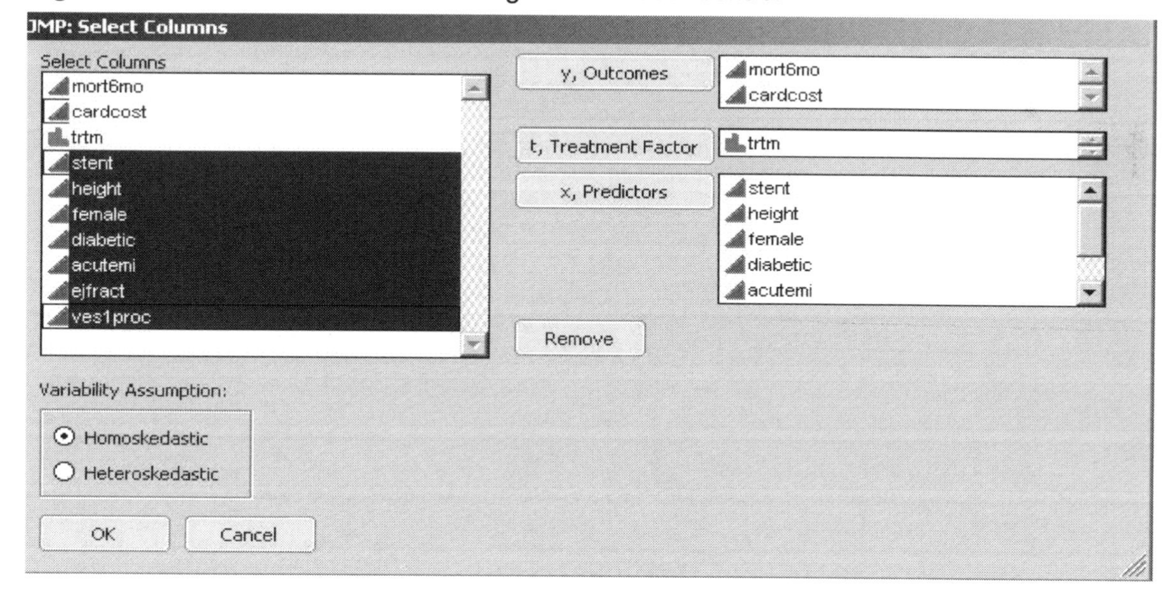

My JMP scripts for local control and artificial LTD distribution have a key restriction. All outcome *y*-variables are analyzed by computing averages, and all *x*-variables are used to cluster patients by computing distances (dissimilarities) between patients. Therefore, all *y*- and *x*-variables need to be declared both numeric and continuous in JMP. In other words, discrete *y*- and *x*-variables need to be first recoded using one or more dummy (0-1) variables, and all other *y*- and *x*-variables need to be coded using only finite, real numbers. A binary (class) variable may be declared nominal (or ordinal) in JMP only if it will be used as the t, treatment factor. Location and scaling of *y*- and *x*-variables input to my JMP script for local control are unimportant because the script re-centers all *x*-variables at 0 and standardizes their scale.

Note that the pair of radio buttons toward the lower left corner of the dialog box in Figure 7.10 allow the user to choose between the assumptions of either homoskedasticity or heteroskedasticity of variances in local control analysis. To be informative about local heteroskedasticity, each patient cluster must contain at least two treated patients plus at least two untreated patients. Because estimated within-cluster variances can be as small as 0, supposedly optimally weighted averages of LTDs across clusters can actually ignore much of the data. Thus the assumption of homoskedasticity is generally recommended for initial local control analyses.

Once the user has clicked on the **OK** box displayed in Figure 7.10, intensive and lengthy calculations are triggered. Depending on the speed of your computer and/or the amount of RAM it contains, somewhere between 15 seconds and 90 seconds are required to compute the full hierarchical clustering tree for the LSIM10K data set.

Eventually, a dendrogram like that displayed in Figure 7.11 is displayed in a JMP window and a dialog box like that in Figure 7.12 appears in the foreground on your screen. The main computational advantages of using hierarchical clustering in local control analysis is that all clusters are strictly nested and (vertical) cuts of the dendrogram tree (as illustrated in Figure 7.11) can yield almost any requested number of terminal clusters.

Figure 7.11 Vertical Cuts of the JMP Clustering Dendrogram Produce a Requested Number of Clusters from the Hierarchy

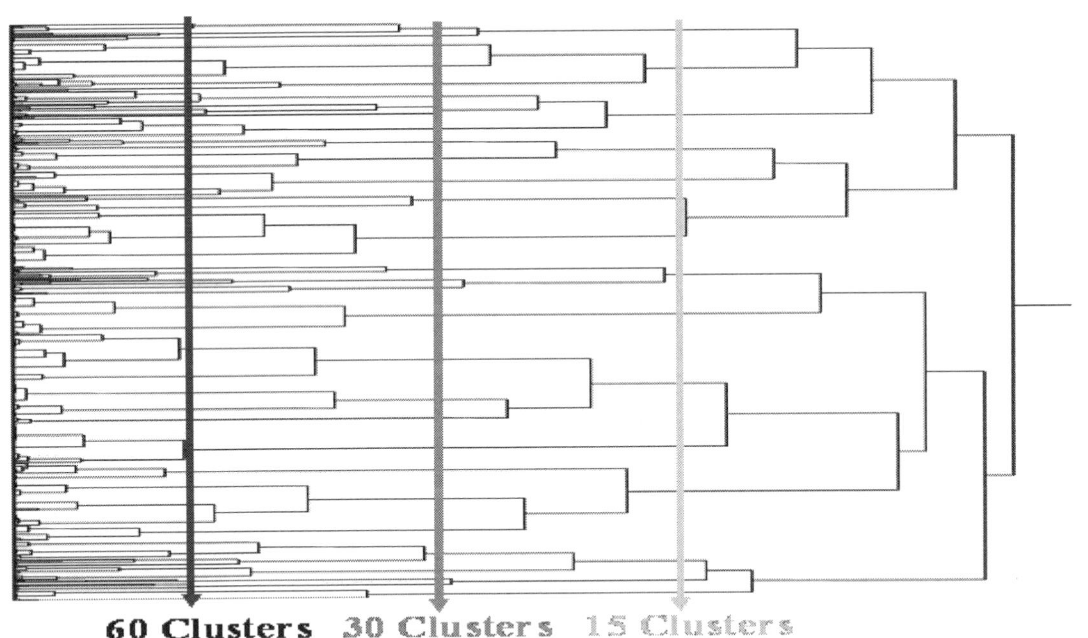

In the Next Number of Clusters dialog box in Figure 7.12, note that the initial default value is 50 clusters. When one cluster is requested, the average outcome from all untreated patients is subtracted from the average outcome for all treated patients to yield the (potentially badly biased) traditional estimate of the main effect of treatment.

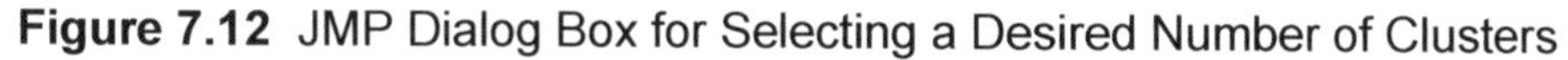

Figure 7.12 JMP Dialog Box for Selecting a Desired Number of Clusters

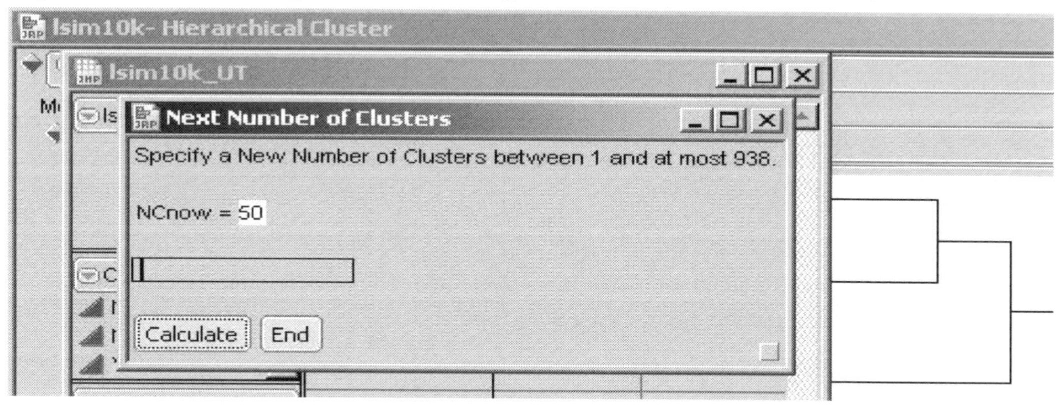

With 10,325 patients and an overall average cluster size of at least 11 patients, the number of clusters would be constrained to be at most 938, as noted in this dialog box. It is possible that clusters as small as only two patients will still be informative. However, my experience is that when the average cluster size dips to 10 or fewer patients, there is usually a wasteful abundance of clusters that are uninformative; so many clusters have been requested that some clusters have essentially been forced to be too small.

To change the number of clusters (NCnow) being requested, use your cursor to move the slider right or left. In response, the displayed value of NCnow usually changes in jumps of 10 patients or 100 patients. To select values of NCnow that are not in such a sequence, highlight the displayed value of NCnow using your cursor and edit that value using the number keys and the DELETE or BACKSPACE key. Once the desired value of NCnow is displayed, click **Calculate** in the dialog box.

Caution: My local control JMP script does not verify that the number of clusters specified is actually a new number (that is, a value different from all previously specified values of NCnow). Specifying the same number of final clusters more than once produces unnecessary and undesirable duplication of effort. On the other hand, the user can always simply delete duplicate rows in the unbiasing TRACE table as well as any duplicate tables created unintentionally.

Once you have clicked **Calculate** at least three times, the local control script starts displaying the LC unbiasing TRACE display(s) of LTD main effects *(*± two sigma*)*, as in Figures 7.13 and 7.14, respectively. At each such iteration within phase one, the user should examine these trace displays to help decide whether to

- extend the graph to the left
- extend it to the right
- fill in gaps between displayed values for the number of clusters

Figure 7.13 LC Unbiasing TRACE for the LTD Main Effect in the First Outcome

First Outcome: Y1 = Mortality within Six Months

Y1 = Across Cluster *Average* LTD Outcome ± Two *Sigma*

NCreq = Number of Clusters Requested

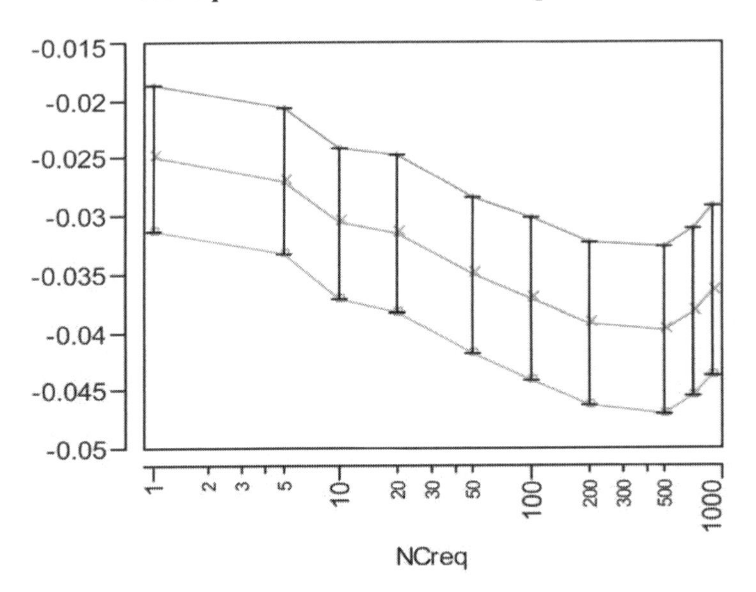

Table 7.3 Across Cluster Summary Statistics Displayed in Figure 7.13

NCreq	NCinfo	Y1 LTD MAIN	Y1 Local Std Err	Y1 Lower Limit	Y1 Upper Limit
1	1	–0.0250	0.00313	–0.0313	–0.0188
5	5	-0.0270	0.00319	-0.0333	-0.0206
10	10	-0.0306	0.00326	-0.0371	-0.0241
20	20	-0.0315	0.00338	-0.0383	-0.0248
50	50	-0.0351	0.00340	-0.0419	-0.0283
100	100	-0.0372	0.00346	-0.0441	-0.0302
200	199	-0.0393	0.00351	-0.0463	-0.0322
500	492	-0.0398	0.00360	-0.0470	-0.0326
700	660	-0.0383	0.00363	-0.0456	-0.0311
900	816	-0.0365	0.00363	-0.0438	-0.0293

NCreg = Number of Clusters Requested
NCinfo = Number of Informative Clusters Found

Figure 7.14 LC Unbiasing TRACE for the LTD Main Effect in the Second Outcome

Second Outcome: Six-Month Cumulative Cardiac-Related Cost

Y2 = Across Cluster *Average* LTD Outcome ± Two *Sigma*

NCreq = Number of Clusters Requested

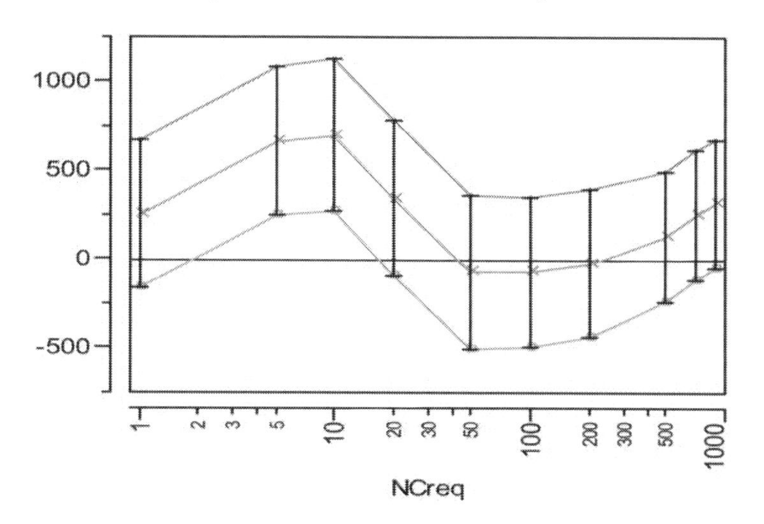

Once you decide to stop exploring different numbers of clusters, click **End**, also shown in Figure 7.12. While this action terminates the automated sequence of iterations within phase one, you will still want to explore one or more of the individual JMP data tables that were created for each specified number of clusters. As we see here, each of these tables has one or more built-in scripts to generate detailed data visualizations and/or to perform further analyses.

For example, the JMP table LSIM10K_UT contains the statistics displayed in the LC unbiasing TRACE graphics for LTD main effects on outcome(s). This table also contains script(s), named UTsumy1 and UTsumy2, for redisplaying these graphics. This allows the graphs to be customized. For example, the user can change the tic-mark spacing, orientation of tic-mark labels, and specification of descriptive axis labels. The resulting graphs and tables can then be saved in a JMP journal file and, ultimately, written to the user's hard disk as, say, RTF or DOC files.

In Figure 7.13 and its corresponding table (numerical listing), note that negative values for the mean of the LTD distribution (main effect of treatment) on the `Y1=mort6mo` outcome imply that treated patients have a lower expected 6-month mortality rate than untreated patients. Furthermore, this mean difference initially becomes more negative in the unbiasing TRACE as patient comparisons are made more and more local (by using more or smaller clusters). After all, the initial global result (treated minus untreated mort6mo rates = –0.025) essentially assumes that all available patients are in the same, single cluster, In fact, as shown on the left side of Figure 7.15, the LTD distribution is nowhere near to being smoothly continuous. For example, it has a point mass of probability 0.690 at LTD = 0 when 900 clusters are requested (and 816 informative clusters are found). In other words, there is strong evidence that treatment selection and confounding were biasing the mean of the nonlocal comparisons of mort6mo outcomes in a way unfavorable to treatment. The mean of the LTD distribution for mort6mo thus shifts mostly left (from –0.0250 to –0.0398 at NCreq = 500 to –0.0365 at NCreq = 900) as its comparisons become more local, but this LTD distribution remains rather complicated (unsmooth) but bounded on [–1.00, +1.00].

The second unbiasing TRACE of Figure 7.14 for the **Y2=cardcost** outcome suggests some potentially confusing and complicated possibilities. In fact, the mean of the cardcost LTD distribution (main effect of treatment on cardcost) bounces around, first sharply up, then distinctly down, and then partially back up again. As seen on the right side of Figure 7.15, the LTD distribution of cardcost contains some obvious outliers (–$38K, –$21K, +$28K, +$29K, +$34K, +$82K, and +$98K). On the other hand, the LTD distribution for cardcost is much smoother than the LTD distribution for mort6mo.

In summary, there is no real evidence that treatment selection and confounding are biasing mean cardcost either up or down in the LSIM10K data set. In fact, a relatively wide range of LTD cardcost point estimates of main effect (ranging from +$699 to –$74) are all supported by Figure 7.14. Note that the point estimates of uncertainty (sigma) displayed in Figure 7.14, which are computed at fixed values for the number of clusters, are clearly underestimating the true uncertainty about the cardcost main effect that is revealed by varying the number of clusters.

Table 7.4 Across Cluster Summary Statistics Displayed in Figure 7.14

NCreq	NCinfo	Y2 LTD MAIN	Y2 Loc Std Err	Y2 Low Limit	Y2 Upr Limit
1	1	255.08	206.21	-157.33	667.50
5	5	664.94	208.99	246.96	1082.92
10	10	698.80	214.19	270.42	1127.19
20	20	341.77	220.48	-99.19	782.74
50	50	-71.92	214.84	-501.59	357.75
100	100	-73.59	212.71	-499.02	351.83
200	199	-24.28	209.32	-442.93	394.37
500	492	127.11	184.59	-242.08	496.30
700	660	248.93	183.97	-119.01	616.87
900	816	312.96	181.35	-49.74	675.66

NCreg = Number of Clusters Requested
NCinfo = Number of Informative Clusters Found
All results expressed in 1998 US Dollars ($)

To create the graphs displayed in Figure 7.15, open the LC_900 data table created by the LocalControl script. This table contains 900 rows for clusters (numbered 1 to 900) but only 816 non-missing values for the LTD estimates, Y1LTD and Y2LTD, from informative clusters. The table also contains script(s), named LTDdist1 and LTDdist2, for displaying detailed graphics that describe the LTD distributions (for mort6mo and cardcost) using histograms, normal probability plots, and tabulated summary statistics, as shown in Figure 7.15. The script Y12dist generates the graphic displayed in Figure 7.16, while the fourth script, LTDjoin, is useful in phase two (and four) local control analyses.

Figure 7.15 LTD Graphics and Summary Stats for 816 Informative Clusters

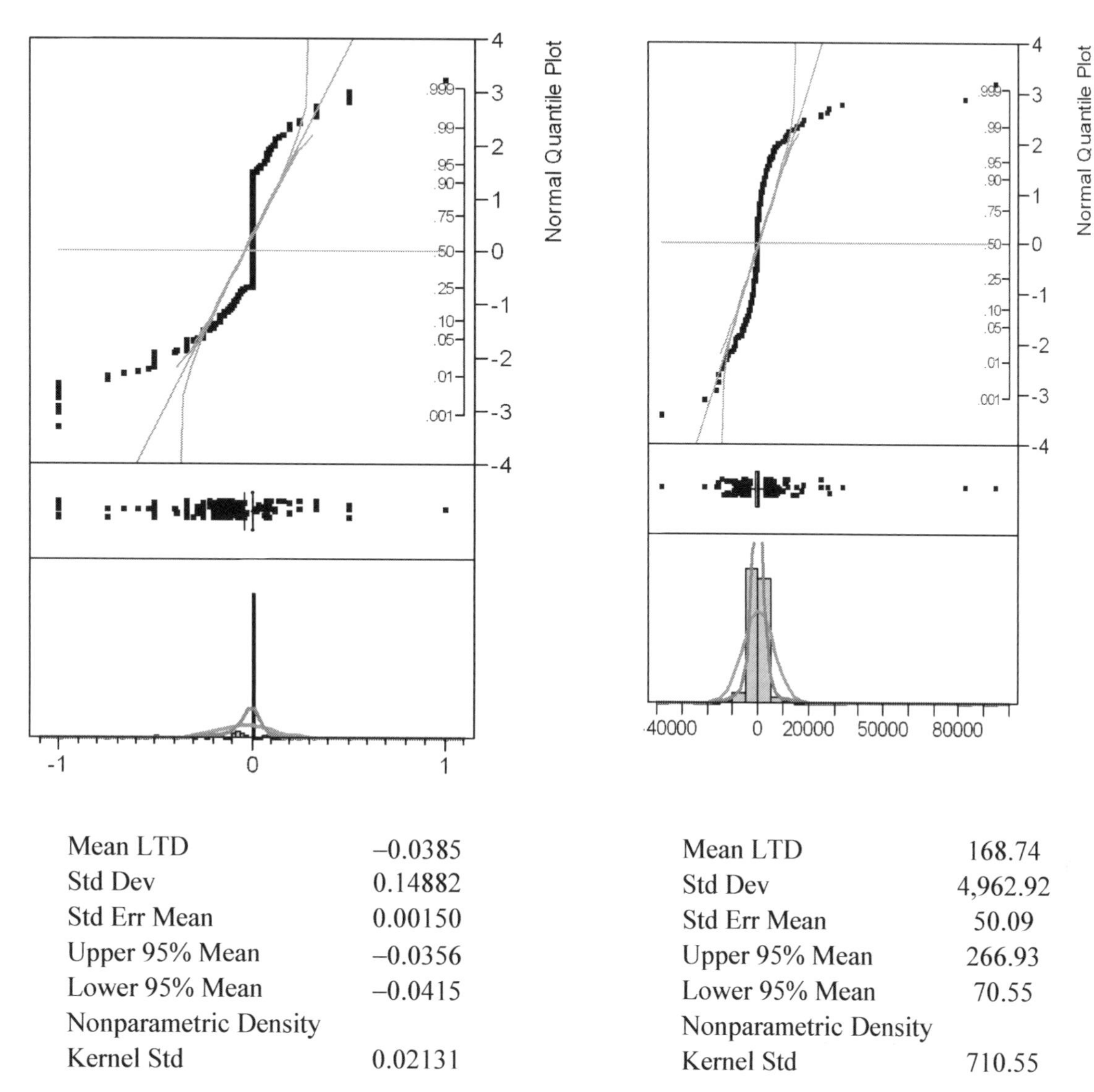

Note also that both of these LTD distributions tend to be more leptokurtic than the best fitting normal distributions in the histograms and probability plots.

Note that point-masses in the mort6mo LTD distribution at –1 and 0 are clearly visible on the left-hand side of Figure 7.15. Furthermore the LTD mean for the 2,332 patients (23.7%) like those predicted to have better mort6mo average outcomes when treated was –0.1957, while the corresponding mean LTD for the 718 patients (7.3%) like those predicted to have better average mort6mo outcomes when untreated was +0.1350. In other words, the mort6mo LTD main effect of –0.0365 is not descriptive or representative of this LTD distribution, where 69.0% of patients have an expected mort6mo LTD of exactly 0.0. In fact, –0.0385 could also be viewed as the mort6mo LTD main effect for only the 31.0% of patients with non-zero LTDs, and (again) the LTDs for these patients still range all from –1 to +1.

Figure 7.16 Bivariate LTD Scatter for 816 Informative Clusters

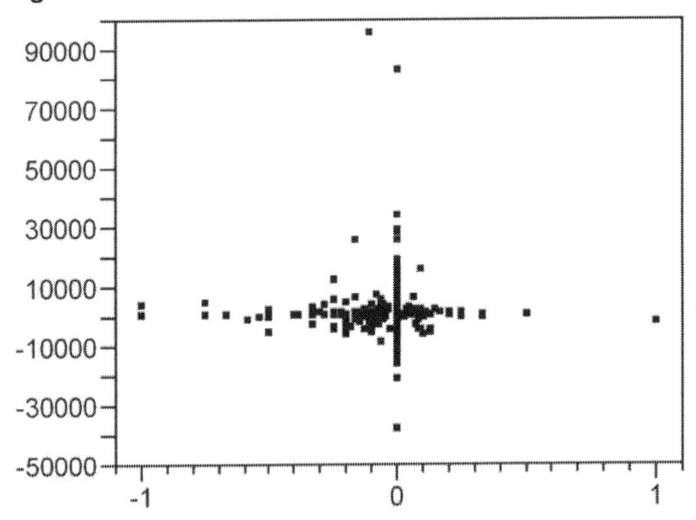

Finally, as is clear from Figure 7.9, there is little or no association (correlation) between mort6mo and cardcost LTD outcomes within their (bivariate) joint distribution. In fact, note that the patients with the most extreme cardcost LTDs tend to have mort6mo LTDs of 0. Similarly, patients with extreme mort6mo LTDs tend to have relatively small cardcost LTDs.

7.3.3 Phase Two: Determining Whether an LTD Distribution Is Salient

Suppose that a researcher has used phase one local control tactics to define a set of clusters from patient baseline characteristics and has estimated the corresponding LTD distribution. This distribution cannot be meaningful unless it is different from the artificial LTD distribution that results from purely random assignment of patients to clusters. In other words, when these two distributions are not different, the measures of patient similarity or dissimilarity used to form clusters are really no more informative than random patient characteristics!

Specifically, the objective of phase two local control tactics is to ask whether observed *x*-covariates are predictive of true patient similarity in the sense that their observed LTD distribution is indeed different from the corresponding artificial (completely random) LTD distribution. When these two LTD distributions are different, the observed LTD distribution is said to be salient (statistically meaningful). Importantly, the artificial LTD distribution can be estimated with increased precision using replicated Monte Carlo simulations. One simply uses repeated, random resampling without replacement for the same fixed number of clusters and the same treatment fractions within each cluster as in the observed clusters.

Due to heteroskedasticity of LTD estimates from clusters of different sizes with different local treatment fractions, the sufficient statistic that characterizes both the observed and the artificial LTD distributions is the (weighted) empirical cumulative distribution function (eCDF). The observed and artificial LTD distributions can also be compared in many revealing alternative ways, but comparison of LTD sCDFs (observed vs. artificial) is key for establishing saliency.

If no (open) data set is currently selected in JMP when the artificial LTD distribution script is selected, JMP again displays a dialog box for opening a *.JMP or *.SAS7BDAT data set, as illustrated in Figure 7.9. On the other hand, this script is usually invoked when the target JMP table has just been created and opened. Specifically, to follow along with the computations illustrated here, you should first invoke the LTDjoin script built into the LC_900 data set (for 900 requested clusters) for the LSIM10K data. While the LC_900 table has 900 rows (one for each cluster) and 816 non-missing LTD estimates for the 816 informative clusters, the resulting joinDt table contains 10,325 rows for individual patients, a cluster ID variable (containing an integer from 1 to 900, inclusive, for each patient), and 9,839 non-missing LTD estimates for the patients within the 816 informative clusters. This is the specific type of JMP table that the artificial LTD distribution script is designed to operate upon.

Invoking the JMP aLTD script then displays the customized Select Columns dialog box in Figure 7.17. Here, only one outcome variable (mort6mo), one binary treatment factor, and no patient baseline *x*-characteristics are specified. However, the researcher must also specify

1. the name of the cluster ID variable (C_900 here)
2. a total number of replications (displayed default value is 25)
3. a random number seed value (displayed default value is 12,345)

Figure 7.17 Artificial LTD Distribution Dialog Box

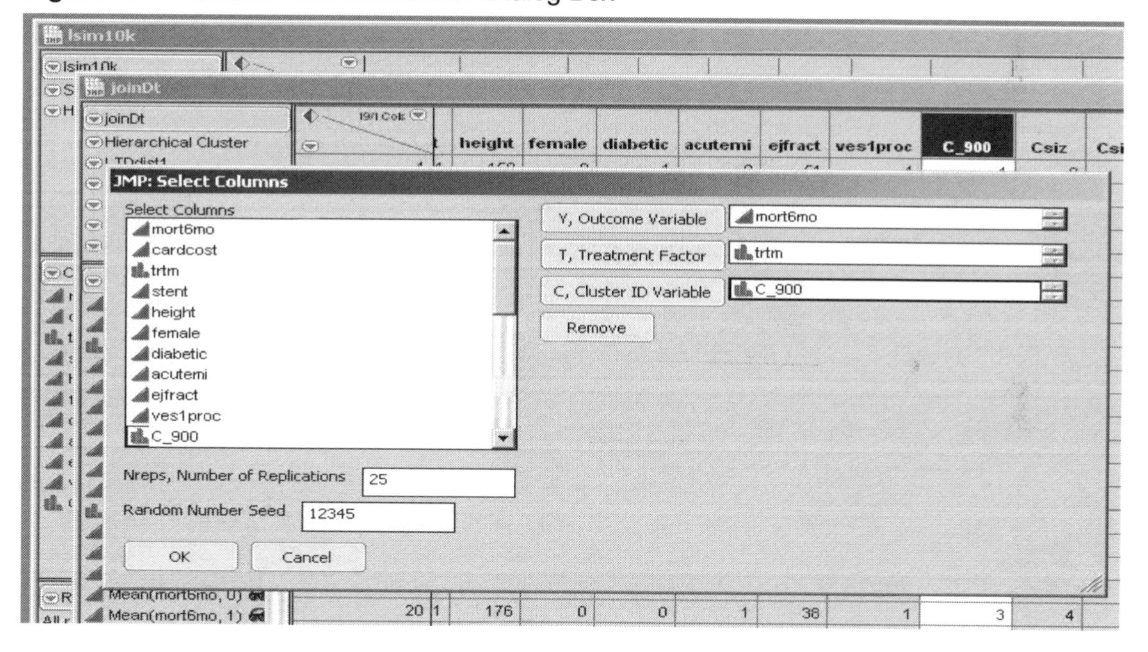

Researchers may wish to first specify a smaller number of replications (for example, three) to estimate how long calculations will take. Whenever a second invocation of the aLTD script is then used to increase precision, be sure to use a different initial seed in the second run so that the two batches of artificial LTD estimates will be independent and can be merged. On the other hand, if a second invocation is used to evaluate a different *y*-outcome, be sure to use the same number of replications and the same initial seed in both runs if you wish to estimate the joint artificial LTD distribution of the two outcomes.

Figure 7.18 illustrates the standard way to compare two unrelated samples (here, of very different sizes) in JMP using the Y by X platform. In Figure 7.18, the Y variable contains estimated LTDs while the binary X variable labels each LTD estimate as either observed or artificial. The observed LTD distribution consists of 816 estimates from the 9,816 patients within informative clusters. Here, the artificial LTD distribution consists of $25 \times 816 = 20{,}400$ non-missing LTD estimates; each set of 816 artificial LTD estimates uses the data from 9,839 patients randomly selected from the original 10,325. On the other hand, because the mort6mo variable is binary, only 254 distinct numerical values for LTDs occur in the merged observed and artificial LTD samples, as seen in Figures 7.18 and 7.19.

Figure 7.18 JMP Side-by-Side Comparison Using the Spread Option of the Artificial and Observed LTD Distributions

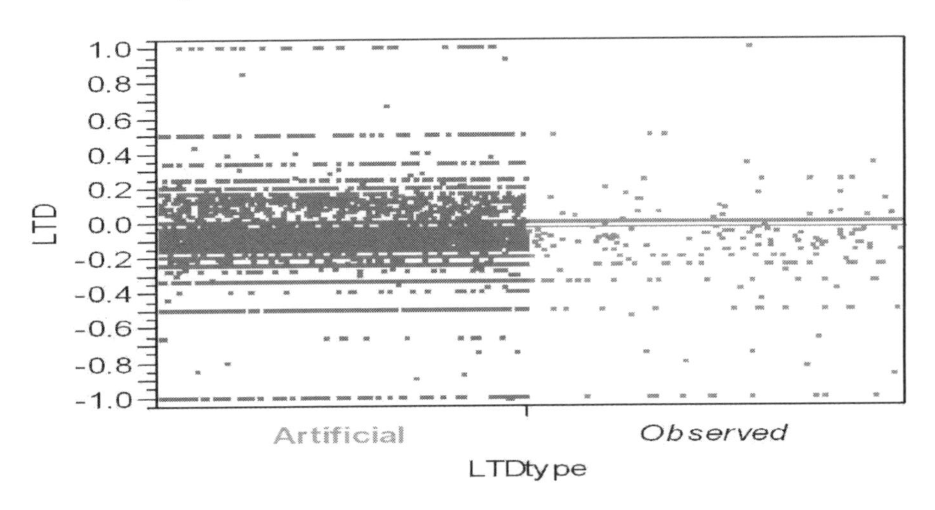

Even when individual patient outcomes are assumed to be homoskedastic, some might argue that LTD estimates need to be weighted because they can still be distinctly heteroskedastic. For an informative cluster containing $n > 1$ patients, let $n \times p$ represent the number of treated patients, where p denotes the local propensity to be treated, and $0 < 1/n \leq p \leq (n-1)/n < 1$. The number of untreated patients is thus $n \times (1-p)$. It follows that the variance of the local difference, $(\bar{Y}_{treated} - \bar{Y}_{untreated})$, would be proportional to $1/[n \times p \times (1-p)]$. Thus a weight could be assigned to the LTD estimate from this cluster that is proportional to $n \times p \times (1-p)$ (that is, inversely proportional to variance). These weights would then need to be renormalized so as to sum to $\Sigma n = 9{,}839$ in this example. Instead, here we simply assign a frequency of n to the LTD computed from an informative cluster of n patients, thereby assuring that $\Sigma f = 9{,}839$.

Unfortunately, Figure 7.19 doesn't strike me as being particularly helpful in comparing the observed and artificial LTD distributions. In addition to several variations on the sort of visualization shown in Figure 7.18, the JMP Y by X platform also contains several alternative ways to test for differences between the distributions represented by (two) samples. Alas, comparisons of the 9,839 observed LTD main effect estimates with the 245,975 artificial LTD main effect estimates are more or less expected to suggest that even small differences are highly significant due to such gigantic sample sizes! For example, Dunnett's method for comparing the aLTD mean with the observed LTD mean yielded a Abs(Dif)–LSD = 0.009 ($p < .0001$); variances of the LTD distributions are different ($p < 0.0001$) using all four tests routinely performed by JMP, and the Welch test assuming unequal variances yields a t-statistic of 7.986 with 10,401 estimated degrees of freedom ($p < 0.0001$). The Wilcoxon/Kruskal-Wallis rank sums test yields a z-score of –5.508 ($p < 0.0001$).

Still, it is clear that the observed LTD distribution has a larger atom of probability at –1 and a smaller atom of probability at 0 than does the artificial LTD distribution:

LTD Estimate	Observed Frequency in 9,839	Observed Fraction of Patients	Artificial Frequency in 20,400	Artificial Fraction of Patients
–1.00	60	0.0061	48	0.0024
0.00	6,789	0.690	15,192	0.745
+1.00	14	0.0014	33	0.0016

Similarly, the comparison of empirical CDFs displayed in Figure 7.19 strongly suggests that the observed LTD distribution for 816 informative clusters is indeed salient. Specifically, the observed LTD distribution has a thicker left-hand tail (of negative LTDs favorable to treatment) and a possibly thinner right-hand tail (of positive LTDs unfavorable to treatment).

Our local control analysis has definitely revealed some bias. After all, the initial observed mean difference in mortality fraction (for 4,679 treated patients minus that for 5,646 untreated patients when all patients are assumed to be within a single cluster) was –0.0250 (that is, –2.5%). The artificial LTD main effect for 816 informative clusters of –2.45% is very slightly larger (less negative), but it is also clearly biased. In sharp contrast, the mort6mo observed LTD main effect of –3.85% is clearly less biased and more favorable to treatment.

Of course, LTD means (main effects) are not particularly descriptive or representative of these sorts of relatively complex (zero-inflated) LTD distributions, where more than 2 out of 3 patients have an expected mort6mo LTD of 0.0. In fact, the –3.85% observed reduction in mort6mo and –2.45% artificial reduction could be viewed as the mort6mo LTD main effects for the fewer than 1 in 3 patients with non-zero LTD estimates. Besides, the LTD distributions for these patients still range from –1.0 to +1.0. In summary, visual comparison of eCDFs provides essential information about saliency, providing insights that are much more relevant and robust than tests for differences in mean values!

Figure 7.19 Visual Comparison of Patient Frequency-Weighted Empirical CDFs for the Observed LTD (Solid) and Artificial LTD (Dotted) Distributions

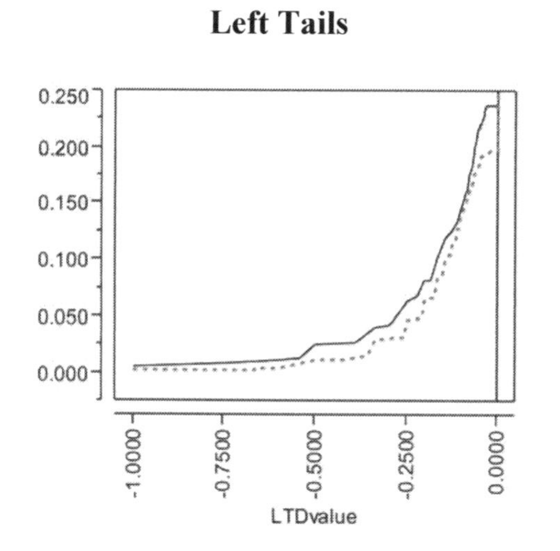

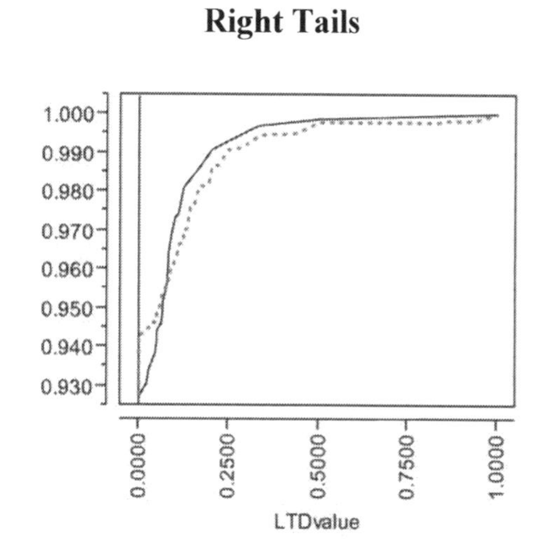

7.3.4 Phase Three: Performing Systematic Sensitivity Analyses

The fundamental concept that forms the basis for phase three of the local control approach is that observed LTD distributions need to be shown to be relatively stable over a range of meaningful, alternative patient clusterings. While the number of clusters is increased in phase one to show that, as comparisons are forced to become more and more local, they typically also become more and more different from—and more interesting than—simplistic overall comparisons. In contrast, careful and systematic sensitivity analyses are badly needed in phase three to illustrate that a range of alternative clusterings can yield realistic, salient LTD distributions that actually have much in common.

This third phase of local control calls for rather tedious and repetitive calculations best done using some sort of batch mode processing. Unlike the interactive approach implemented in my local control and alternative LTD distribution scripts in JMP that implement tactics for phases one and two, no automatic implementation for the phase three sensitivity analyses currently exists. Thus, I describe here some alternative clusterings for the LSIM10K data that the reader may find interesting and then review the basic clustering concepts that should be used in phase three sensitivity analyses.

7.3.4.1 Alternative Clusterings That Readers Can Try on Their Own

The three patient baseline ***x***-characteristics that appear to be most predictive of ***t***-treatment choice and the mortality ***y***-outcome are stent, acutemi, and ejfract. Thus, a local control analysis using only these three patient characteristics is parsimonious. Interestingly, the resulting local control unbiasing trace for mort6mo is similar to Figure 7.13 while the corresponding cardcost trace is much smoother than Figure 7.14. Furthermore, the number of informative clusters drops to only 166 when between 300 and 900 clusters are requested. The 166 informative clusters out of 300 contain 98.4% of the patients, while the 166 informative clusters out of 900 are somewhat smaller (containing 92.6% of all patients, 96.0% of treated patients and 89.9% of untreated patients). Finally, the observed LTD distributions for 900 requested clusters are again salient!

7.3.4.2 Review of Clustering Concepts Useful in Sensitivity Analysis

The objective of cluster analysis is to partition patients into mutually exclusive and exhaustive subgroups. All patients within a cluster should have *x*-vectors that are as similar as possible, while patients in different clusters should have *x*-vectors that are as dissimilar as possible. A metric for measuring similarity or dissimilarity between any two *x*-vectors is needed to do this (Kaufman and Rousseeuw, 1990). My local control JMP script uses the standardize (mean 0 and variance 1) principal co-ordinates of the *x*-covariates to represent patients in Euclidean space, which is equivalent to computing Mahalanobis distances between patients (Rubin, 1980). A variety of distance and similarity measures, such as the Dice coefficient, the Jaccard coefficient, and the cosine coefficient, are also widely used for clustering. All of these unsupervised methods can identify patient closeness relationships that may be impossible to visualize in only two or three Euclidean dimensions.

Suppose that some patient ***x***-characteristics are qualitative factors either with only relatively few levels or with only unordered levels. The analyst may then wish to require that all patients within the same cluster match exactly on these particular ***x***-components. Alternatively, an ***x***-factor with *k* levels can be recoded as *k*–1 dummy (binary) variables.

If certain $\boldsymbol{x}$-covariates are being used primarily as instrumental variables, the analyst may wish to give them extra weight when defining patient dissimilarity. For example, McClellan and colleagues (1994) used approximate distance from the hospital of admission (derived from pairs of ZIP codes) as their initial key variable in clustering 205,021 elderly patients; the only other available $\boldsymbol{x}$-characteristics were age, sex, and race. With such a gigantic number of subjects, the logical strategy is to start by stratifying patients into several distance-from-the-hospital bands. Smaller clusters can be easily formed within these initial strata by, for example1, matching patients on both sex and race and then grouping them into age ranges.

Patient clusterings certainly do not need to be hierarchical, but the resulting dendrogram (tree) can be quite helpful computationally in sensitivity analyses designed to deliberately vary the total number of clusters to study the stability of the observed LTD distribution.

Agglomerative (bottom-up) clustering methods start with each patient in his/her own cluster and iteratively combine individual patients and/or clusters of patients to form larger and larger clusters. This is a "natural" way to do unsupervised, hierarchical analyses, and the vast majority of clustering algorithms work this way.

Divisive (top-down) clustering methods start with a single cluster containing all patients and focus on making the few, very large clusters at the top of the tree more meaningful. The "diana" method of Kaufman and Rousseeuw (1990) is divisive.

To get more compact clusters, it also makes sense to use complete linkage methods that minimize the maximum patient dissimilarity within a cluster rather than single linkage methods.

Again, a cluster is said to be uninformative (pure) if all subjects within that cluster received the same treatment (either all $t = 0$ or all $t = 1$). There is no possibility of observing any local outcome (y) difference between treatments using only subjects from within a pure cluster! In this sense, local control methods automatically discard all information from treated patients who are different from all untreated patients and all information from untreated patients who are different from all treated patients. Again, patients lying outside of the common support of the estimated propensity score distributions for treated and untreated patients are supposed to be excluded from analyses, but this fundamental principle (that is, compare only patients who are comparable) is typically ignored by practitioners of the covariate adjustment augmented with propensity score covariates methods.

To be fully informative about a within-cluster local treatment difference without assuming homoskedasticity of patient outcomes (equal variances), a cluster must contain at least two patients on each treatment. These patients are needed first to compute the heteroskedastic standard errors of the two treatment outcome means and then to compute the conventional standard error of the resulting local treatment difference.

7.3.5 Phase Four: Identifying Baseline Patient Characteristics Predictive of Differential Treatment Response

The objective of the fourth and final phase of local control analysis is to answer questions such as, "Do the differential benefits and/or risks of treatment vary systematically with observed patient characteristics?" and "Which types of patients are better off being treated rather than left untreated?" The first three phases of local control analysis pave the way to answering these ultimate questions by addressing a more fundamental question: "Do important differences in outcomes due to treatment exist?" Specifically, phase one identifies LTD distributions, phase two determines whether an LTD distribution is salient, and phase three establishes which salient LTD distributions are most typical. Before phase four even starts, results from the first three phases may have rendered the ultimate questions (that is, the prediction of differential benefit / risk variation) essentially moot because little or no evidence of any form of patient differential response to treatment has been uncovered.

Phase four analyses can use conventional covariate adjustment methods to predict LTD variables constructed by assigning the (salient and typical) LTD value for a cluster to all patients within that cluster (whether treated or untreated). Similarly, the LTD outcome for each patient that fell into an uninformative cluster is set to missing. This tactic allows researchers to address questions such as, "How do the patients in the left-hand and right-hand tails of an observed LTD distribution differ in their baseline *x*-characteristics?" and "Which types of patients are least likely (or most likely) to make their optimal treatment choice?"

Given my personal distrust of smooth, global models, my favorite phase four local control strategy for predictive modeling is to rely on local, semi-parametric methods like regression (partition) tree models to the LTD variable from patient baseline *x*-characteristics. The tree model of Figure 7.20 can be fit using the Partition option on the JMP **Analyze: Modeling** menu and is, as usual, easy to interpret.

Figure 7.20 JMP Partition (Regression) TREE for Predicting mort6mo LTDs from Seven Baseline Patient *x*-Characteristics

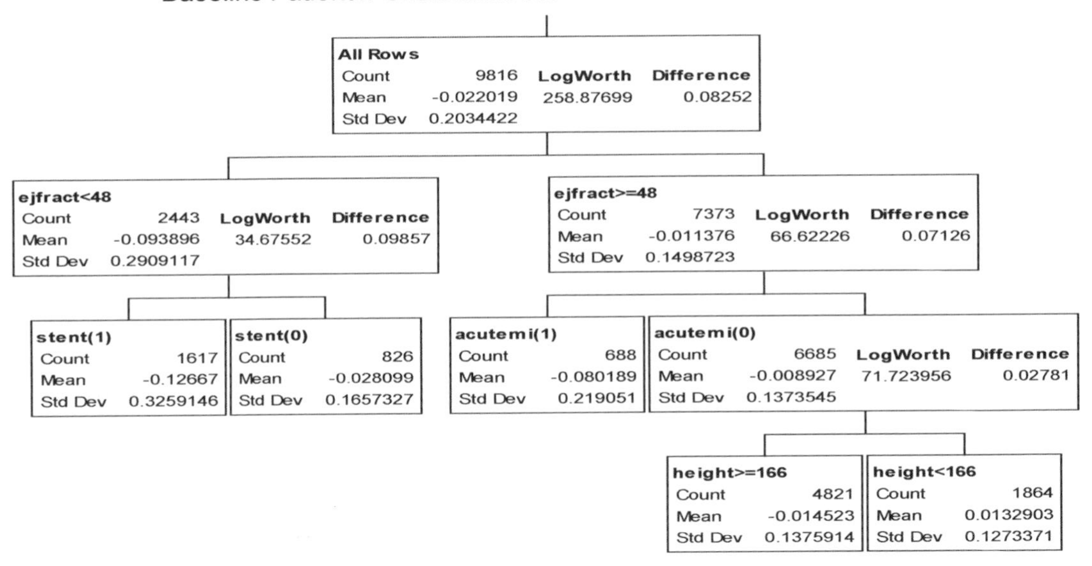

Treatment is most highly effective for the 16.5% of patients with a left-ejection fraction less than 48% and who are to receive a stent; these patients experience a 12.7% absolute reduction in 6-month mortality. Similarly, the 7% of patients who have suffered an acute myocardial infarction within the previous 7 days but have a left-ejection fraction of at least 48% experience an 8.0% reduction in 6-month mortality when treated. In fact, treatment is expected to yield a numerically lower 6-month mortality rate for 81% of all patients; patients expected to do better when untreated tend to be short (height < 166 cm or 5 feet, 5 inches).

Also as usual, the global, multivariable model for predicting mort6mo LTD described in Figure 7.21 is complicated and, thus, not particularly easy to interpret or visualize. I used the JMP effect screening platform to fit a factorial to degree 2 model in the seven available patient *x*-characteristics. Like the regression tree model, this model has an R-squared statistic of only 14%, so it too has considerable lack of fit. For example, the mort6mo LTDs vary from –1.0 to +1.0, but the estimates from this covariate adjustment model range only from –0.4 to +0.14 (see Figure 7.21). Furthermore, many terms are significant primarily because the data set contains so many observations (9,816 non-missing values of LTDs for patients within informative clusters). Having such a large number of terms in the prediction equation greatly hampers use of such a model in practical applications, where an expected LTD typically needs to be computed for each individual patient to make a treatment recommendation.

Figure 7.21 JMP Multivariable Model for Predicting mort6mo LTDs from Seven Baseline Patient *x*-Characteristics

Summary of Fit

RSquare	0.144396
RSquare Adj	0.141948
Root Mean Square Error	0.188451

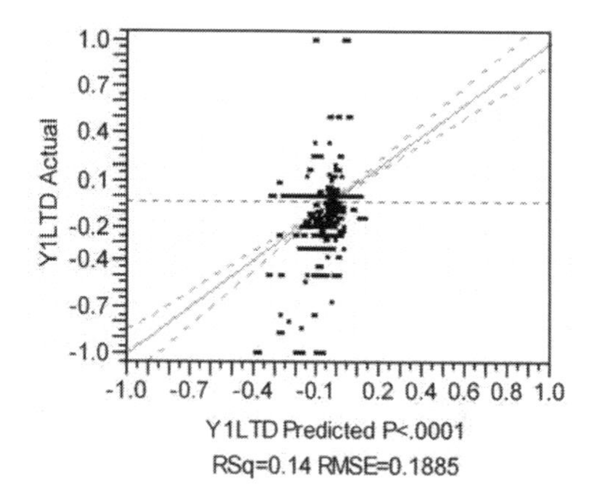

Analysis of Variance

Source	DF	Sum of Squares	Mean Square	F Ratio
Model	28	58.65786	2.09492	58.9892
Error	9787	347.57256	0.03551	**Prob > F**
C. Total	9815	406.23042		<.0001

Sorted Parameter Estimates

Term	Estimate	Std Error	t Ratio	Prob>|t|
stent[0]*(ejfract-53.3258)	-0.002267	0.000151	-14.97	<.0001
diabetic[0]*(ves1proc-1.15983)	0.0309841	0.00346	8.96	<.0001
(height-173.388)*(ejfract-53.3258)	0.0001851	2.255e-5	8.21	<.0001
ejfract	0.0030098	0.000375	8.04	<.0001
acutemi[0]*(ves1proc-1.15983)	-0.042697	0.005336	-8.00	<.0001
diabetic[0]*(ejfract-53.3258)	-0.001307	0.000171	-7.66	<.0001
stent[0]*acutemi[0]	0.0187662	0.002453	7.65	<.0001
acutemi[0]	0.0313478	0.004146	7.56	<.0001
female[0]*(ejfract-53.3258)	-0.001634	0.00023	-7.11	<.0001
female[0]	-0.029563	0.004364	-6.77	<.0001
female[0]*acutemi[0]	0.0202919	0.003597	5.64	<.0001

Term	Estimate	Std Error	t Ratio	Prob>|t|
(height-173.388)*diabetic[0]	-0.001409	0.000276	-5.11	<.0001
stent[0]*diabetic[0]	-0.008277	0.001828	-4.53	<.0001
acutemi[0]*(ejfract-53.3258)	0.0014733	0.000344	4.28	<.0001
height	0.0012274	0.00038	3.23	0.0012
stent[0]	-0.007796	0.002929	-2.66	0.0078
female[0]*diabetic[0]	0.0071039	0.002721	2.61	0.0091
(height-173.388)*acutemi[0]	-0.000705	0.000301	-2.34	0.0194
female[0]*(ves1proc-1.15983)	0.0078406	0.003395	2.31	0.0209
stent[0]*female[0]	-0.004199	0.001942	-2.16	0.0306
(ejfract-53.3258)*(ves1proc-1.15983)	0.0005172	0.000272	1.90	0.0572
(height-173.388)*(ves1proc-1.15983)	-0.000434	0.00033	-1.32	0.1882
(height-173.388)*female[0]	0.0001881	0.000197	0.95	0.3400
diabetic[0]*acutemi[0]	-0.00349	0.003981	-0.88	0.3806
ves1proc	0.005063	0.006262	0.81	0.4188
stent[0]*(ves1proc-1.15983)	0.0004261	0.002269	0.19	0.8510
diabetic[0]	-0.000365	0.004074	-0.09	0.9287
stent[0]*(height-173.388)	-5.615e-6	0.000193	-0.03	0.9767

In summary, I find it interesting that the local control approach can generate LTD distributions that are sufficiently rich and detailed that they actually are difficult to model using conventional regression techniques (parametric or semi-parametric). Clearly, LTD distributions can capture both signal and (considerable) noise from raw data!

7.4 Conclusion

We have seen that the fundamental concepts of *blocking* and *randomization* that play such important roles in the prospective design of experiments (DoE) have variations that can play similarly fundamental roles in the analysis of data on human subjects. These variations are retrospective *local control* and *resampling* (with or possibly without replacement). Use of these highly flexible, post-data collection tools is typically avoided when study objectives are primarily confirmatory (that is, when the study's statistical analysis plan needs to be completely pre-specified and deterministic).

Table 7.5 gives brief definitions of the five basic alternative approaches to analysis of observational data and also discusses their major advantages and disadvantages.

Table 7.5 Five General Approaches to Analysis of Observational Data

Covariate Adjustment (CA) Using Multivariable Models	**History:** Generalization of ANOVA and regression models. **Advantages:** Ubiquitous; widely taught and well accepted; implemented in all statistical analysis packages. **Disadvantages:** Essentially ignores imbalance (for example, always uses all available data); global, parametric models are difficult to visualize and thus may be unrealistic; results are frustratingly sensitive to model specification details; *p*-values can be small simply due to large sample sizes.
Inverse Probability Weighting (IPW)	**History:** Heuristic modification of CA somewhat similar to Horvitz-Thompson adjustment in sample surveys. **Advantages:** As easy to perform as CA; does attempt to adjust for local variation in treatment selection fraction (imbalance); requires software for (diagonally) weighted regression. **Disadvantages:** Basically the same as CA; IPW focuses on up-weighting rarely observed outcomes (never really ignores observations from uninformative clusters); basic variance assumptions somewhat counterintuitive (least frequently observed outcomes are treated as being more precise).
Propensity Score (PS) Matching and Subgrouping	**History:** Fundamental PS theory has attracted more and more attention over the last 25 some years; motivates use of traditional matching and subclassifying approaches. **Advantages:** Intuitive, weak assumptions; widely applicable; many results easily displayed using histograms. **Disadvantages:** Results may be less precise than they appear (are reported) to be; no built-in sensitivity analyses; not a standard method implemented in current commercial statistical software.
Instrumental Variable (IV) Methods	**History:** Adding IV variable(s) to structural equation models can identify causal effects when the given *x*-covariates are correlated with model error terms due to endogenous effects, omitted covariates, or errors in variables. Newest IV approaches use patient clustering and nonparametric, local PS estimates. **Advantages:** Near the top of the theoretical pecking order. **Disadvantages:** IV assumption is very strong and not testable; implemented only in some commercial statistical packages.
Local Control Methods Using Patient *x*-clusterings (Unsupervised Learning)	**History:** Generalization of nested ANOVA (treatment within cluster) and hierarchical models. **Advantages:** Intuitive, weak assumptions; widely applicable; guaranteed asymptotic balancing scores finer than propensity scores; inferences based upon bootstrap confidence or tolerance intervals; built-in sensitivity analyses. **Disadvantages:** Quite new; completely different focus from that of traditional parametric models; not a standard method implemented in current statistical software packages.

The local control approach is interesting primarily because it directly addresses the highly relevant subject of the distribution of LTDs in an almost non-parametric way (using nested cell-means models, as in Row 2 of Table 7.1). In fact, the only obvious down sides of this approach are that taking this local difference essentially doubles the variance of the resulting outcome point estimates and that LTDs definitely are not identically distributed because they have local means and variances that depend upon cluster size and local treatment fractions.

In contrast, the IV plotting approach (based upon Row 1 of Table 7.1) of McClellan, McNeil, and Newhouse (1994) requires parametric modeling across clusters on the plot of LATEs versus observed within-cluster treatment fractions (local propensity score estimates). By averaging outcomes over both treated and untreated patients within clusters, at least IV methods do avoid doubling the variance in outcome point estimates. However, doing only a pure IV analysis (and thus failing to examine LTDs) strikes me as an extremely high price to pay!

Randomized studies will probably long remain the gold standard for scientific research on humans. I think that this is unfortunate, especially in health outcomes research and pharmacoeconomic settings, where performing prospective experiments within otherwise general medical practice settings typically implies imposing strong enrollment / participation incentives that result in unrealistic (unnatural) behaviors from both patients and clinicians. If you want to develop real insight into what happens when new treatments become available, shouldn't you use real data from actual experience? There is absolutely nothing wrong with using real-world data to try to realistically answer real-world questions. On the other hand, it is quite obvious that more and much better insights could be developed if researchers had access to better (much more complete) observational data and to better local control software, especially for phase three local control systematic sensitivity analyses.

All of the five basic approaches covered by Table 7.4 address the problem of unobserved confounders only obliquely. After all, the unknown and unobserved could actually represent anything. Still, observed variables that are surrogates for those unobserved (that is, those that are correlated with them) can be used in all of these approaches. The strength of the local control approach in this regard is that it directly addresses the question of whether the observed LTD distribution is salient. While one can never know how much better they could do with better data, it is essential to be confident that at least some progress has been made.

In any case, the good news is that much more sensitive, robust, and data-driven methods for assessing treatment effects in observational data are practical. Meanwhile, the bad news is that these approaches will rely heavily on unsupervised learning methods (clustering and density estimation) that address the most challenging / difficult computational problems in statistics.

Acknowledgments

The author wishes to thank Gerhardt Pohl and Stan Young for helpful discussions of many of the topics addressed in this chapter.

Appendix: Propensity Scores and Blocking/Balancing Scores

A.1 Review of the Fundamental Theorem of Propensity Scoring

For a patient with a given $\boldsymbol{x}$–vector of baseline characteristics, that patient's propensity score is their conditional probability of receiving the first of, say, two treatments, $\boldsymbol{t} = 1$. This conditional probability is denoted in equation (A.1) by the symbol "p." Thus, by definition, p is a function only of the given $\boldsymbol{x}$–vector of patient baseline characteristics.

$$p \equiv \Pr(\boldsymbol{t} = 1 \mid \boldsymbol{x}) \tag{A.1}$$

A simple four-line proof of the fundamental conditional independence theorem of propensity scoring (Rosenbaum and Rubin, 1983) is displayed in equation (A.2). The $\Pr(\boldsymbol{x}, \boldsymbol{t} \mid p)$ factor on the left-hand side of the first line denotes the conditional joint distribution of a patient's baseline $\boldsymbol{x}$-vector and their treatment choice, $\boldsymbol{t}$, given that patient's (possibly unknown, true) propensity score, p. The factoring of the right-hand side of the first line then follows from the very definition (≡) of conditional probability. In the second line, the second factor on the right-hand side is simplified by noting that p is a function of $\boldsymbol{x}$ and, thus, conditioning upon both $\boldsymbol{x}$ and p is really no stronger than conditioning on $\boldsymbol{x}$ alone. The third line then follows because equation (A.1) shows that $\Pr(\boldsymbol{t} \mid \boldsymbol{x})$ is either p or $(1 - p)$. Finally, the fourth line follows because the third line result shows that conditioning on the distribution of $\boldsymbol{t}$ given $\boldsymbol{x}$ is no stronger than conditioning on only p.

$$\begin{aligned} \Pr(x, t \mid p) &\equiv \Pr(x \mid p)\Pr(t \mid x, p) \\ &= \Pr(x \mid p)\Pr(t \mid x) \\ &= \Pr(x \mid p)\,p \quad \text{or} \quad \Pr(x \mid p)(1 - p) \\ &= \Pr(x \mid p)\Pr(t \mid p) \end{aligned} \tag{A.2}$$

In summary, equation (A.2) establishes that the joint conditional distribution of x and t given the true p must necessarily factor into the product of the conditional distribution of x given p times the conditional distribution of t given p. In statistics and probability theory, this factoring has profound implications. The distribution of baseline patient $\boldsymbol{x}$-characteristics has thereby been shown to be statistically independent of the distribution of treatment choice, where both distributions are conditional upon the given (possibly unknown, true) p.

Technically, the first, $\Pr(x \mid p)$ factor in the fourth line of equation (A.2) actually shows that conditioning on a fixed value of p defines a block of patients. To avoid forming too many blocks, p can be rounded to two or at most three decimal places. The conditional distribution of $\boldsymbol{x}$ for a given, rounded value of p may be rather complicated, but at least one knows (due to independence) that this distribution will be the same for both treated and untreated patients within each block (defined by a single, rounded value of p). On the other hand, the fact that the $\boldsymbol{x}$-distribution can vary across block*s* (that is, as p varies) provides ample motivation and justification for calling these patient subgroupings blocks.

Similarly, the second, $\Pr(t \mid p)$ factor in the fourth line of equation (A.2) defines local treatment balance (or imbalance) on the local fraction treated. Specifically, the local (within-block) ratio of treated to untreated patients is expected to be very close to 1:1 only within the block with $p =$ 0.50.

In data sets where p does not appear to vary with x, there is, for all practical purposes, only one block in the entire data set! In randomized clinical trials (RTCs), p is typically not only known but also usually does not vary with x. In observational (nonrandomized) studies, the true value of p is typically unknown. Furthermore, p must vary with x whenever patient differential treatment selection is present.

A.2 Practical Problems with Estimated Propensity Scores

The result expressed by equation (A.2) is really rather profound and yet requires only relatively weak assumptions to be valid. Unfortunately, the true propensity score, p, for a given $\boldsymbol{x}$–vector is unknown in observational studies, and estimates of p can easily be sufficiently poor (unrealistic) that treated and untreated patients matched on rounded propensity score estimates can actually have rather different $\boldsymbol{x}$–vector distributions. Any such patients may really belong in different true conditional blocks rather than within the same block.

An illustration of how this can happen when propensity scores are estimated using logistic regression and the space of x–vectors is three-dimensional is depicted in Figure A.1. This model uses a linear functional (vector inner product) of the form $x'\beta$ to estimate the logit transform, $\{\log[p/(1-p)]\}$, of propensity to be treated. Two different patients then have the same rounded propensity score estimate if and only if their corresponding $\boldsymbol{x}$–vectors lie strictly on or between a pair of parallel, two–dimensional planes (depicted as a thin slab in Figure A.1) that are orthogonal to the three–dimensional estimated β–hat vector (depicted in Figure A.1).

Note that, because the thin slab extends out to infinity in all directions strictly orthogonal to the estimated β–hat vector, two patients with essentially the same fitted propensity score can actually be very far apart in $\boldsymbol{x}$–space. In other words, all of the $\boldsymbol{x}$–vectors for treated patients might possibly be well separated from the corresponding $\boldsymbol{x}$–vectors for untreated patients. Thus, there is absolutely no assurance that the conditional $\boldsymbol{x}$–distributions for given rounded propensity score estimates will be identical (or even similar).

When using estimated propensity scores, it is absolutely essential to verify that conditioning upon such estimates does yield blocks that behave, at least approximately, like those resulting from conditioning upon true propensity scores. This sort of validation process, which is described and illustrated here in Section 7.2.3 and in publications like Kereiakes and colleagues (2000) and Yue (2007), can be rather tedious and frustrating.

Figure A.1 The x-Space Geometry of Linear Functionals from Logistic Regression

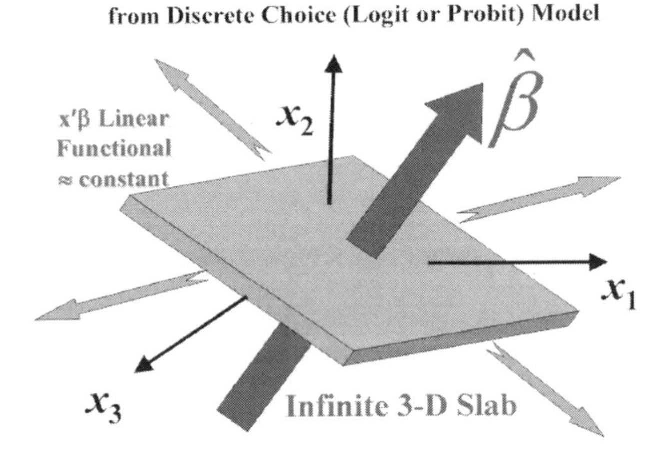

As we will see in Section A.4, a major practical advantage of the local control approach is that it can be performed without either modeling propensity or validating propensity scores estimates!

A.3 Range of Blocking/Balancing Scores: From Most Fine to Most Coarse

Rosenbaum and Rubin (1983) proposed calling any statistic, such as φ, a *balancing score* if the conditional distributions of $\boldsymbol{x}$-covariates and treatment choice are independent given φ, as in equation (A.2). Here, we will call any such statistic, φ, a blocking/balancing (or B/B) score because, again, $\Pr(\, x \mid \varphi\,)$ characterizes the within-block conditional $\boldsymbol{x}$-distribution independently from the $\Pr(\, t \mid \varphi\,)$ factor that describes treatment fraction balance (or imbalance) within that block.

A patient's true propensity score, p, is clearly a B/B score due to equation (A.2). However, unlike true propensity scores that are well defined as conditional probabilities, φ statistics can apparently be specified in many alternative ways.

Rosenbaum and Rubin (1983) established that the patient $\boldsymbol{x}$–vector of baseline characteristics is the most detailed possible B/B score. They accomplished this by simply noting that

$$\Pr(\, \boldsymbol{x}, \boldsymbol{t}\,) \equiv \Pr(\, \boldsymbol{x}\,)\Pr(\, \boldsymbol{t} \mid \boldsymbol{x}\,), \tag{A.3}$$

where $\Pr(\, x\,)$ denotes a degenerate distribution (point mass at the given x). When the given x–vectors contain continuous measures and/or many components, the bad news here is simply that there may be no exact matches and only few relatively good matches within the entire data set!

Even more importantly, Rosenbaum and Rubin (1983) also successfully argued (by contradiction) that true propensity scores are also extreme in the sense that they are always the most coarse (least detailed) B/B scores.

A.4 Cluster Membership Is an Asymptotic Blocking/Balancing Score

A simple two-line proof of our desired approximate conditional independence result is displayed in equation (A.4). The $\Pr(\, x, t \mid \mathrm{C})$ factor on the left-hand side of the first line denotes the conditional joint distribution of a patient's baseline $\boldsymbol{x}$–vector and their treatment choice, t, given that the patient is a member of cluster C. The factoring of the right-hand side of the first line then again follows from the very definition ($\equiv$) of conditional probability. In the second line, the first factor on the right-hand side is then simplified by noting that $\Pr(\, x \mid t, \mathrm{C}\,)$ and $\Pr(\, x \mid \mathrm{C}\,)$ are approximately equal ($\approx$) whenever clusters are small and information about treatment choice, t, is not used to help define clusters. Unfortunately, $\Pr(\, x, t \mid \mathrm{C}\,) = \Pr(\, x \mid \mathrm{C}\,)\Pr(\, t \mid \mathrm{C}\,)$ cannot possibly hold when clusters are large because cluster membership would then be a B/B score that is more coarse than the propensity score. What we will be able to argue is that $\Pr(\, \boldsymbol{x}, t \mid \mathrm{C}\,)$ does approximately factor as shown in the limit as clusters become small, compact, and numerous.

$$\begin{aligned} \Pr(\, x, t \mid \mathrm{C}\,) &\equiv \Pr(\, x \mid t, \mathrm{C}\,)\Pr(\, t \mid \mathrm{C}\,) \\ &\approx \Pr(\, x \mid \mathrm{C}\,)\Pr(\, t \mid \mathrm{C}\,) \end{aligned} \tag{A.4}$$

Note that the last factor, $\Pr(\, t \mid \mathrm{C}\,)$, on both lines of equation (2.4) has an extremely natural, non-parametric estimator: namely, the observed fractions of treated and untreated patients within cluster C. Furthermore, $\Pr(\, t{=}1 \mid \mathrm{C}\,)$ can be as extreme as 0 or 1, and cluster C is then said to be pure or uninformative about the corresponding local treatment difference (LTD). After all, such a cluster then contains either only treated patients or only untreated patients.

Consider the following heuristic argument that the Pr(x | t, C) factor in the first line of equation (A.4) is asymptotically well represented by the Pr(x | C) factor in the second line. First of all, observed treatment assignment is used in the approaches known as *optimal matching*, (Rosenbaum, 2003) or full matching (Hansen, 2004) that are designed specifically to prevent creating uninformative clusters. Supposing that a potential cluster contains only, for example, treated patients, full matching would then distort and extend that cluster until it includes at least one untreated patient (that is, the clustering algorithm is primarily based on observed x-vectors but is semi-supervised by t). On the other hand, even when clustering does not depend upon t-assignment, Pr(x | t, C) and Pr(x | C) can still be quite different whenever cluster C is large.

For example, the distribution of x–vectors within a very large cluster can be quite inelegant, with large separation of all treated patients from all untreated patients having occurred simply by accident. Furthermore, a large cluster might contain patients with a wide range of values for their true p = Pr(t=1 | x). If Pr(x | t, C) and Pr(x | C) were equal in this case, cluster membership would again be a B/B score more coarse than the true p, which is impossible.

At the opposite extreme, where all clusters contain only one patient, C = x and Pr(x | t, x) = Pr(x | x) is a degenerate distribution with unit mass at x. Thus, the smallest possible clusters are clearly exact B/B scores.

OK, so when *is* cluster membership an approximate B/B score? When clusters are small, compact, and numerous, patients with the same rounded propensity scores could be in different clusters. For all practical purposes, this means that cluster membership has become an approximate B/B score finer than p but clearly coarser than individual x–vectors. Furthermore, this situation is likely to occur whenever Pr(t = 1 | x) tends to be a smooth function of x and clusters have small x-space volume. Meanwhile, when these small clusters have not been distorted to prevent creation of uninformative clusters, the conditional distribution of x given both t and C is also clearly less dependent upon t-assignment. When all of this happens, one would certainly not need to confirm blocking (x-distribution balance between treatment groups within informative clusters); their local B/B properties will have been assured. This concept is illustrated in Figure A.2.

First, note that the three-dimensional cubes depicted in Figure A.2 represent relatively small, compact, and numerous clusters. Here, the displayed clusters just happen to intersect a thin slab of rounded propensity score estimates from a fitted logistic regression model for treatment choice. Suppose now that the white cubes denote uninformative clusters while each dark cube contains at least one treated patient as well as at least one untreated patient. If the rounded propensity score estimates satisfied equation (A.2), then all of these clusters would need to have nearly the same within-cluster treatment fraction, namely the rounded estimate of p. Fortunately, there is no such restriction when using clusters to define B/B scores; the within-cluster treatment fraction is simply the observed local fraction. Furthermore, because each cluster is small and compact, the local x-distributions for treated and untreated patients must necessarily be quite similar, and the resulting B/B scores must be finer than propensity scores.

Figure A.2 The *x*-Space Geometry of Small, Compact, and Numerous Clusters that Intersect a Thin Slab of Rounded Propensity Score Estimates from Logistic Regression

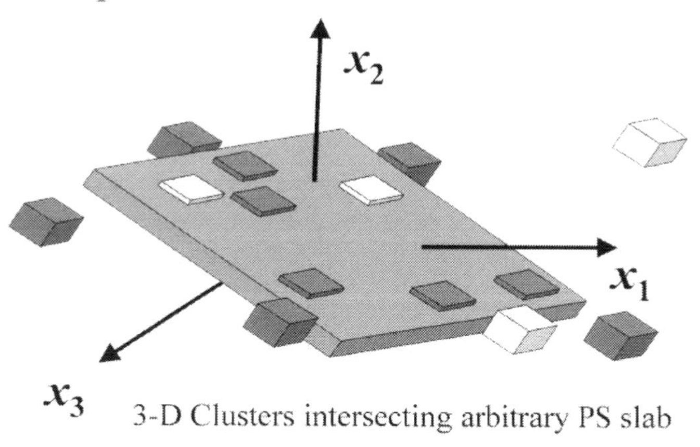

References

Angrist, J. D., G. W. Imbens, D. B. Rubin, J. M. Robins, et al. 1996. "Identification of causal effects using instrumental variables." *Journal of the American Statistical Association* 91: 444–472.

Bang, H., and J. M. Robins. 2005. "Doubly robust estimation in missing data and causal inference models." *Biometrics* 61(4): 962–973.

Barlow, H. B. 1989. "Unsupervised learning." *Neural Computation* 1(3): 295–311.

Board on Life Sciences. 2003. *Sharing Publication-Related Data and Materials: Responsibilities of Authorship in the Life Sciences*. Washington, DC: The National Academies Press. Available at http://www.nap.edu/books/0309088593/html.

Box, G. E. P. 1979. "Robustness Is the Strategy of Scientific Model Building." *Robustness in Statistics: Proceedings of a Workshop*, 202. Edited by R. L. Launer and G. N. Wilkinson. New York: Academic Press.

Cochran, W. G. 1965. "The planning of observational studies of human populations (with discussion)." *Journal of the Royal Statistical Society A: (Statistics in Society)* 128: 234–266.

Cochran, W. G. 1968. "The effectiveness of adjustment by subclassification in removing bias in observational studies." *Biometrics* 24: 295–313.

Concato, J., N. Shah, and R. I. Horwitz. 2000. "Randomized, controlled trials, observational studies, and the hierarchy of research designs." The *New England Journal of Medicine* 342: 1887–1892.

D'Agostino, Jr., R. B. 1998. "Propensity score methods for bias reduction in the comparison of a treatment to a non-randomized control group. *Statistics in Medicine* 17: 2265–2281.

D'Agostino, Jr., R. B., and D. B. Rubin. 2000. "Estimating and using propensity scores with partially missing data." *Journal of the American Statistical Association* 95: 749–759.

D'Agostino, Jr., R. B., W. Lang, M. Walkup, T. Morgan, and A. Karter. 2001. "Examining the impact of missing data on propensity score estimation in determining the effectiveness of self-monitoring of blood glucose (SMBG)." *Health Services and Outcomes Research Methodology* 2: 291–315.

Diaconis, P., S. Holmes, and R. Montgomery. 2007. "Dynamical bias in the coin toss." *SIAM Journal* 49: 211–235.

Efron, B. 1979. "Computers and the theory of statistics: thinking the unthinkable." *SIAM Review* 21: 460–480.

Efron, B., and R. J. Tibshirani. 1993. *An Introduction to the Bootstrap.* London: Chapman & Hall/CRC.

Federal Judicial Center. 2000. *Reference Manual on Scientific Evidence*. 2d ed. Available at http://www.fjc.gov/public/pdf.nsf/lookup/sciman00.pdf/$file/sciman00.pdf.

Fisher, R. A. 1925. *Statistical Methods for Research Workers.* Edinburgh: Oliver and Boyd.

Fraley, C., and A. E. Raftery. 2002. "Model-based clustering, discriminant analysis, and density estimation." *Journal of the American Statistical Association* 97: 611–631.

Gelman, A., and D. Nolan. 2002. "You can load a die but you can't bias a coin." *The American Statistician* 56: 308–311.

Gu, C. 2002. *Smoothing Spline ANOVA Models.* New York: Springer-Verlag.

Hansen, B. B. 2004. "Full matching in an observational study of coaching for the SAT." *Journal of the American Statistical Association* 99: 609–618.

Hayward R. A., D. M. Kent, S. Vijan, and T. P. Hofer. 2005. "Reporting clinical trial results to inform providers, payers and consumers." *Health Affairs* 24(6): 1571–1581.

Holland, P. W. 1986. "Statistics and causal inference." *Journal of the American Statistical Association* 81: 945–960.

Horvitz, D. G., and D. J. Thompson. 1952. "A generalization of sampling without replacement from a finite universe." *Journal of the American Statistical Association* 47(260): 663–685.

Imbens, G. W., and J. D. Angrist. 1994. "Identification and estimation of local average treatment effects." *Econometrica* 62: 467–475.

Ioannidis, J. P. A. 2005. "Contradicted and initially stronger effects in highly cited clinical research." The *Journal of the American Medical Association* 294: 218–229.

Ioannidis, J. P. A. 2005. "Why most published research findings are false." *PLoS Medicine* 2(8): e124. Available at 10.1371/journal.pmed.0020124.

Kaufman, L., and P. J. Rousseeuw. 1990. *Finding Groups in Data: An Introduction to Cluster Analysis*. New York: John Wiley & Sons, Inc.

Kent, D. M., and R. A. Hayward. 2007. "Limitations of applying summary results of clinical trials to individual patients: the need for risk stratification." The *Journal of the American Medical Association* 298(10): 1209–1212.

Kent, D. M., and R. A. Hayward. 2007. "When averages hide individual differences in clinical trials." *American Scientist* 95(1): 60–68.

Kereiakes, D. J., R. L. Obenchain, B. L. Barber, A. Smith, M. McDonald, T. M. Broderick, J. P. Runyon, T. M. Shimshak, J. F. Schneider, C. R. Hattemer, E. M. Roth, D. D. Whang, D. L. Cocks, and C. W. Abbottsmith. 2000. "Abciximab provides cost-effective survival advantage in high volume interventional practice." *American Heart Journal* 140(4): 603–610.

Leamer, E. E. 1978. *Specification Searches: Ad Hoc Inference with Nonexperimental Data.* New York: John Wiley & Sons, Inc.

McClellan, M., B. J. McNeil, and J. P. Newhouse. 1994. "Does more intensive treatment of acute myocardial infarction in the elderly reduce mortality? Analysis using instrumental variables." The *Journal of the American Medical Association* 272:859–866.

McEntegart, D.J. 2003. "The pursuit of balance using stratified and dynamic randomization techniques: an overview." *Drug Information Journal* 37: 293–308.

Müllner, M., H. Matthews, and D. G. Altman. 2002. "Reporting on statistical methods to adjust for confounding: a cross-sectional survey." [Brief Communication] *Annals of Internal Medicine* 136(2): 122–126.

Newhouse, J. P., and M. McClellan. 1998. "Econometrics in outcomes research: the use of instrumental variables." Annual Review of Public Health 19: 17–34.

Obenchain, R. L. 2004. "Unsupervised propensity scoring: NN and IV plots. In *ASA Proceedings of the Joint Statistical Meetings*. Alexandria, VA: American Statistical Association, 1899–1906.

Obenchain, R. L. 2005. "USPS: R package for unsupervised and supervised propensity scoring and instrumental variable adjustment." Available at http://www.r-project.org.

Obenchain, R. L. 2006. "Identifying meaningful patient subgroups via clustering—sensitivity graphics." In *ASA Proceedings of the Joint Statistical Meetings*. Alexandria, VA: American Statistical Association.

Obenchain, R. L. 2009. JMP scripts for local control and artificial LTD distribution. Available at http://members.iquest.net/~softrx/other/LC_aLTD.zip.

Obenchain, R. L., and C. A. Melfi. 1997. "Propensity score and Heckman adjustments for treatment selection bias in database studies." In *ASA Proceedings* in the *Biopharmaceutical Section*. Alexandria, VA: American Statistical Association, 297–306.

Pocock, S. J., S. E. Assmann, L. E. Enos, and L. E. Kasten. 2002. "Subgroup analysis, covariate adjustment and baseline comparisons in clinical trial reporting: current practice and problems." *Statistics in Medicine* 21: 2917–2930.

Rao, C. R. 1973. *Linear Statistical Inference and Its Applications*. 2d ed. New York: John Wiley & Sons, Inc.

Robins, J. M., M. A. Hernan, and B. Brumback. 2000. "Marginal structural models and causal inference in epidemiology." *Epidemiology* 11: 550–560.

Rosenbaum, P. R. 2002. *Observational Studies*. 2d ed. New York: Springer-Verlag.

Rosenbaum, P. R., and D. B. Rubin. 1983. "The central role of the propensity score in observational studies for causal effects." *Biometrika* 70: 41–55.

Rosenbaum, P. R., and D. B. Rubin. 1984. "Reducing bias in observational studies using subclassification on the propensity score." *Journal of the American Statistical Association* 79: 516–524.

Rubin, D. B. 1980. "Bias reduction using Mahalanobis-metric matching." *Biometrics* 36: 293–298.

Rubin, D. B. 1997. "Estimating causal effects from large data sets using propensity scores." *Annals of Internal Medicine* 127: 757–763.

Salsburg, D. 2002. *The Lady Tasting Tea: How Statistics Revolutionized Science in the Twentieth Century.* New York: Owl Books.

Shah, B. R., A. Laupacis, J. E. Hux, and P. C. Austin. 2005. "Propensity score methods gave similar results to traditional regression modeling in observational studies: a systematic review." *Journal of Clinical Epidemiology* 58(6): 550–559.

Stürmer, T., M. Joshi, R. J. Glynn, J. Avorn, K. J. Rothman, and S. Schneeweiss. 2006. "A review of the application of propensity score methods yielded increasing use, advantages in specific settings, but not substantially different estimates compared with conventional multivariable methods." *Journal of Clinical Epidemiology* 59(5): 437.e1–437.e24.

Wainer, H., M. Gessaroli, and M. Verdi. 2006. "Finding what is not there through the unfortunate binning of results: the Mendel effect." *Chance* 19: 49–52.

Wegman, E. J., and Q. Luo. 2002. "On methods of computer graphics for visualizing densities." *Journal of Computational and Graphical Statistics* 11: 137–162.

Yue, L. Q. 2007. "Statistical and regulatory issues with the application of propensity score analysis to nonrandomized medical device clinical studies." *Journal of Biopharmaceutical Statistics* 17: 1–13.

Part 3

Longitudinal Bias Adjustment

Chapter 8

A Two-Stage Longitudinal Propensity Adjustment for Analysis of Observational Data

Andrew C. Leon
Donald Hedeker
Chunshan Li

Abstract

A two-stage longitudinal propensity adjustment is described for treatment effectiveness analyses of observational data. The propensity score is estimated in a mixed-effects logistic regression model. Treatment effectiveness is then examined with quintile-stratified mixed-effects grouped-time survival models. Tests of model assumptions are described, including representativeness of treatments in each quintile, treatment by quintile interaction, and balance between treatment groups. An application that evaluates the effectiveness of antidepressants is presented for illustration.

8.1 Introduction

Treatment effectiveness evaluations of observational data face several fundamental challenges. First, because of non-randomized treatment assignment, there is the clear possibility of non-equivalent comparison groups. This is because selection biases often play a role in the particular treatment that is received by those in need. For instance, those who seek and receive treatment are likely to be more severely ill than those who do not. As a consequence, unadjusted effectiveness analyses would likely find that untreated subjects have better outcomes. In part, this is because the factors that contribute to treatment choices are confounding variables because they are also associated with outcome. Second, a longitudinal observation study will have repeated measures on many of the subjects. Third, unlike randomized controlled clinical trials, the duration of treatment is not standardized in a research protocol but instead determined by the clinician and the patient.

Rosenbaum and Rubin (1983) proposed the propensity score as a balancing score for comparison of non-equivalent comparison groups. They defined the propensity score as the conditional probability of assignment to receive a particular treatment given a vector of observed covariates (x):

$$e(x_i) = P(T_i = 1 \mid x_i),$$

for subject i ($i = 1, \ldots, N$), for T_i, which represents treatment.

The propensity adjustment is used to reduce the impact of confounding variables on effectiveness analyses and, thus, the propensity score can reduce bias in estimates of treatment effect in an observational study (Rosenbaum and Rubin, 1983, 1984). They proposed implementation through matching, subclassification, or covariate adjustment, yet discussed caveats regarding use of the latter. Here we use subclassification, also called stratification.

8.2 Longitudinal Model of Propensity for Treatment

A strategy to implement the propensity for longitudinal, observational data has been proposed. It was a dynamic adaptation of the propensity adjustment for ordinal doses (Leon et al., 2001, 2003). For simplicity, here we simply consider the longitudinal propensity adjustment for binary treatment. It is a two-stage, longitudinal data analytic strategy that includes a model of propensity for treatment and a model of treatment effectiveness. In the first stage, the propensity model examines repeated observations of binary treatment over time. The model can include multiple treatment intervals per subject over time and variations in both within-subject propensity for treatment and within-subject treatment over the course of the study. The model characterizes those who either did or did not receive treatment over time based on covariates such as clinical and demographic features. In the second stage, a treatment effectiveness model examines the time from the start of each treatment until a prespecified event. In this chapter we examine the time until recurrence.

The mixed-effects framework accounts for the correlated recurrence times that represent the successive within-subject treatment intervals. A mixed-effects logistic regression model examines treatment as a function of these characteristics, whether time-invariant or time-varying:

$$e(x_{ij}, \upsilon_i) = P(T_{ij} = 1 \mid \upsilon_i, x_{ij}),$$

for subject i ($i = 1, \ldots, N$), at time j ($j = 1, \ldots, J_i$), and where υ_i is a subject-specific random intercept. Assuming this mixed-effects logistic model, the propensity score, which ranges in value from 0 to 1, can be expressed using the logistic response function for subject i at time j as:

$$e(x_{ij}, \upsilon_i) = \frac{\exp(\alpha + x_{ij}'\beta + \upsilon_i)}{1 + \exp(\alpha + x_{ij}'\beta + \upsilon_i)},$$

A subject with a low propensity score presents as someone unlikely to receive treatment at time point j, whereas a subject with a high propensity score has characteristics of someone more likely to receive treatment.

8.3 Longitudinal Propensity-Adjusted Treatment Effectiveness Analyses

The propensity adjustment is implemented in the treatment effectiveness analyses through stratification. This is based on the assumption that treatment assignment is ignorable within a propensity score stratum. (Here we stratify into quintiles.) Stated differently, within a quintile subjects who do and do not receive treatment will not differ on the covariates (x) that are included in the propensity score. Next, we discuss a method to examine the extent to which balance between groups has been achieved with the adjustment. Based on the ignorability assumption, causal inferences can be drawn regarding direct effects of treatment, conditioned on the random intercept.

8.3.1 Propensity-Based Quintile Classification

Based on the distribution of the propensity score, each observation of subject i at time j is classified into one propensity quintile, $q_{(1)} \ldots q_{(5)}$. The propensity score $e(x_{ij}, \upsilon_i)$ comprises both time-varying and time-invariant variables. Therefore, each subject's propensity score varies over time and, consequently, the subject's propensity quintile could also vary in a longitudinal study. Quintile classification is conducted so that treatment effectiveness analyses can be conducted separately for each quintile. The rationale is that this approach will remove much of the confounding effect of each variable that is included in the propensity score. However, before quintile-specific analyses can be conducted, the representation of each treatment group in each quintile must be examined. If a treatment is not well-represented in a particular quintile, of course, treatment effectiveness analyses cannot be conducted for that quintile. Quintile representation is evaluated by examining cell frequencies in a propensity quintile by treatment contingency table.

8.3.2 Longitudinal Treatment Effectiveness Analyses

The effectiveness of treatment is examined using survival analysis methods in which the time until recurrence of disease is the dependent variable. In the example used in this chapter, the measurement of survival is ascertained in time intervals, examining whether the event occurred since the prior follow-up visit. Therefore, a grouped-time approach to survival analysis is used. Furthermore, in an effort to incorporate all data throughout follow-up, which typically involves multiple observations per subject (for example, multiple recurrences), a mixed-effects grouped-time survival analysis model is used (Hedeker et al., 2000). The model examines the probability of *recurrence* up to, and including, time interval t for observation j of subject i as:

$$P_{ijt} = Pr(t_{ij} \leq t)$$

Using a complementary log-log link function, the model is a proportional hazards regression model that describes the cumulative probability of recurrence as a function of treatment:

$$P_{ijt} = 1 - exp(-exp(\alpha_t + x'_{ij}\beta + \upsilon_i))$$

where α_t represents the intercept term (that is, the baseline hazard), x is an indicator variable to represent the treatment group, and υ_i represents a random subject effect. Of note, marginal structural models, which we do not consider here, provide an alternative approach to evaluating time-varying treatments in which inverse probability weighting attempts to produce between-group balance in covariates. (See Chapter 9.)

8.3.3 Effectiveness Analysis Stratification

As stated earlier, the treatment effectiveness analyses are conducted separately for each propensity quintile. This is based on the work of Cochran (1968), who showed that quintile-stratification on a confounding variable removes a substantial proportion of the bias associated with that variable. The quintile-specific estimates of treatment effectiveness are then pooled to obtain one unified estimate of the treatment effect.

8.3.4 Pooling the Quintile-Specific Effectiveness Results

The quintile-specific results are pooled using the Mantel-Haenszel (1959) procedure as described by Fleiss (1981). Using this strategy, each quintile-specific parameter estimate is weighted by the inverse of its squared standard error and the pooled estimate is calculated as a weighted mean. The strategy assumes that there is not a treatment by propensity interaction (that is, that the treatment effect does not differ across quintiles). We assess this assumption in analyses of the pooled data set, which includes all observations from the five quintiles. A likelihood ratio test compares two mixed-effects models:

1. main effects terms for treatment and quintile (expressed with indicator variables)
2. main effects and the interaction of treatment and quintile

A significant interaction would indicate that the effect of treatment varies across propensity quintiles. In such a case, pooling of quintile-specific results is not indicated. Instead, treatment effectiveness conclusions must be reported at the quintile-specific level. In contrast, if there is no treatment by propensity interaction, the focus of the hypothesis test is the pooled treatment effect: H_0: $\beta = 0$.

8.4 Application

This application examines data from the National Institute of Mental Health Collaborative Depression Study. The study enrolled subjects with affective disorders from 1978–1981 who sought treatment for one of the major affective disorders at five medical centers in the United States (Boston, Chicago, Iowa City, New York, and St. Louis). Each subject provided written informed consent. The design and objectives of this longitudinal, observational study have been described elsewhere (Katz and Klerman, 1979). Subjects were followed with semi-annual assessments for the first five years and annual assessments for as much as 23 additional years. We examine somatic antidepressant treatment effectiveness for relapse prevention among those who recovered from unipolar major depression as defined by the Research Diagnostic Criteria (RDC) (Spitzer et al., 1978). The data that were used in the analyses reported here include up to 20 years of follow-up assessments.

8.4.1 Data Analytic Procedures

The analyses proceeded in two stages, as previously described. Initially, the model of propensity for treatment examined the magnitude of the association of demographic and clinical variables that were hypothesized to be associated with receiving somatic antidepressant treatment. In this example, treatment was the binary dependent variable. (An ordinal treatment intensity variable, described in Keller, 1988, and Leon et al., 2003, was dichotomized so that a treatment intensity of 0 was compared with intensities of 2, 3, and 4 combined. Intensity levels of 1 were excluded in the analyses for this application.) A mixed-effects logistic regression model was used because many subjects had multiple observations of treatment over time. A subject-specific random intercept was included in this model to account for the within-subject clustering of the repeated observations within subjects.

The second stage involved a mixed-effects grouped-time survival model of antidepressant treatment effectiveness that examined the time from the start of the course of treatment until the recurrence of an affective episode. The survival variable, time until recurrence, represented the number of consecutive weeks during which treatment status (yes/no) remained unchanged during a well period. The survival intervals could terminate in one of three ways:

1. recurrence of an affective episode
2. change in treatment status
3. end of follow-up

The latter two were classified as censored. In these analyses, it was assumed that censoring due to the end of follow-up was unrelated to time until recurrence. Subjects accrued additional survival intervals, also referred to here as *treatment intervals*, with each new episode and each change in treatment status while in episode. Treatment intervals were the unit of analysis for both the propensity and effectiveness models. Thus the data set included multiple observations per subject, one observation for each treatment interval. The intervals represent the distinct courses of treatment, including no treatment, that each subject received. Separate propensity scores were calculated for each of the treatment intervals.

8.4.2 Results

8.4.2.1 Subjects

Four hundred thirty-one subjects had major depressive disorder at study intake (Keller et al., 1992). Eighty-two of those subjects were excluded from the analyses because they developed bipolar disorder and another 46 of them did not recover from their intake episode and, therefore, were also excluded. Of those who otherwise met criteria for these analyses, 19 were excluded due to missing covariate data required for calculating a propensity score. Therefore, the analyses described here include 284 subjects with 1,319 observations.

8.4.2.2 Propensity for Treatment

The propensity models includes five variables: symptom severity (Psychiatric Status Rating, PSR, which ranges from 0–6: variable name *meanpsr*), symptom trajectory over the prior 8 weeks (increasing vs. decreasing vs. stable: *symdec* and *syminc*), educational status (*colgrad, somecol,* and *highsch)*, age category (*agelt30, age40t49, age50t59,* and *agege60*), and study site (*site1, site3, site4,* and *site5*). (See Program 8.1.) Three of the findings in the model are highlighted. (See Output from Program 8.1.) Subjects with more severe symptoms were significantly more likely to receive treatment (odds ratio [OR]: 1.99; 95% confidence interval [CI]: 1.70–2.34). Those whose symptom severity decreased in the 8 weeks prior to the interval were marginally less likely to get treated (OR: 0.70; 95% CI: 0.49–1.02). Similarly, subjects from three of the study sites (New York, Iowa, and Chicago) were more likely to get treatment than were subjects from the other sites. Whether or not a subject received treatment, across the multiple treatment intervals, was moderately consistent over time (intraclass correlation coefficient=0.305).

Program 8.1 Computing the Propensity Score with Mixed-Effects Logistic Regression

```
TITLE1 'Performing Mixed-effects Logistic Regression of Propensity
Model';

/* Propensity Analysis for Binary tx    */
/* Binary LOGISTIC RANDOM-INTERCEPT MODEL */

Data data1;
   SET "c:\uniint.sas7bdat";


PROC NLMIXED;
PARMS b0=0 b1=0 b2=0 b3=0 b4=0 b5=0 b6=0 b7=0 b8=0 b9=0 b10=0 b11=0
b12=0 b13=0 b14=0 sd=1;
z = b0 + b1*meanpsr + b2*colgrad + b3*somecol + b4*highsch + b5*site1
+ b6*site3 + b7*site4 + b8*site5 + b9*agelt30 + b10*age40t49 +
b11*age50t59
         + b12*agege60 + b13*symdec + b14*syminc + sd*u;
IF (tx=0) THEN
  p = 1 - (1 / (1 + EXP(-z)));
ELSE IF (tx=1) THEN
  p = 1 / (1 + EXP(-z));
like = LOG(p);
MODEL tx ~ GENERAL(like);
RANDOM u ~ NORMAL(0,1) SUBJECT=id;
PREDICT z OUT=zest;
ESTIMATE 'ICC' sd*sd/((((ATAN(1)*4)**2)/3)+sd*sd);
RUN;
```

Output from Program 8.1

The NLMIXED Procedure

Observations Used	1319
Observations Not Used	0
Total Observations	1319
Subjects	284
Max Obs Per Subject	27
Parameters	16
Quadrature Points	5

NOTE: GCONV convergence criterion satisfied.

Fit Statistics

-2 Log Likelihood	1537.3
AIC (smaller is better)	1569.3
AICC (smaller is better)	1569.8
BIC (smaller is better)	1627.7

Parameter Estimates

Parameter	Estimate	Standard Error	DF	t Value	Pr > |t|	Alpha	Lower	Upper	Gradient
b0	-3.5115	0.4758	283	-7.38	<.0001	0.05	-4.4481	-2.5749	0.003336
b1	0.6898	0.08074	283	8.54	<.0001	0.05	0.5309	0.8487	0.008001
b2	0.6704	0.3528	283	1.90	0.0584	0.05	-0.02410	1.3649	0.000295
b3	-0.1628	0.3320	283	-0.49	0.6241	0.05	-0.8162	0.4906	-0.00037
b4	0.4327	0.3210	283	1.35	0.1788	0.05	-0.1992	1.0645	0.003104
b5	1.3591	0.4779	283	2.84	0.0048	0.05	0.4185	2.2997	0.001145
b6	0.4026	0.3673	283	1.10	0.2739	0.05	-0.3203	1.1255	-0.00018
b7	1.1222	0.3770	283	2.98	0.0032	0.05	0.3802	1.8642	0.000473
b8	1.0876	0.4245	283	2.56	0.0109	0.05	0.2520	1.9232	0.0013
b9	-0.5782	0.2439	283	-2.37	0.0184	0.05	-1.0584	-0.09803	0.000034
b10	0.3813	0.2100	283	1.82	0.0705	0.05	-0.03206	0.7946	0.002361
b11	0.2037	0.2979	283	0.68	0.4948	0.05	-0.3827	0.7900	0.000226
b12	0.5608	0.3100	283	1.81	0.0715	0.05	-0.04930	1.1710	0.00244
b13	-0.3508	0.1889	283	-1.86	0.0644	0.05	-0.7226	0.02108	0.000302
b14	0.3339	0.2110	283	1.58	0.1148	0.05	-0.08154	0.7493	0.001543
sd	1.2023	0.1390	283	8.65	<.0001	0.05	0.9287	1.4759	0.001859

Additional Estimates

Label	Estimate	Standard Error	DF	t Value	Pr > |t|	Alpha	Lower	Upper
ICC	0.3053	0.04903	283	6.23	<.0001	0.05	0.2088	0.4018

The results of the propensity model (see Output from Program 8.1) were used to calculate a propensity score for each observation. Note that because time-varying covariates (that is, symptom severity and symptom trajectory) are included in the propensity score, the propensity score itself is time-varying. Each observation was then classified into one of the propensity score quintiles. (See Program 8.2.) A contingency table is displayed to evaluate the representativeness of treatments in each quintile. (See Output from Program 8.2.) It is clear that subjects in the lower quintiles were less likely to receive treatment, whereas those in higher quintiles were more likely to receive treatment. This lends some support to the validity of the model. Importantly, each treatment group is represented in each quintile and, therefore, quintile-specific treatment effectiveness analyses can be used to compare the groups.

Program 8.2 Quintile Stratification

```
/* Generate QUINTILE values (0 to 4) based on estimates from above model */
DATA data2 (Keep = id event tx meanpsr colgrad somecol highsch site1
site3 site6 site7 agelt30 age40t49 age50t59 agege60 symdec syminc surv2
pred ppred);
MERGE data1 zest;

/* convert to probability scale */
ppred =  1 / (1 + EXP(-pred));

PROC RANK GROUPS=5 OUT=rankout;
     VAR ppred;
     RANKS QUINT;

DATA all; SET rankout;
q1=0;q2=0;q3=0;q4=0;
if quint eq 1 then q1 = 1;
if quint eq 2 then q2 = 1;
if quint eq 3 then q3 = 1;
if quint eq 4 then q4 = 1;

/* Table of Quintile by tx */
PROC FREQ;
TABLES tx*QUINT;
RUN;
```

Output from Program 8.2

```
The FREQ Procedure

Table of tx by QUINT

tx(Treated yes/no)     QUINTILE(Rank for Variable ppred)

Frequency|
Percent  |
Row Pct  |
Col Pct  |       0|       1|       2|       3|       4|  Total
---------+--------+--------+--------+--------+--------+
       0 |    247 |    224 |    169 |    104 |     24 |    768
         |  18.73 |  16.98 |  12.81 |   7.88 |   1.82 |  58.23
         |  32.16 |  29.17 |  22.01 |  13.54 |   3.13 |
         |  93.92 |  84.85 |  64.02 |  39.39 |   9.09 |
---------+--------+--------+--------+--------+--------+
       1 |     16 |     40 |     95 |    160 |    240 |    551
         |   1.21 |   3.03 |   7.20 |  12.13 |  18.20 |  41.77
         |   2.90 |   7.26 |  17.24 |  29.04 |  43.56 |
         |   6.08 |  15.15 |  35.98 |  60.61 |  90.91 |
---------+--------+--------+--------+--------+--------+
Total          263      264      264      264      264     1319
             19.94    20.02    20.02    20.02    20.02   100.00
```

8.4.3 Treatment Effectiveness Analyses

Initially, the treatment by propensity interaction was evaluated with a likelihood ratio test that compared the fit of the main effect model (–2 log likelihood = 3203.7; see Output from Program 8.5) with that of the main effects and interaction model (–2 log likelihood = 3197.3; see Output from Program 8.6). The interaction is not statistically significant (χ^2=6.40, df=4, p=0.171). Therefore, results from the quintile-specific treatment effectiveness analyses were pooled as described previously. The pooled results show that when subjects received somatic antidepressant therapy, they were 35% less likely to have a recurrence than when they did not receive somatic treatment (OR: exp [–0.427] = 0.65; 95% CI: 0.50–0.85; see Output from Program 8.4), after controlling for propensity for treatment.

Program 8.3 Quintile-Specific Treatment Effectiveness Analyses

```
/* Analysis for Grouped-Time Survival - QUINTILE-SPECIFIC ANALYSES
*/
/* Binary Complementary Log-Log RANDOM-INTERCEPT MODEL with censoring
*/
PROC SORT; BY QUINT ID;
PROC NLMIXED;
PARMS b0=0 b1=0 sd=1 t2=1 t3=1.25 t4=1.5 t5=1.75 t6=2 t7=2.25;
ODS OUTPUT ParameterEstimates=estb;
z = b0 + b1*tx + sd*u;
IF (event = 1) THEN
DO;                                          /* event occurred */
  IF (surv2=1) THEN
    p = 1 - EXP(0 - EXP(0+z));
  ELSE IF (surv2=2) THEN
    p = (1 - EXP(0 - EXP(t2+z))) -  (1 - EXP(0 - EXP(0+z)));
  ELSE IF (surv2=3) THEN
    p = (1 - EXP(0 - EXP(t3+z))) -  (1 - EXP(0 - EXP(t2+z)));
  ELSE IF (surv2=4) THEN
    p = (1 - EXP(0 - EXP(t4+z))) -  (1 - EXP(0 - EXP(t3+z)));
  ELSE IF (surv2=5) THEN
    p = (1 - EXP(0 - EXP(t5+z))) -  (1 - EXP(0 - EXP(t4+z)));
  ELSE IF (surv2=6) THEN
    p = (1 - EXP(0 - EXP(t6+z))) -  (1 - EXP(0 - EXP(t5+z)));
  ELSE IF (surv2=7) THEN
    p = (1 - EXP(0 - EXP(t7+z))) -  (1 - EXP(0 - EXP(t6+z)));
END;
IF (event = 0) THEN
DO;                            /* event did not occur - censored */
  IF (surv2=1) THEN
    p = 1 - (1 - EXP(0 - EXP(0+z)));
  ELSE IF (surv2=2) THEN
    p = 1 - (1 - EXP(0 - EXP(t2+z)));
  ELSE IF (surv2=3) THEN
    p = 1 - (1 - EXP(0 - EXP(t3+z)));
  ELSE IF (surv2=4) THEN
    p = 1 - (1 - EXP(0 - EXP(t4+z)));
  ELSE IF (surv2=5) THEN
    p = 1 - (1 - EXP(0 - EXP(t5+z)));
  ELSE IF (surv2=6) THEN
    p = 1 - (1 - EXP(0 - EXP(t6+z)));
  ELSE IF (surv2=7) THEN
    p = 1 - (1 - EXP(0 - EXP(t7+z)));
END;
```

```
like = LOG(p);
MODEL surv2 ~ GENERAL(like);
RANDOM u ~ NORMAL(0,1) SUBJECT=id;
ESTIMATE 'ICC' sd*sd/((((ATAN(1)*4)**2)/6)+sd*sd);
BY QUINT;
RUN;
```

Program 8.4 Pooling Quintile-Specific Treatment Effectiveness Results

```
/* Generate pooled results based on results from the above quintile-
   specific models */
DATA estw; SET estb;
w = 1 / StandardError**2;
west = Estimate*w;

PROC SORT; BY Parameter;

PROC MEANS NOPRINT; CLASS Parameter; VAR west w;
OUTPUT OUT=sums SUM = sumwest sumw;

DATA poolest; SET sums; IF _TYPE_ EQ 1;
poolest = sumwest / sumw;
poolse  = 1 / sqrt(sumw);
poolz   = poolest / poolse;
poolp   = 2*(1 - probnorm(abs(poolz)));

/* Print the pooled results */
PROC PRINT;
VAR Parameter poolest poolse poolz poolp;
RUN;
```

Output from Program 8.4

Obs	Parameter	poolest	poolse	poolz	poolp
1	b0	-3.84229	0.23478	-16.3656	0.00000
2	**b1**	**-0.42659**	**0.13324**	**-3.2016**	**0.00137**
3	sd	0.13043	0.09210	1.4161	0.15674
4	t2	0.50464	0.13715	3.6795	0.00023
5	t3	0.89581	0.16553	5.4118	0.00000
6	t4	1.60004	0.19464	8.2204	0.00000
7	t5	2.45576	0.21083	11.6482	0.00000
8	t6	2.86478	0.21645	13.2354	0.00000
9	t7	4.10759	0.23911	17.1784	0.00000

Program 8.5 Treatment Effectiveness Analyses Pooled across All Subjects: Main Effects

```
/* Analysis for Grouped-Time Survival - all subjects - all QUINTILES
   main effects */
/* Binary Complementary Log-Log RANDOM-INTERCEPT MODEL with censoring   */
PROC NLMIXED;
PARMS b0=0 b1=0 b2=0 b3=0 b4=0 b5=0  sd=1
      t2=1 t3=1.25 t4=1.5 t5=1.75 t6=2 t7=2.25;
z = b0 + b1*tx + b2*q1 + b3*q2 + b4*q3 + b5*q4 + sd*u;

...more SAS statements...

like = LOG(p);
MODEL surv2 ~ GENERAL(like);
RANDOM u ~ NORMAL(0,1) SUBJECT=id;
ESTIMATE 'ICC' sd*sd/((((ATAN(1)*4)**2)/6)+sd*sd);
RUN;
```

Output from Program 8.5

```
NOTE: GCONV convergence criterion satisfied.

             Fit Statistics

-2 Log Likelihood               3203.7
AIC (smaller is better)         3229.7
AICC (smaller is better)        3230.0
BIC (smaller is better)         3277.2
```

Program 8.6 Treatment Effectiveness Analyses Pooled across All Subjects: Main Effects and Interactions

```
/* Analysis for Grouped-Time Survival - all subjects - all QUINTILES
main effects and interactions */
/* Binary Complementary Log-Log RANDOM-INTERCEPT MODEL with censoring
*/
PROC NLMIXED;
PARMS b0=0 b1=0 b2=0 b3=0 b4=0 b5=0 b6=0 b7=0  b8=0 b9=0 sd=1
      t2=1 t3=1.25 t4=1.5 t5=1.75 t6=2 t7=2.25;
z = b0 + b1*tx + b2*q1 + b3*q2 + b4*q3 + b5*q4
       + b6*tx*q1 + b7*tx*q2 + b8*tx*q3 + b9*tx*q4 + sd*u;

...more SAS statements...


like = LOG(p);
MODEL surv2 ~ GENERAL(like);
RANDOM u ~ NORMAL(0,1) SUBJECT=id;
ESTIMATE 'ICC' sd*sd/((((ATAN(1)*4)**2)/6)+sd*sd);
RUN;
```

Output from Program 8.6

```
NOTE: GCONV convergence criterion satisfied.


             Fit Statistics

-2 Log Likelihood               3197.3
AIC (smaller is better)         3231.3
AICC (smaller is better)        3231.7
BIC (smaller is better)         3293.3
```

8.4.4 Evaluating Balance across Treatment Groups

The propensity score is a balancing score that, if assumptions are fulfilled, allows for comparison of non-equivalent groups. The extent to which balance has been achieved can be examined. In an effort to parallel the propensity adjustment that has been described, balance is examined here by using a quintile-stratification strategy in each of a series of mixed-effects models for the time-varying variables that comprise the propensity score. In this case, however, the independent variable is the treatment group and the respective dependent variables in the successive models are the variables that were included in the propensity score. (Contrast this with the propensity model described previously in which the dependent variable is the treatment and the independent variables are those that are components of the propensity score.) If the primary objective of the propensity adjustment has been achieved, there would not be substantial differences between treatment groups on each variable included in the propensity score. We illustrate this for one time-varying continuous variable, symptom severity (PSR). The results show that the magnitude of the association between treatment group and symptom severity has been muted (B=.589 and p<.0001 [in Output from Program 8.7] vs. B=0.037 and p=0.425 [in Output from Program 8.8]) and therefore, in the case of symptom severity, the objective has been achieved. Note that this examination must focus not simply on whether the statistical significance of the association has been attenuated but also on the reduction in the magnitude of the bivariate association between treatment and symptom severity.

Program 8.7 Evaluating Balance of Psychiatric Status Rating (PSR) across Treatment Groups with No Propensity Adjustment

```
Title2 "Compare the treatment groups on PSR using unadjusted model";
PROC SORT DATA=ALL; BY ID;
RUN;
PROC MIXED data =ALL;
MODEL meanpsr = tx / S;
RANDOM INTERCEPT / SUB=id;
RUN;
```

Output from Program 8.7

```
Compare the treatment groups on PSR using unadjusted model

The Mixed Procedure

                    Solution for Fixed Effects

                              Standard
Effect         Estimate          Error       DF     t Value     Pr > |t|

Intercept        2.4170        0.04891      283       49.42       <.0001
tx               0.5889        0.06359     1034        9.26       <.0001
```

Program 8.8 Evaluating Balance of Psychiatric Status Rating across Treatment Groups with a Propensity Adjustment

```
Title2 "Compare the treatment groups on PSR using quintile
adjustment";
/*Linear random intercept model*/
PROC SORT DATA=ALL; BY QUINT ID;

PROC MIXED data=ALL;
ODS OUTPUT SolutionF=estc1;
MODEL meanpsr = tx / S;
RANDOM INTERCEPT / SUB=id;
BY QUINT;
RUN;

/* Generate pooled results based on results from the above quintile-
specific models */
DATA estw1; SET estc1;
w = 1 / StdErr**2;
west = Estimate*w;

PROC SORT; BY Effect;

PROC MEANS NOPRINT; CLASS Effect; VAR west w;
OUTPUT OUT=sums1 SUM = sumwest sumw;
```

```
DATA poolest1; SET sums1; IF _TYPE_ EQ 1;
poolest = sumwest / sumw;
poolse  = 1 / sqrt(sumw);
poolz   = poolest / poolse;
poolp   = 2*(1 - probnorm(abs(poolz)));

/* Print the pooled results */
PROC PRINT;
VAR Effect poolest poolse poolz poolp;
RUN;
```

Output from Program 8.8

```
Compare the treatment groups on PSR using quintile adjustment.

Obs    Effect        poolest      poolse        poolz      poolp

 1     Intercept     2.47631     0.044452     55.7073    0.00000
 2     tx           -0.03650     0.045767     -0.7976    0.42512
```

This approach is not necessary for time-invariant components of the propensity score (for example, ethnicity). Instead, a simpler approach (not shown here) is to compare the strength of the association of each (time-invariant) component of the propensity score (in this case, the independent variable) with treatment (in this case, the dependent variable). Results from two models, the unadjusted model and a propensity-adjusted model that includes four quintile indicator variables as covariates, can be compared (for example, see Leon et al., 2007). If balance is achieved, the propensity-adjusted models will show substantially attenuated, and presumably nonsignificant, associations.

8.5 Summary

A two-stage longitudinal propensity adjustment has been described for treatment effectiveness analyses of observational data. A mixed-effects logistic regression model is used to estimate the propensity for treatment, and quintile-stratified, mixed-effects, grouped-time survival models are used to estimate the treatment effect. Tests of three of the model assumptions have been described, including the representativeness of treatments in each quintile, the treatment by quintile interaction, and the balance.

Finally, we mention two topics that have not been considered here. First, the impact of model propensity misspecification on cross-sectional and longitudinal analyses has been examined in simulation studies (Drake, 1993; Leon and Hedeker, 2007b). Sensitivity analyses to evaluate propensity model misspecification have been described in detail elsewhere (Rosenbaum, 2002). Second, the sample size required for the propensity adjustment has not been discussed. The choice of sample size is guided by statistical power analyses and the *N* needed for stable estimates in mixed-effects models, which each have been examined in simulation studies (Leon and Hedeker, 2005; Leon et al., 2007). The sample size is also driven by the stratification process, which necessitates analyses of five quintile-specific effectiveness models, each of which contains only 20% of the observations.

Acknowledgments

The National Institute of Mental Health Collaborative Depression Study was conducted with current participation of the following investigators: M.B. Keller, M.D. (Chairperson, Providence); W. Coryell (Co-Chair Person, Iowa City); D.A. Solomon, M.D. (Providence); W.A. Scheftner, M.D. (Chicago); W. Coryell, M.D. (Iowa City); J. Endicott, Ph.D., A.C. Leon, Ph.D., J. Loth, M.S.W. (New York); and J. Rice, Ph.D. (St. Louis). Other current contributors include: H.S. Akiskal, M.D.; J. Fawcett, M.D.; L.L. Judd, M.D.; P.W. Lavori, Ph.D.; J.D. Maser, Ph.D.; and T.I. Mueller, M.D. This manuscript has been reviewed by the Publication Committee of the Collaborative Depression Study, and has its endorsement. The data for this manuscript came from the National Institute of Mental Health (NIMH) Collaborative Program on the Psychobiology of Depression-Clinical Studies (Katz and Klerman, 1979). The Collaborative Program was initiated in 1975 to investigate nosologic, genetic, family, prognostic, and psychosocial issues of mood disorders, and is an ongoing, long-term multidisciplinary investigation of the course of mood and related affective disorders. The original principal and co-principal investigators were from five academic centers and included Gerald Klerman, M.D. (Co-Chairperson), Martin Keller, M.D., and Robert Shapiro, M.D. (Massachusetts General Hospital, Harvard Medical School); Eli Robins, M.D., Paula Clayton, M.D., Theodore Reich, M.D., and Amos Wellner, M.D. (Washington University Medical School); Jean Endicott, Ph.D., and Robert Spitzer, M.D. (Columbia University); Nancy Andreasen, M.D., Ph.D., William Coryell, M.D., and George Winokur, M.D. (University of Iowa); and Jan Fawcett, M.D., and William Scheftner, M.D. (Rush-Presbyterian-St. Luke's Medical Center). The NIMH Clinical Research Branch was an active collaborator in the origin and development of the Collaborative Program with Martin M. Katz, Ph.D., Branch Chief as the Co-Chairperson, and Robert Hirschfeld, M.D., as the Program Coordinator. Other past contributors include: J. Croughan, M.D.; M.T. Shea, Ph.D.; R. Gibbons, Ph.D.; M.A. Young, Ph.D.; and D.C. Clark, Ph.D.

This research was supported, in part, by NIH grants MH60447 and MH49762.

References

Cochran, W. G. 1968. "The effectiveness of adjustment by subclassification in removing bias in observational studies." *Biometrics* 24: 295–313.

Drake, C. 1993. "Effects of misspecification of the propensity score on estimators of the treatment effect." *Biometrics* 49: 1231–1236.

Fleiss, J. L. 1981. *Statistical Methods for Rates and Proportions*. New York: John Wiley & Sons.

Hedeker, D., O. Siddiqui, and F. B. Hu. 2000. "Random-effects regression analysis of correlated grouped-time survival data." *Statistical Methods in Medical Research* 9: 161–179.

Katz, M. M., and G. L. Klerman. 1979. "Introduction: overview of the clinical studies program." *The American Journal of Psychiatry* 136(1): 49–51.

Keller, M. B. 1988. "Undertreatment of major depression." *Psychopharmacology Bulletin* 24(1): 75–80.

Keller, M. B., P. W. Lavori, T. I. Mueller, J. Endicott, W. Coryell, R. M. Hirschfeld, T. Shea. 1992. "Time to recovery, chronicity, and levels of psychopathology in major depression: A five-year prospective follow-up of 431 subjects. "*Archives of General Psychiatry* 49(10):809-816.

Leon, A. C., and D. Hedeker. 2005. "A mixed-effects quintile-stratified propensity adjustment for effectiveness analyses of ordered categorical doses." *Statistics in Medicine* 24: 647–658.

Leon, A. C., and D. Hedeker. 2007a. "A comparison of mixed-effects quantile stratification propensity-adjustment strategies for longitudinal treatment effectiveness analyses of continuous outcomes." *Statistics in Medicine* 26: 2650–2665.

Leon, A. C., and D. Hedeker. 2007b. "Quintile stratification based on a misspecified propensity score in longitudinal treatment effectiveness analyses of ordinal doses." *Computational Statistics and Data Analysis* 51(12): 6114–6122.

Leon, A. C., D. Hedeker, and J. J. Teres. 2007. "Bias reduction in effectiveness analyses of longitudinal ordinal doses with a mixed-effects propensity adjustment." *Statistics in Medicine* 26: 110–123.

Leon, A. C., T. L. Mueller, D. A. Solomon, and M. B. Keller. 2001. "A dynamic adaptation of the propensity score adjustment for effectiveness analyses of ordinal doses of treatment." *Statistics in Medicine* 20(9/10): 1487–1498.

Leon, A. C., D. A. Solomon, T. I. Mueller, J. Endicott, J. P. Rice, J. D. Maser, W. Coryell, and M. B. Keller. 2003. "A 20-year longitudinal, observational study of somatic antidepressant treatment effectiveness." *The American Journal of Psychiatry* 160: 727–733.

Mantel, N., and W. Haenszel. 1959. "Statistical aspects of the analysis of data from retrospective studies of disease." *Journal of the National Cancer Institute* 22(4): 719–748.

Rosenbaum, P. R. 2002. *Observational Studies*. 2d ed. New York: Springer.

Rosenbaum, P. R., and D. B. Rubin. 1983. "The central role of the propensity score in observational studies for causal effects." *Biometrika* 70(1): 41–55.

Rosenbaum, P. R., and D. B. Rubin. 1984. "Reducing bias in observational studies using subclassification on the propensity score." *Journal of the American Statistical Association* 79(387): 516–24.

Spitzer, R. L., J. Endicott, and E. Robins. 1978. Research diagnostic criteria: rationale and reliability." *Archives of General Psychiatry* 35(6): 773–782.

Chapter 9

Analysis of Longitudinal Observational Data Using Marginal Structural Models

Douglas E. Faries
Zbigniew A. Kadziola

Abstract

Assessing treatment effectiveness in longitudinal, observational data can be complex because in observational treatment patients can change medications at any time. In addition to the need to control for selection bias at baseline due to the lack of randomization, time-varying confounders can influence treatment changes over time and, thus, affect treatment group effectiveness comparisons. One approach to producing causal treatment effect estimates—even in the presence of treatment switching, missing data, and time-varying confounders—is to use marginal structural models. To illustrate, simulated data based on an observational schizophrenia study were analyzed using a marginal structural model approach. SAS code for performing the analysis is provided, and output using data from the schizophrenia study is examined.

9.1 Introduction

Assessing the causal effect of medications in longitudinal, observational (naturalistic) data presents analytical challenges—including the need to address selection bias; missing data; and switching, stopping, and augmenting medications. Addressing the issue of selection bias is critical because treatment groups likely differ in aspects other than treatment choice, and adjustment in the analysis is necessary (Rosenbaum and Rubin, 1983; Grimes and Schulz, 2002; Haro et al., 2006). In addressing data that are both longitudinal and observational, the issue of selection bias also extends to treatment switching over time (Robins et al., 2000, Hernán et al., 2000) as patients may switch, stop, augment, or otherwise not comply for a variety of reasons. In addition, such patient/physician choices are typically based upon stochastic and/or time-varying factors that may well differ among treatments. Because of such issues, statistical methods commonly used for longitudinal analyses of randomized clinical trial data, such as intent-to-treat

(ITT) last observation carried forward (LOCF) or repeated measures models, may not be appropriate.

ITT analyses group patients based only on their initial treatment assignment and ignore all information on other medications prescribed or taken. Patient dropout in such studies is often addressed by utilizing a LOCF approach. Clearly, such a technique does not directly address treatment effectiveness when there has been a substantial amount of switching among treatments. ITT analyses certainly have their place in longitudinal, observational research, such as in studies to compare policies or treatment strategies where one is not primarily interested in the effects of individual medications (Tunis et al., 2006).

While utilizing repeated measures models with treatment as a time-dependent variable may seem to provide a simple solution, Hernán and colleagues (2004, 2005) explain that such an approach does not provide estimates with a causal interpretation (see the following) in the presence of time-dependent confounders (a predictor of subsequent outcome and subsequent treatment) that are also affected by prior treatment. For instance, any longitudinal measure of disease severity would likely be problematic because it could be associated with the outcome measure, it could predict subsequent treatment, and it could have been affected by prior treatment. Thus, even if treatment is randomized at the beginning of a study, the result of usual-care treatment over time will ultimately result in imbalance in key patient characteristics among treatment groups. To address the switching of treatments, one could ignore the data after the medication switch and use standard repeated measures mixed models that have proven very useful in longitudinal data analyses (Verbeke and Molenberghs, 2000; Mallinckrodt et al., 2003). Such an approach treats the data after the switch as missing data but clearly does not make use of the information gathered after the medication switch.

In this chapter, we examine the use of marginal structural models (MSMs) for longitudinal, observational data. To explain the potential benefits of the MSM approach, we first must briefly review the notions of counterfactual outcomes and causal effect. We will follow the notation provided by Hernán and colleagues (2002). Let $\bar{a}$ denote the treatment history for a patient over a period of time (for example, $\bar{a}$ = [a(1), a(2), …,a(t)], where a(1) denotes the treatment used at time 1). A counterfactual outcome for patient *i* on treatment sequence $\bar{a}$ denotes that patient's outcome if, possibly contrary to fact, the patient received treatment $\bar{a}$. It is denoted by $Y_{\bar{a},i}(t)$. Each patient has an unknown counterfactual outcome for each treatment he did not receive, plus an observed outcome for the treatment actually received. On an individual basis, treatment is said to have a causal effect on a patient's outcome if $Y_{\bar{a},i}(t) \neq Y_{\bar{a}',i}(t)$ for some time point *t* and treatment patterns $\bar{a}$ and $\bar{a}'$. That is, the outcome for the patient differs based on the treatment taken. On a population basis, treatment is said to have a causal effect on outcome if the mean outcome had all patients followed a particular treatment pattern ($\bar{a}$ for example) differs from the mean outcome had all patients followed a different treatment pattern ($\bar{a}'$ for example) (that is, $E[Y_{\bar{a}}(t)] \neq E[Y_{\bar{a}'}(t)]$ for some time point and treatment pattern).

Robins and colleagues (1999) demonstrated that MSMs, under a set of assumptions discussed here, produce consistent estimates of the average causal treatment effects—even in the presence of treatment changes, time-dependent confounders, and missing at random study dropout. In this chapter, we first describe the MSM approach (Section 9.2) and then present the MSM analysis of a longitudinal schizophrenia study (Section 9.3). SAS code is provided, and SAS output is discussed to allow readers to understand the implementation of the analysis and to modify the code for their own use. Faries and colleagues (2007) also summarize data from this study using a variety of methods, including MSMs. Some other applications of MSMs in the literature include Hernán and colleagues (2000, 2002), Ko and colleagues (2003), Brumback and colleagues (2004), and Cole and colleagues (2005), who examined time to event outcomes for HIV patients; and Bodnar and colleagues (2004), Yamaguchi and Ohashi (2004a and 2004b), Mortimer and colleagues (2005), Suarez and colleagues (2006), Peterson and colleagues (2007), and Vansteeldandt and colleagues (2009), who assessed other applications.

9.2 MSM Methodology

An MSM analysis is basically a weighted repeated measures approach – using treatment as a time-varying covariate. Weights, based on inverse probability of treatment weighting, control for time-dependent confounders and essentially produce a pseudo-population with balance in both time-invariant and time-varying covariates allowing for causal treatment comparisons using standard repeated measure models. The weighting can also be adjusted to incorporate adjustments for missing data—providing validity under missing at random (MAR; missing data may depend upon observed but not unobserved measures) and missing completely at random (MCAR; missing data does not depend upon observed or unobserved measures) data.

Conducting an MSM analysis is a two-step process. First, one estimates two weights for each observation (patient visit): one adjusting for treatment selection and one adjusting for study discontinuation. Computation of these estimated weights can incorporate time-independent and time-dependent factors. The stabilized weight is recommended by Hernán (2002), and we use the notation from that manuscript (here for the treatment selection weight),

$$SW = \prod_{k=0}^{t} \frac{f[A(k) \mid \overline{A}(k-1), V]}{f[A(k) \mid \overline{A}(k-1), \overline{L}(k)]}$$

where $A(k)$ represents the treatment at time k and $\overline{A}(k-1)$ represents the treatment history prior to time k, V represents a vector of time-independent variables (baseline covariates), and $\overline{L}(k)$ represents a vector of time-varying covariates through time k—which includes baseline variables V. The numerator of the weight is the probability a patient is on the observed treatment at time k, given the prior treatment history and baseline covariates. The denominator is basically the same factor, except it incorporates time-varying covariates as predictors. Thus, one can see that observations where the time-varying factors are strong predictors of the current treatment selection are down-weighted in the analyses (because such observations are over-represented in the observed data).

To incorporate adjustment for early patient dropout, the same stabilized weight approach is used—except the outcome is not treatment selection but a flag variable denoting whether the patient remained in the study. The final weight for each patient's observation is obtained by multiplying the treatment selection weights and the censoring weights.

For the second step of the MSM analysis, one simply conducts a weighted repeated measures model analysis using generalized estimating equations. In this second stage, time-dependent confounders are not included in the repeated measures model—as their effects have been incorporated into the weights. Treatment is included as a time-dependent factor, and time-invariant covariates may also be included as appropriate (just as in a cross-sectional analysis where variables may be included in a propensity model and in the analysis model).

As mentioned previously, MSMs can produce consistent estimates of the average causal treatment effects—even in the presence of treatment changes, time-dependent confounders, and missing at random study dropout. The assumptions necessary for causal inference from an MSM correspond to the same assumptions necessary for common cross-sectional bias control methods such as propensity scoring:

1. no unmeasured confounders—that is, all variables that relate to treatment assignment and outcome were collected and utilized in the analysis; called *conditional exchangeability*; formally: $Y_{\bar{a}}(t+1) \coprod A(k) | \bar{A}(k-1), \bar{L}(k)$, for all $\bar{a}$ and $t \geq k$.
2. positivity—there is a positive probability of each treatment for each set of covariates (no perfect confounding); formally $f[\bar{a}(k-1), \bar{l}(k)] > 0 \Rightarrow f[a(k) | \bar{a}(k-1), \bar{l}(k)] > 0$.
3. use of the correct models (weighting and analysis models).

As strong assumptions are necessary, assessing the appropriateness of the assumptions and performing sensitivity analyses are critical to a quality analysis. The no unmeasured confounders and correct models assumptions can never be fully proven and are discussed here. The positivity assumption basically says that all treatment options are possible given any combination of covariate values. Mortimer and colleagues (2005) recommended assessing this by computing predicted probabilities of treatment selection using the covariates from the models across the entire study (looking for 0 or 1 predicted probabilities). Mortimer and colleagues (2005) also provide an example of assessing the correctness of the models used in an MSM analysis using test and training data sets.

To limit the possibility of unmeasured confounding, every effort should be made to identify and collect data on potential confounders by searching the literature, examining relevant data, having discussions with experts, and utilizing potential confounding variables in the analysis. Such diligence will still never allow one to completely conclude no bias is unaccounted for, but an analyst first needs to make sure that all known confounders are addressed. Robins and colleagues (1999) and Brumback and colleagues (2004) have also provided a more formal method to study the sensitivity of an MSM analysis to unmeasured confounding. They quantify such confounding through a sensitivity parameter (alpha) and confounding function and assess the amount of unmeasured confounding that can be present before inferences would change. The confounding function (or alpha itself when a simple constant function is used) represents the difference in potential outcomes between patients in the different treatment groups. We use a simple constant function in our analysis, referring the reader to Brumback and colleagues (2004) for more options.

9.3 Example: MSM Analysis of a Simulated Schizophrenia Trial

9.3.1 Study Description

To illustrate the implementation of an MSM analysis, we simulated data based on a study of the effectiveness of medications for patients with schizophrenia in usual-care settings. A brief description of the design for the actual study follows, though the reader is referred to Tunis and colleagues (2006) for details. This was a one-year study of patients with schizophrenia, schizoaffective disorder, or schizophreniform disorder who were randomized to one of three different treatment regimens. After randomization, the remainder of the study was observational in the sense that physicians/patients were allowed to stop or switch medications as deemed necessary in usual practice. Data on a variety of domains were captured at five post-baseline visits (approximately 2 weeks and 2, 5, 8, and 12 months post-baseline). The outcome measure of interest for this analysis was the Brief Psychiatric Rating Scale (BPRS) total score, a measure of schizophrenia symptom severity where lower scores indicate lesser symptom severity. For demonstrative purposes, we simulated data for this analysis (see Tunis et al., 2006, for actual data results) maintaining the design and data structure and focused the final comparison between two groups rather than three. These groups are referred to as *treatment* and *control* during this example analysis. However, each treatment is considered as a separate treatment in the analytical steps until the final model to demonstrate how one can handle more than two groups with the MSM approach.

9.3.2 Data Analysis

9.3.2.1 Data Overview

Before conducting the MSM analysis, we provide a brief summary of the simulated data pertaining to medication changes and the steps taken to prepare the data set for analysis. The treatment groups were balanced with respect to demographics and baseline patient characteristics due to the randomization. After randomization, study discontinuation was similar across the treatment groups though rates of switching medication differed, with almost half (47.7%) of the control group (treatment C) switching medications during the study with a lower rate for the treatment group (treatment groups A and B pooled; 20.4%). At each visit, patients were considered to be on a particular medication if they had been treated with that medication for at least the previous 14 days. Given this definition, on 41.6% of the 2,548 patient visits during the study, patients were taking treatment A, 25.1% were taking treatment B, 23.8% were taking treatment C, 4.8% were taking both A and C, and 4.8% were not taking any antipsychotic medication. A total of 17 patient visits were excluded from the analysis due to small sample sizes for certain treatment combinations (A and B n=16; A and B and C n=1). In addition, approximately 4% of the patient visits had missing covariate information (see the list of covariates later) that was imputed using a LOCF approach. Outcome data were not imputed, only covariate data and only when the outcome measure was available. The analysis data set, INPDS, used a one observation per patient per visit format. A description of the key variables follows.

Table 9.1 Description of Key Variables in MSM Analysis

Variable	Description	Variable	Description
INVSC	Investigator number	BPRS	BPRS at this visit
PATSC	Patient number	GAFC	GAF at this visit
AGEYRS	Age in years	EVNT	Events during visit
GENDER	Gender	HOSP	Hosp. during visit
ORIGIN2	Race	PR1TRTA	Trt A previous visit
THERAPY	Randomized trtmnt	PR1TRTB	Trt B previous visit
VIS	Visit number	PR1TRTC	Trt C previous visit
BAVAR	Baseline BPRS total	PR1BPRS	Previous vis BPRS
BGAF	Baseline GAF score	PR1GAF	Previous vis GAF
BEVNT	Baseline adv events	PR1EVNT	Previous vis event
BHOSP	Baseline hospitaliz.	PR1HOSP	Previous vis hosp

(continued)

Table 9.1 *(continued)*

Variable	Description	Variable	Description
TRTA	On Trt A during vis		
TRTB	On Trt B during vis		
TRTC	On Trt C during vis		
TRT	Treatment during vis		

9.3.2.2 Computation of Inverse Weights

Step one in conducting the MSM analysis requires estimation of the treatment selection and censoring weights (using the formula for stabilized weights [SW] from Section 9.2). For estimating the treatment selection weights, separate multinomial models for the numerator and denominator were implemented using PROC LOGISTIC with the LINK= GLOGIT option (see Program 9.1). Treatment was the dependent variable for both models and the GLOGIT option was used because the treatment choice at each visit had five potential outcomes (three individual treatments, no treatment, and one combination). Output from the LOGISTIC procedure contains the predicted probabilities of treatment selection (data sets PREDTRT0 and PREDTRT1). In addition to previous treatment, the following time-varying covariates were included in this model:

- BPRS total
- global assessment of functioning (GAF)
- events (the presence or absence of at least one moderate or severe adverse event)
- hospitalization

These variables were chosen a priori to cover the domains of symptom severity, functioning, tolerability, and resource utilization. Time-independent variables included in this initial model included age, gender, ethnicity, and baseline value for each of the time-dependent variables. Macro variables could be utilized to input all model parameters at the beginning of the code; however, we chose to simplify the understanding of the process by simply showing the models directly in the LOGISTIC statements. In addition, output from the weight models is suppressed for simplification of the output. However, one can easily remove the restriction to evaluate the weight model in more detail.

PROC GENMOD was used to compute the estimated stabilized weights to adjust for censoring using a logistic regression model (see Program 9.1). The dependent variable for the censoring weight model was a binary flag for remaining in the study. The independent variables for this model were the same as for the treatment selection weight model—though the time-varying covariates were offset by one visit due to the structure of the data as censoring looked forward (did the patient return for a following visit?) relative to treatment (what was the treatment assigned in the previous time period?). The Logit LINK function was used here because the outcome measure was binomial. The GENMOD approach could be used for both weight calculations in studies where only two treatment groups are assessed.

Partial output from the multinomial and logistic regression denominator weights models is provided in the Output from Program 9.1. Previous treatment was the strongest predictor of present treatment. None of the time-varying covariates were strong predictors of treatment changes—suggesting bias in treatment selection over time may not be particularly strong in these data. Along with previous treatment, higher (time-varying) symptom severity was found to be a predictor of censoring. Patients with more severe symptoms were more likely to discontinue from the study.

Program 9.1 Computing Treatment Selection and Censoring Weights

```
/* This section of code computes the treatment selection and censoring
weights. This is accomplished in 4 steps:
1) multinomial model to compute numerator of treatment selection weights;
2) multinomial model to compute denominator of treatment selection weights;
3) binomial model to compute numerator of censoring adjustment weights;
4) binomial model to compute denominator of censoring adjustment weights.*/

/* treatment selection weights:  numerator calculation
(probability of treatment using only baseline covariates) */
PROC LOGISTIC DATA = INPDS;
  CLASS VIS THERAPY PR1TRTA PR1TRTB PR1TRTC GENDER ORIGIN2 BHOSP BEVNT;
  MODEL TRT = VIS THERAPY PR1TRTA PR1TRTB PR1TRTC GENDER ORIGIN2 BHOSP
  BEVNT AGEYRS BGAF BBPRS
    /LINK=GLOGIT;
  OUTPUT OUT=PREDTRT0(WHERE=(TRT=_LEVEL_)) PRED=PREDTRT0;
run;

/* treatment selection weights:  denominator calculation
(probability of treatment with baseline covariates and time-dependent
covariates) */
PROC LOGISTIC DATA = INPDS;
  CLASS VIS THERAPY PR1TRTA PR1TRTB PR1TRTC GENDER ORIGIN2 BHOSP BEVNT
        PR1EVNT PR1HOSP;
  MODEL TRT = VIS THERAPY PR1TRTA PR1TRTB PR1TRTC GENDER ORIGIN2 BHOSP
           BEVNT AGEYRS BGAF BBPRS PR1EVNT PR1HOSP PR1BPRS PR1GAFC
    /LINK=GLOGIT;
  OUTPUT OUT=PREDTRT1(WHERE=(TRT=_LEVEL_)) PRED=PREDTRT1;
run;

/* censoring adjustment weights:  numerator calculation
(probability of censoring using only baseline covariates) */
ODS LISTING EXCLUDE OBSTATS;
PROC GENMOD DATA = INPDS;
  CLASS PATSC   VIS THERAPY TRTA TRTB TRTC GENDER ORIGIN2 BHOSP BEVNT;
  MODEL CFLAG = VIS THERAPY TRTA TRTB TRTC GENDER ORIGIN2 BHOSP BEVNT
                AGEYRS BGAF BBPRS
    /DIST = BIN LINK = LOGIT TYPE3 OBSTATS;
  REPEATED SUBJECT = PATSC / TYPE = EXCH;
  ODS OUTPUT OBSTATS = PREDCEN0(RENAME=(PRED=PREDCEN0));
run;
ODS LISTING SELECT ALL;

/* censoring adjustment weights:  denominator calculation
(probability of censoring using baseline covariates and time-dependent
covariates) */
ODS LISTING EXCLUDE OBSTATS;
PROC GENMOD DATA = INPDS;
  CLASS PATSC VIS THERAPY TRTA TRTB TRTC GENDER ORIGIN2 BHOSP BEVNT
  EVNT HOSP;
  MODEL CFLAG = VIS THERAPY TRTA TRTB TRTC GENDER ORIGIN2 BHOSP BEVNT
          EVNT HOSP AGEYRS BGAF BBPRS BPRS GAFC
    /DIST = BIN LINK = LOGIT TYPE3 OBSTATS;
  REPEATED SUBJECT = PATSC / TYPE = EXCH;
  ODS OUTPUT OBSTATS = PREDCEN1(RENAME=(PRED=PREDCEN1));
run;
ODS LISTING SELECT ALL;
```

Output from Program 9.1

```
weight denominator model: treatment weights

      Type 3 Analysis of Effects

                              Wald
Effect          DF      Chi-Square      Pr > ChiSq

VIS             16        124.2743          <.0001
THERAPY          8         11.8349          0.1587
PR1TRTA          4        229.7185          <.0001
PR1TRTB          4        100.6526          <.0001
PR1TRTC          4        269.8939          <.0001
GENDER           4          3.3971          0.4937
ORIGIN2          8         10.4911          0.2322
BHOSP            4          0.4611          0.9772
BEVNT            4          3.0900          0.5429
AGEYRS           4          1.4473          0.8359
BGAF             4          1.9736          0.7406
BBPRS            4          2.2390          0.6919
PR1EVNT          4          7.5905          0.1078
PR1HOSP          4          4.6487          0.3253
PR1BPRS          4          2.5962          0.6275
PR1GAFC          4          2.5983          0.6271

weight denominator model: censoring weights

  Score Statistics For Type 3 GEE Analysis

                                 Chi-
Source              DF          Square     Pr > ChiSq

VIS                  4           13.21         0.0103
THERAPY              2            9.04         0.0109
TRTA                 1            3.95         0.0468
TRTB                 1            3.74         0.0532
TRTC                 1            0.39         0.5346
GENDER               1            0.15         0.6964
ORIGIN2              2            0.99         0.6087
BHOSP                1            0.88         0.3473
BEVNT                1            0.93         0.3338
EVNT                 1            0.61         0.4338
HOSP                 1            0.05         0.8163
AGEYRS               1            4.89         0.0270
BGAF                 1            0.04         0.8431
BBPRS                1            0.67         0.4115
BPRS                 1           12.21         0.0005
GAFC                 1            0.32         0.5726
```

To produce the overall weights for each observation (patient visit) in this analysis, the inverse probability weights for treatment selection and censoring computed here were multiplied together cumulatively in a DATA step based on the formula for SW in Section 9.2 (see Program 9.2). In the SAS code, the SQL procedure gathers data from the four output data sets from the treatment selection and weight models (PREDTRT0, PREDTRT1, PREDCENS0, and PREDCENS1) and produces the stabilized weights. Variable STABWT is the final estimate of SW. Output from Program 9.2 displays the distribution of the final weights across all patient visits in box plot form. The mean is near 1 (mean = 1.002, SD = 0.1555), as would be expected from the average of weights, and no major outliers were noted in the box plot.

Program 9.2 Merging Output from Program 9.1

```
/* This section of code performs the steps necessary to merge the output
from the weight models (Program 9.1) to allow for computation of a single
adjustment for each observation in the analysis data set (stabilized
weight). This is followed by code to produce summaries of the final
weights.   */

PROC SQL;
  /*ratio of probabilities for treatment*/
  CREATE TABLE PREDTRT AS
    SELECT *,PREDTRT0/PREDTRT1 AS PREDTRT
    FROM PREDTRT1(KEEP=PATSC VIS PREDTRT1)
         NATURAL FULL JOIN
         PREDTRT0(KEEP=PATSC VIS PREDTRT0)
    ORDER PATSC,VIS
  ;
  /*ratio of probabilities for censoring*/
  CREATE TABLE PREDCEN AS
    SELECT *,PREDCEN0/PREDCEN1 AS PREDCEN
    FROM (SELECT INPUT(PATSC,BEST.) AS PATSC, INPUT(VIS,BEST.) AS VIS,
PREDCEN0 FROM PREDCEN0)
         NATURAL FULL JOIN
         (SELECT INPUT(PATSC,BEST.) AS PATSC, INPUT(VIS,BEST.) AS VIS,
PREDCEN1 FROM PREDCEN1)
    ORDER PATSC,VIS;
QUIT;

/*calculate stabilized weight*/
PROC SORT DATA=INPDS OUT=WEIGHTS;
  BY PATSC VIS;
RUN;

DATA WEIGHTS;
  MERGE WEIGHTS PREDTRT PREDCEN;
  BY PATSC VIS;
  VWT=PREDTRT*PREDCEN;
  IF FIRST.PATSC THEN STABWT=VWT;
                 ELSE STABWT=VWT*DUM;
  RETAIN DUM;
  DROP DUM;
  DUM=STABWT;
RUN;

/*diagnostic plot for weights*/
DATA GRPH;
  SET WEIGHTS; /*assignment of months to visits is study-specific*/
  IF VIS = 3 THEN MONTH = 0.5;
  IF VIS = 4 THEN MONTH = 2;
  IF VIS = 5 THEN MONTH = 5;
  IF VIS = 6 THEN MONTH = 8;
  IF VIS = 7 THEN MONTH = 12;

  IF MONTH = 0.5 THEN DELETE; /*simplify plot by focusing on months
     with greater switching and thus greatest variability in weights */
RUN;

PROC SORT DATA = GRPH;
  BY MONTH;
RUN;
```

```
ODS RTF FILE="%SYSFUNC(PATHNAME(WORK))\FIG1.RTF";

FILENAME FIGURE "%SYSFUNC(PATHNAME(WORK))\SASGRAPH.EMF";

GOPTIONS RESET=ALL TARGET=SASEMF DEVICE=SASEMF FTEXT=DUPLEX HTEXT=.75
   CBACK=WHITE XMAX=6IN XPIXELS=1200 YMAX=5IN YPIXELS=1000
   GSFNAME=FIGURE GSFMODE=REPLACE;

SYMBOL1 COLOR=BLACK INTERPOL=JOIN
        WIDTH=2 VALUE=SQUARE
        HEIGHT=1;

AXIS1 MINOR = NONE COLOR = BLACK LABEL=("STABILIZED WEIGHT" ANGLE=90
ROTATE=0);

PROC BOXPLOT DATA=GRPH;
  PLOT STABWT*MONTH / CFRAME = WHITE
                      CBOXES = DAGR
                      CBOXFILL = WHITE
                      VAXIS = AXIS1;
  TITLE "SUMMARY OF VISITWISE WEIGHT VALUES";
  TITLE2 "(box and whiskers: min, 1st quartile, median, 3rd quartile, max;
square: mean)";
RUN;

GOPTIONS RESET=ALL;

ODS RTF CLOSE;
```

Output from Program 9.2

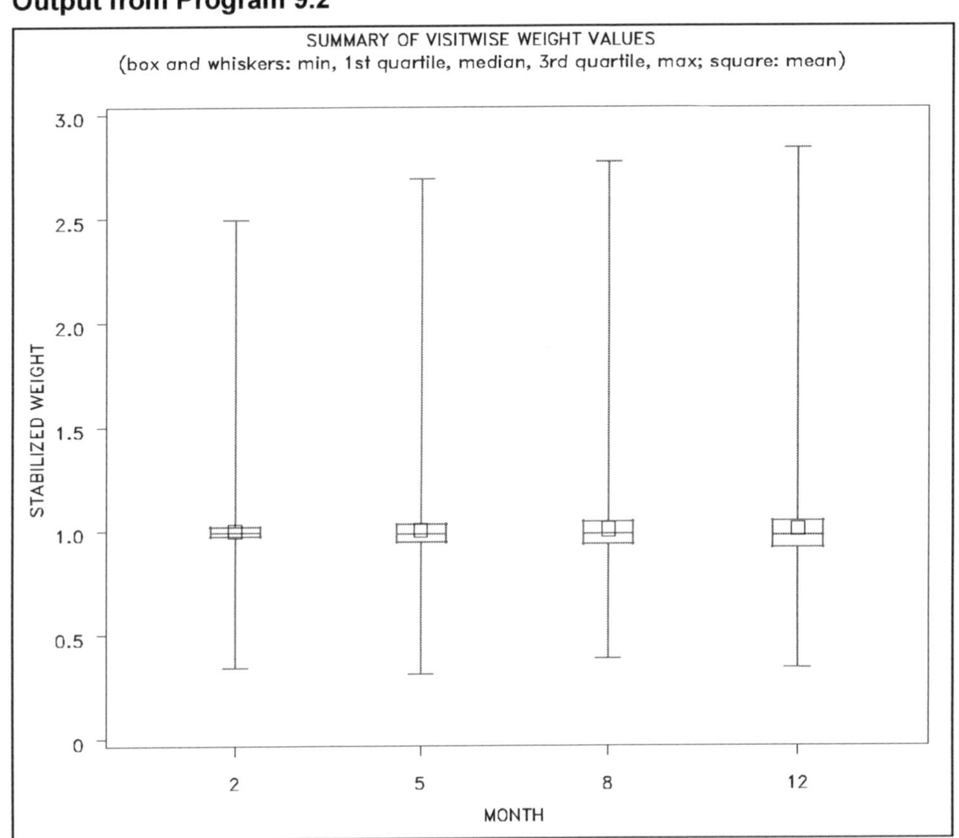

9.3.2.3 Treatment Effectiveness Analysis Model

The final step of the MSM analysis is to estimate causal treatment effects using a weighted repeated measures model with generalized estimating equations (PROC GENMOD—see Program 9.3) and an exchangeable correlation matrix. Change from baseline BPRS total score was the dependent measure in the analysis model. Independent variables for the analysis model were investigational site, age, gender, race, baseline BPRS, visit, time-varying treatment, and the treatment-by-visit interaction. The WEIGHT statement in PROC GENMOD incorporates the inverse probability weighting, which allows for the causal treatment effect estimates. The ESTIMATE statement utilized in PROC GENMOD pooled individual treatments together and produced estimated mean group differences for pooled groups (as opposed to comparing individual treatment groups). This portion of the code is not necessary for many applications. Output from Program 9.3 displays a summary of the final model results and a figure displaying the least squares means at each visit. Results showed a statistically significant treatment difference favoring the treatment group (pooled treatments A and B) relative to the control group, with an estimated average treatment difference in BPRS changes of 1.8 [0.4, 3.2], p=.015 across the 1-year period. Though treatment differences grew numerically over time, the treatment-by-visit interaction term was not statistically significant (p=.158).

Program 9.3 Running Final Analysis Model

```
/* This section of code runs the final analysis model using a weighted
repeated measures approach. The results are presented graphically using
PROC GPLOT.*/

/*final analysis model*/
PROC GENMOD DATA = WEIGHTS;
  CLASS VIS PATSC GENDER ORIGIN2 INVSC TRT;
  WEIGHT STABWT;
  MODEL CAVAR = INVSC BAVAR VIS AGEYRS GENDER ORIGIN2 TRT VIS*TRT
              / DIST=NORMAL LINK=ID TYPE3;
  REPEATED SUBJECT = PATSC / TYPE=EXCH;
  LSMEANS TRT VIS*TRT / PDIFF;
  TITLE 'MSM FINAL ANALYSIS MODEL';
  ESTIMATE 'A+B VS C'
    TRT 0 .5 .5 -1 0;
  ESTIMATE 'A+B VS C AT VIS 3'
    TRT 0 .5 .5 -1 0
    VIS*TRT 0 .5 .5 -1 0     0 0 0 0 0     0 0 0 0 0
            0  0  0  0 0     0 0 0 0 0;
  ESTIMATE 'A+B VS C AT VIS 4'
    TRT 0 .5 .5 -1 0
    VIS*TRT 0 0 0 0 0           0 .5 .5 -1 0       0 0 0 0 0
            0 0 0 0 0           0  0  0  0 0;
  ESTIMATE 'A+B VS C AT VIS 5'
    TRT 0 .5 .5 -1 0
    VIS*TRT 0 0 0 0 0           0 0 0 0 0         0 .5 .5 -1 0
            0 0 0 0 0           0 0 0 0 0;
  ESTIMATE 'A+B VS C AT VIS 6'
    TRT 0 .5 .5 -1 0
    VIS*TRT 0 0 0 0 0           0 0 0 0 0         0 0 0 0 0
            0 .5 .5 -1 0   0 0 0 0 0;
  ESTIMATE 'A+B VS C AT VIS 7'
    TRT 0 .5 .5 -1 0
    VIS*TRT 0 0 0 0 0           0 0 0 0 0         0 0 0 0 0
            0 0 0 0 0           0 .5 .5 -1 0;
  ODS OUTPUT LSMEANS=LSMEANS;
RUN;
```

```
/*LS means plot for the final model*/
DATA LSMEANS2;
  SET LSMEANS;
  WHERE TRT IN ('A__','_B_','__C');
  IF TRT IN ('A__','_B_') THEN TRT2='A+B';
                           ELSE TRT2='C  ';
RUN;

PROC SQL;
  CREATE TABLE LSMEANS3 AS
    SELECT TRT2 AS TRT, VIS, MEAN(ESTIMATE) AS ESTIMATE
    FROM LSMEANS2
    GROUP TRT2, VIS;
QUIT;

ODS RTF FILE="%SYSFUNC(PATHNAME(WORK))\FIG2.RTF";

FILENAME FIGURE "%SYSFUNC(PATHNAME(WORK))\SASGRAPH.EMF";

GOPTIONS RESET=ALL TARGET=SASEMF DEVICE=SASEMF FTEXT=DUPLEX HTEXT=.75
CBACK=WHITE
         XMAX=6IN XPIXELS=1200 YMAX=5IN YPIXELS=1000 GSFNAME=FIGURE
GSFMODE=REPLACE;

AXIS1 MINOR = NONE COLOR = BLACK LABEL=(ANGLE=90 ROTATE=0 "CHANGE IN BPRS
TOTAL SCORE");

SYMBOL1 I=JOIN W=2 L=1 C=RED   V=SQUARE;
SYMBOL2 I=JOIN W=2 L=2 C=BLACK V=CIRCLE;

PROC GPLOT DATA=LSMEANS3;
  PLOT ESTIMATE*VIS=TRT/VAXIS=AXIS1;
  TITLE "MSM ESTIMATED MEAN CHANGE FROM BASELINE BPRS SCORES";
  LABEL VIS="VISIT";
  LABEL TRT="TREATMENT";
RUN;

GOPTIONS RESET=ALL;

ODS RTF CLOSE;
```

Output from Program 9.3

MSM FINAL ANALYSIS MODEL
Score Statistics For Type 3 GEE Analysis

Source	DF	Chi-Square	Pr > ChiSq
INVSC	19	84.25	<.0001
BAVAR	1	71.12	<.0001
VIS	4	37.69	<.0001
AGEYRS	1	0.80	0.3725
GENDER	1	0.09	0.7624
ORIGIN2	2	0.86	0.6500
TRT	4	11.70	0.0197
VIS*TRT	16	21.57	0.1576

Contrast Estimate Results

Label	Estimate	Standard Error	Alpha	Confidence Limits		Chi-Square	Pr > ChiSq
A+B VS C	-1.7852	0.7321	0.05	-3.2201	-0.3504	5.95	0.0147
A+B VS C AT VIS 3	-0.7336	0.9615	0.05	-2.6181	1.1509	0.58	0.4455
A+B VS C AT VIS 4	-1.1225	0.9417	0.05	-2.9682	0.7232	1.42	0.2333
A+B VS C AT VIS 5	-1.7746	1.2532	0.05	-4.2307	0.6815	2.01	0.1567
A+B VS C AT VIS 6	-2.1785	1.2752	0.05	-4.6778	0.3208	2.92	0.0876
A+B VS C AT VIS 7	-3.1169	1.3185	0.05	-5.7012	-0.5327	5.59	0.0181

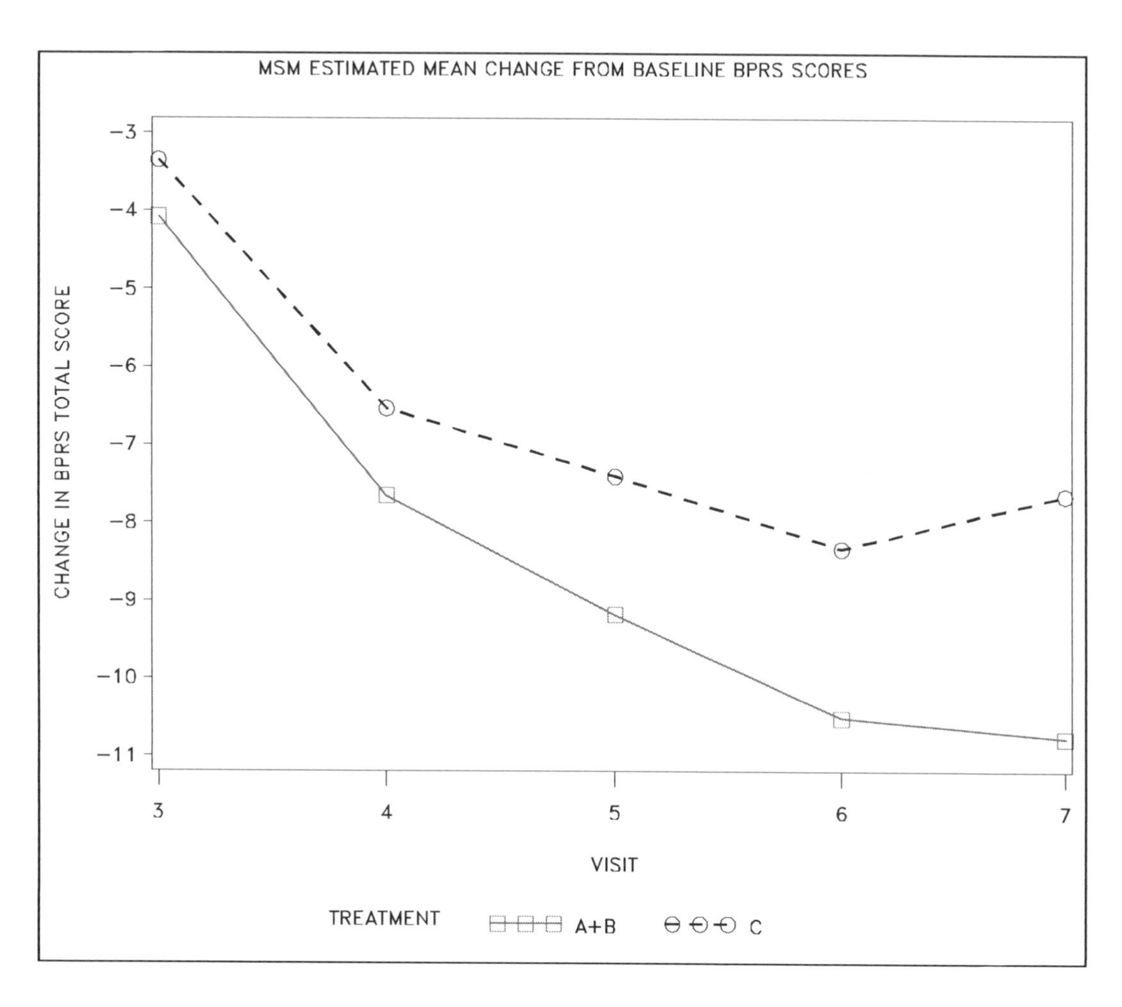

9.3.2.4 Sensitivity Analysis

To assess the robustness of the findings, one should evaluate the plausibility of the three main assumptions for causality (no unmeasured confounding, positivity, correct model) as well as implementing other statistical methods that are based on different assumptions. Regarding the unmeasured confounding assumption, effort was made to collect and incorporate information from experts and the literature on potential confounders prior to the analysis. The variables included in the model were selected in order to cover the domains of symptom severity, functioning, tolerability, and resource use burden. To assess the potential impact of unmeasured confounding on the results, we implemented a simple, unmeasured confounding function (we chose a constant function alpha) based on Brumback and colleagues (2004). Using this function, a missing confounder resulting in a shift of 0.45 (in BPRS total score) in potential outcomes on the BPRS scale favoring patients with high probability of being in the treatment group would result in a loss of the statistically significant finding. In other words, our finding of a significant difference between groups depends upon the assumption that such a confounder (or a group of confounders combining to have the same effect) does not exist. Multiple constants were evaluated using the ALPHA=c statement in the SAS code (see Program 9.4). The value of 0.45 was retained because this was the smallest value producing a p-value of approximately 0.05. While it is challenging to interpret the implications of a particular alpha, such an effect (<1 point on BPRS) does not appear to be extremely large, and the existence of such a confounder is certainly possible in an actual application. However, it is greater than the observed confounding (the difference between unweighted and weighted analyses) of 0.29 in the opposite direction observed in this study. Regardless of the sensitivity analysis results, one can simply not dismiss the possibility of unaccounted for factors that would result in this analysis failing to produce an estimate of a causal treatment effect. Thus, one must view the results with some caution. Different sensitivity functions can easily be tested using the provided SAS code by altering the calculation of the variables CAVAR_SENS and SAPT.

Program 9.4 Finding Level of Confounding That Would Eliminate Treatment Difference

```
/* This section of code examines the sensitivity of the results to
unmeasured confounding by finding the level of confounding that would
eliminate the observed treatment difference.*/

/*sensitivity analysis per Brumback et al. (2004) - constant
function alpha is used*/
DATA WEIGHTSS;
  SET WEIGHTS;
  BY PATSC VIS;
  IF TRT IN ('A  ',' B ') THEN SNSTRT = 1;
                          ELSE SNSTRT = -1;
  SAVT = -SNSTRT*(1 - PREDTRT1);
  IF FIRST.PATSC THEN SAPT = SAVT;
                 ELSE SAPT = SAVT + DUM;
  RETAIN DUM;
  DROP DUM;
  DUM=SAPT;
  ALPHA = 0.45;
  CAVAR_SENS = CAVAR - ALPHA*SAPT;
RUN;

PROC GENMOD DATA = WEIGHTSS;
  CLASS VIS PATSC GENDER ORIGIN2 INVSC TRT;
  WEIGHT STABWT;
  MODEL CAVAR_SENS = INVSC BAVAR VIS AGEYRS GENDER ORIGIN2 TRT VIS*TRT
              / DIST=NORMAL LINK=ID TYPE3;
  REPEATED SUBJECT = PATSC / TYPE=EXCH;
  LSMEANS TRT VIS*TRT / PDIFF;
  TITLE 'MSM SENSITIVITY ANALYSIS: ALPHA = 0.45';
```

```
    ESTIMATE 'A+B VS C'
      TRT 0 .5 .5 -1 0;
    ESTIMATE 'A+B VS C AT VIS 3'
      TRT 0 .5 .5 -1 0
      VIS*TRT 0 .5 .5 -1 0      0 0 0 0 0     0 0 0 0 0
              0  0  0  0 0      0 0 0 0 0;
    ESTIMATE 'A+B VS C AT VIS 4'
      TRT 0 .5 .5 -1 0
      VIS*TRT 0 0 0 0 0         0 .5 .5 -1 0      0 0 0 0 0
              0 0 0 0 0         0  0  0  0 0;
    ESTIMATE 'A+B VS C AT VIS 5'
      TRT 0 .5 .5 -1 0
      VIS*TRT 0 0 0 0 0         0 0 0 0 0         0 .5 .5 -1 0
              0 0 0 0 0         0 0 0 0 0;
    ESTIMATE 'A+B VS C AT VIS 6'
      TRT 0 .5 .5 -1 0
      VIS*TRT 0 0 0 0 0         0 0 0 0 0         0 0 0 0 0
              0 .5 .5 -1 0      0 0 0 0 0;
    ESTIMATE 'A+B VS C AT VIS 7'
      TRT 0 .5 .5 -1 0
      VIS*TRT 0 0 0 0 0         0 0 0 0 0         0 0 0 0 0
              0 0 0 0 0         0 .5 .5 -1 0;
  RUN;
```

Output from Program 9.4

MSM SENSITIVITY ANALYSIS: ALPHA = 0.45

Contrast Estimate Results

Label	Estimate	Standard Error	Alpha	Confidence Limits		Chi-Square	Pr > ChiSq
A+B VS C	-1.3911	0.7303	0.05	-2.8224	0.0402	3.63	0.0568
A+B VS C AT VIS 3	-0.6203	0.9615	0.05	-2.5048	1.2642	0.42	0.5188
A+B VS C AT VIS 4	-0.8879	0.9417	0.05	-2.7335	0.9577	0.89	0.3457
A+B VS C AT VIS 5	-1.3184	1.2534	0.05	-3.7750	1.1383	1.11	0.292
A+B VS C AT VIS 6	-1.6479	1.2726	0.05	-4.1422	0.8464	1.68	0.1954
A+B VS C AT VIS 7	-2.4810	1.3143	0.05	-5.0569	0.0950	3.56	0.0591

To assess the positivity assumption, we followed the ideas of Mortimer and colleagues (2005) and estimated the probability of selection of each of the five treatment possibilities using all possible covariates across all study visits. The CATMOD procedure is used here in order to generate predicted probabilities for all possible treatment options. While theoretically there were no issues with the positivity assumption in this study (all patients had the opportunity of being switched from and to any combination of treatments at any time), the goal was to assess whether any observed set of covariates produced a predicted probability of 0 or 1 for this set of data. This was done as shown with Program 9.5 where we computed the predicted probabilities of treatment for each observed set of covariates and then summarized the predicted probabilities (summary statistics using PROC MEANS by treatment). We observed that the smallest (nonzero but <.00015) probabilities were for the theoretical switch from no treatment to the combination of treatments A and C at earlier study visits. In general, the smaller probabilities were associated with the no treatment and combination treatment groups—as would be expected given their observed frequencies. Sensitivity analyses were then performed without the more extreme records and then with combination patients re-assigned to the initial randomized single treatment (for example, a patient randomized to treatment A but treated with A and C would be counted as being treated only with treatment A). No major changes in the inferences were observed from these sensitivity analyses and these results are not shown.

Program 9.5 Examining Positivity Assumption for Causal Inference

```
/* This section of code examines the positivity assumption for causal
inference by examining the predicted values of all possible treatment
changes. Summary statistics are presented as well as a listing to allow
examination of outliers.*/

/*positivity check Mortimer (2005) - generate predicted probabilities*/
ODS LISTING CLOSE;
PROC CATMOD DATA = INPDS;
  DIRECT AGEYRS BGAF BBPRS PR1BPRS PR1GAFC;
  MODEL TRT = VIS THERAPY PR1TRTA PR1TRTB PR1TRTC GENDER ORIGIN2 BHOSP
           BEVNT AGEYRS BGAF BBPRS PR1EVNT PR1HOSP PR1BPRS PR1GAFC
                 /PRED=PROB;
  ODS OUTPUT PREDICTEDPROBS=PREDTRT1POS(KEEP=VIS TRT THERAPY PR1TRTA
             PR1TRTB PR1TRTC GENDER ORIGIN2 BHOSP BEVNT AGEYRS BGAF
          BBPRS PR1EVNT PR1HOSP PR1BPRS PR1GAFC
             SAMPLE OBSFUNCTION PREDFUNCTION
              RENAME=(PREDFUNCTION=PREDTRT1));
RUN;
ODS LISTING;

ODS RTF FILE="%SYSFUNC(PATHNAME(WORK))\FIG3.RTF";

FILENAME FIGURE "%SYSFUNC(PATHNAME(WORK))\SASGRAPH.EMF";

GOPTIONS RESET=ALL TARGET=SASEMF DEVICE=SASEMF FTEXT=DUPLEX HTEXT=.75
         CBACK=WHITE XMAX=6IN XPIXELS=1200 YMAX=5IN YPIXELS=1000
GSFNAME=FIGURE GSFMODE=REPLACE;

PROC UNIVARIATE DATA = PREDTRT1POS;
  VAR PREDTRT1;
  HISTOGRAM;
  PROBPLOT;
  TITLE 'SUMMARY STATS ON PREDICTED VALUES';
RUN;

GOPTIONS RESET=ALL;

ODS RTF CLOSE;

PROC MEANS DATA = PREDTRT1POS;
  CLASS TRT;
  VAR PREDTRT1;
  TITLE 'Positivity Check: Summary Stats on Predicted Values by Observed
Treatment';
RUN;

PROC SORT DATA = PREDTRT1POS;
  BY PREDTRT1;
RUN;

PROC PRINT DATA = PREDTRT1POS;
  TITLE 'Positivity Check: Sorted Listing of Predicted Values';
RUN;

   * (PROC PRINT output not shown but is used to identify individual
patients with combinations of covariates with extreme values *;
```

Output from Program 9.5

Positivity Check: Summary Stats on Predicted Values by Observed Treatment

The MEANS Procedure

Analysis Variable : PREDTRT1 Predicted: Probability

TRT	N Obs	N	Mean	Std Dev	Minimum	Maximum
A_C	2547	2547	0.0475067	0.1254780	0	0.9758886
A__	2547	2547	0.4157827	0.4165088	4.0755123E-7	0.9999826
_B_	2547	2547	0.2508929	0.3999598	1.8471036E-8	0.9999993
__C	2547	2547	0.2383188	0.3699969	3.4082211E-7	0.9998542
___	2547	2547	0.0474988	0.1179316	0	0.9817690

In addition to the assessment of the no unmeasured confounders and positivity assumptions, the appropriateness of the models was assessed by adding interactions, quadratic terms, and other potential confounder variables to the models. No significant changes to the outcome were noted. The model assessment was done by adjusting the appropriate models in the SAS code—which could be automated by putting the model variables as macro variables at the top of the code. In addition, we analyzed the data using other methods: an ITT LOCF analysis (using all data), a repeated measures model (excluding data after a medication switch) and an epoch analysis (see Chapter 8). Analysis of these simulated data using a simple ITT LOCF analysis failed to show a significant difference between treated and control groups (estimated difference of 1.16, p=.334). The repeated measures mixed model (discarding the data after switching) and epoch analyses results were fairly similar to the MSM approach. The disagreement between the ITT analysis and other analyses appears to be a result of ignoring treatment information for the data after a treatment switch, as discussed by Faries and colleagues (2007). Switchers from treatment C performed well after the switch to treatments A and B, information not attributed to treatments A and B in the ITT analysis.

9.4 Discussion

This chapter has presented the issue of assessing the effects of treatment in longitudinal, observational data—with a focus on addressing treatment switching using MSM. We were interested in the performance of MSM because this approach utilizes all of the study data and produces consistent estimates of the causal effect of treatments, even when there are treatment switching, missing data, and time-varying confounders. Validity of the MSM analysis rests on three key assumptions:

1. no unmeasured confounding
2. positivity
3. correct models

Also, the missing data are assumed to follow a missing completely at random (MCAR) or missing at random (MAR) pattern. Thus, well-planned sensitivity analyses are important. This should include an assessment of the assumptions supporting the causal effect estimation by the MSM as well as use of other methodology supported by differing assumptions. In addition, presentation of results should make it clear to the reader that causal interpretation of the results rests on unverifiable assumptions as well as being transparent about which steps were taken to assess the robustness of the results.

In summary, marginal structural models are a promising approach for estimating the causal effects of treatment in longitudinal, observational data. Other chapters in this book provide details on alternative methodologies.

References

Bodnar, L. M., M. Davidian, A. M. Siega-Riz, A. A. Tsiatis. 2004. "Marginal structural models for analyzing causal effects of time-dependent treatments: an application in perinatal epidemiology." *American Journal of Epidemiology*. 159: 926–934.

Brumback, B. A., M. A. Hernán, S. J. Haneuse, and J. M. Robins. 2004. "Sensitivity analyses for unmeasured confounding assuming a marginal structural model for repeated measures." *Statistics in Medicine* 23(5): 749–767.

Cole, S. R., M. A. Hernán, J. B. Margolick, M. H. Cohen, and J. M. Robins. 2005. "Marginal structural models for estimating the effect of highly active antiretroviral therapy initiation on CD4 cell count." *American Journal of Epidemiology* 162: 471–478. Epub 2005 Aug 2.

Faries, D., H. Ascher-Svanum, and M. Belger. 2007. "Analysis of treatment effectiveness in longitudinal observational data." *Journal of Biopharmaceutical Statistics* 17(5): 809–826.

Grimes, D. A., and K. F. Schulz. 2002. "Bias and causal associations in observational research." The *Lancet* 359: 248–252.

Haro, J. M., S. Kontodimas, M. A. Negrin, M. Ratcliffe, D. Suarez, and F. Windmeijer. 2006. "Methodological aspects in the assessment of treatment effects in observational health outcomes studies." *Applied Health Economics & Health Policy* 5(1): 11–25.

Hernán, M. A., B. Brumback, and J. M. Robins. 2000. "Marginal structural models to estimate the causal effect of zidovudine on the survival of HIV-positive men." *Epidemiology* 11: 561–570.

Hernán, M. A., B. Brumback, and J. M. Robins. 2002. "Estimating the causal effect of zidovudine on CD4 count with a marginal structural model for repeated measures." *Statistics in Medicine* 21: 1689–1709.

Hernán, M. A., J. M. Robins, and L. A. Garcia Rodrigues. 2005. Comment on: Prentice, R. L., M. Pettinger, and G. L. Anderson. Discussion on "Statistical issues arising in the women's health initiative." *Biometrics* 61: 922–941.

Hernán, M. A., S. Hernández-Díaz, and J. M. Robins. 2004. "A structural approach to selection bias." *Epidemiology* 15(5): 615–625.

Ko, H., J. W. Hogan, and K. H. Mayer. 2003. "Estimating causal treatment effects from longitudinal HIV natural history studies using marginal structural models." *Biometrics* 59: 152–162.

Mallinckrodt, C. H., T. M. Sanger, S. Dubé, D. J. DeBrota, G. Molenberghs, R. J. Carroll, W. Z. Potter, and G. D. Tollefson. 2003. "Assessing and interpreting treatment effects in longitudinal clinical trials with missing data." *Biological Psychiatry* 53(8): 754–760.

Mortimer, K. M., R. Neugebauer, M. van der Laan, and I. B. Tager. 2005. "An application of model-fitting procedures for marginal structural models." *American Journal of Epidemiology* 162(4): 382–388. Epub 2005 Jul 13.

Petersen, M. L., S. G. Deeks, J. N. Martin, M. J. van der Laan. 2007. "History-adjusted marginal structural models for estimating time-varying effect modification. *American Journal of Epidemiology* 166: 985–993.

Robins, J. M., A. Rotnitzky, and D. O. Scharfstein. 1999. *Statistical Models in Epidemiology: The Environment and Clinical Trials.* Edited by M.E. Halloran and D. Berry. IMA Volume 116. New York: Springer-Verlag, 1–92.

Robins, J. M., M. A. Hernán, and B. Brumback. 2000. "Marginal structural models and causal inference in epidemiology." *Epidemiology* 11: 550–560.

Rosenbaum, P. R. 2005. "Observational Study." In *Encyclopedia of Statistics in Behavioral Science* 3: 1451–1462. Edited by B. S. Everitt and D. C. Howell. Chichester: John Wiley & Sons, Ltd.

Rosenbaum, P., and D. B. Rubin. 1983. "The central role of the propensity score in observational studies for causal effects." *Biometrika* 70: 41–55.

Suarez, D., J. M. Haro, D. Novick, S. Ochoa. 2008. "Marginal structural models might overcome confounding when analyzing multiple treatment effects in observational studies." Journal of Clinical Epidemiology 61: 525–530.

Tunis, S. L., D. E. Faries, A. W. Nyhuis, B. J. Kinon, H. Ascher-Svanum, and R. Aquila. 2006. "Cost-effectiveness of olanzapine as first-line treatment for schizophrenia: results from a randomized, open-label, 1-year trial." *Value in Health* 9(2): 77–89.

Vansteelandt, S., K. Mertens, C. Suetens, E. Goetghebauer. 2009. "Marginal structural models for partial exposure regimes. *Biostatistics* 10(1): 46–59.

Verbeke, G., and G. Molenberghs. 2000. *Linear Mixed Models for Longitudinal Data*. New York: Springer-Verlag.

Yamaguchi, T., and Y. Ohashi. 2004a. "Adjusting for differential proportions of second-line treatment in cancer clinical trials. Part I: structural nested models and marginal structural models to test and estimate treatment arm effects." *Statistics in Medicine* 23: 1991–2003.

Yamaguchi, T., and Y. Ohashi. 2004b. "Adjusting for differential proportions of second-line treatment in cancer clinical trials. Part II: an application in a clinical trial of unresectable non-small-cell lung cancer." *Statistics in Medicine* 23: 2005–2022.

Chapter 10

Structural Nested Models

Daniel Almirall
Cynthia J. Coffman
Will S. Yancy, Jr.
Susan A. Murphy

Abstract

This chapter reviews Robins' Structural Nested Mean Model (SNMM) for assessing the effect of predictors that vary over time. The SNMM is used to study the effects of time-varying predictors (or treatments) in the presence of time-varying covariates that are moderators of these effects. We describe a SAS implementation of a maximum likelihood (ML) estimator of the parameters of an SNMM using PROC NLP. The proposed ML estimator requires correct model specification of the distribution of the primary outcome given the history of time-varying moderators and predictors, including proper specification of both the causal and non-causal portions of the SNMM. The estimator also relies on correct model specification of the observed data distribution of the putative time-varying moderators given the past. We illustrate the methodology and SAS implementation using data from a weight loss study. In the empirical example, we assess the impact of early versus later weight loss (or gain) on end-of-study health-related quality of life as a function of prior weight loss and time-varying covariates thought to be moderators of these effects.

10.1 Introduction

Longitudinal randomized trials are now commonplace in clinical research. This, together with the growing number of health-outcomes databases and improved access to medical records for research purposes, has given rise to an abundance of data sets in which patients contribute measures on a large number of variables repeatedly over time. This wealth of longitudinal data, in turn, has allowed researchers to examine more varied and detailed scientific questions concerning, for example, the etiology of diseases or the different causal pathways through which behavioral and other medical interventions produce positive health effects. Due to the ample availability of longitudinal data, these questions often involve time-varying predictors or treatments of interest (in addition to possibly longitudinal outcomes). Because the primary time-varying predictors (or treatments) of interest—that is, the primary independent or right-hand side variables of interest—often are not (or, as in the case of this chapter's motivating example, cannot be) randomized or directly manipulated by experimentation, empirical longitudinal studies of this sort are often termed *observational studies*.

The methodology we discuss in this chapter focuses on a particular type of question involving time-varying predictors (or treatments). Specifically, we are interested in conceptualizing and estimating scientific questions concerning time-varying causal effect moderation (Petersen et al., 2007; Almirall et al., 2009).

To illustrate, informally, what we mean by time-varying effect moderation, consider a simplification of our motivating example (described in more detail in Section 10.4) in which repeated measures of body weight (Z_j) and a dichotomous time-varying covariate (X_j), exercise (yes/no), are available at multiple time points j ($j = 0,1,2,...,T$) over the course of a study. We define measures of body weight change between successive time points as $D_j = Z_j - Z_{j-1}$ ($j=1, 2,..., T$). Suppose our outcome is a health-related quality of life measure (QOL = Y), available at the end of study (at or after time T). Using these data, at each time point j we are interested in asking how the impact of weight loss or weight gain (D_j) on end-of-study health-related quality of life (Y) differs as a function of the history of exercise through time $j-1$. In other words, we are interested in the effect of D_j on Y as a function of $(X_0, X_1, ..., X_{j-1})$. Thus, by time-varying causal effect moderation we refer to the way in which the time-varying covariate exercise moderates (changes, tempers, or modifies) the causal effects of the time-varying predictor weight loss or weight gain on end-of-study health-related quality of life (HRQOL).

In our motivating example, identifying and understanding time-varying moderators of the effect of weight change on health-related quality of life is important because it enhances our understanding of the causal pathways by which weight loss (or gain) leads to improved (or decreased) health-related quality of life. The process also can help us to better appreciate the relationship among the outcome (HRQOL), time-varying moderators (for example, exercise), and factors that do not vary with time but may moderate both the outcome and the time-varying moderators. Examples of these factors include patient characteristics (for example, demographics, medical diagnoses) and weight loss intervention type (for example, diet composition, weight loss medication, bariatric surgery) or structure (for example, visit frequency, individual vs. group sessions). This specified knowledge can be used to corroborate old hypotheses or to generate new ideas about the relationships among weight loss, health-related quality of life, and time-varying moderators of both weight loss and HRQOL, including exercise or adherence to the intervention. This additional knowledge, in turn, may help clinicians predict the positive health effects of weight loss given current knowledge about a patient's exercise behavior and/or adherence to diet. It may also serve as a guide that behavioral scientists can use to help develop future interventions for weight loss or body weight management.

In linear regression models, effect moderation (or effect modification) is typically associated with interaction terms between the primary predictor variable and the covariate (or putative moderator) of interest. For example, in the point-predictor setting in which the primary predictor D, weight change, and the covariate of interest, X, do not vary over time, the following regression model could be used to study effect moderation:

$$E(Y \mid X, D) = \gamma_0 + \gamma_1 X + \gamma_2 D + \gamma_3 DX \quad (1)$$

In this model, the cross-product term quantifies the extent to which the impact of D on Y varies according to levels of X. That is, a one-unit increase in weight change corresponds to a $\gamma_2 + \gamma_3 X$ unit change in health-related quality of life at the end of the study, which differs by the levels of X, exercise (yes/no). Thus, in this model, $\gamma_3 = 0$ is evidence that there is no effect moderation by X, or exercise level.

Unfortunately, this regression modeling strategy does not translate straightforwardly to the time-varying setting. Consider the following extended model for the time-varying setting where $T = 2$:

$$E(Y \mid X_0, D_1, X_1, D_2) = \gamma_0 + \gamma_1 X_0 + \gamma_2 D_1 + \gamma_3 D_1 X_0 + \gamma_4 X_1 + \gamma_5 D_2 + \gamma_6 D_2 X_1 + \gamma_7 D_2 X_0 + \gamma_8 X_0 X_1 \quad (2)$$

In this model, X_0 is exercise level prior to baseline ($j=0$), X_1 is exercise level between time $j=0$ and time $j=1$, D_1 is weight change between baseline ($j=0$) and time $j=1$, and D_2 is weight change between time $j=1$ and time $j=2$. Even if (2) is the correct model (that is, the correct functional form) for the conditional expectation (association) of Y given (X_0, D_1, X_1, D_2), the parameters associated with the D_1 and the D_1X_0 cross-product terms may not necessarily represent the conditional causal effect of weight change D_1 on end-of-study quality of life Y within levels of exercise X_0. That is, the function $\gamma_2 + \gamma_3 X_0$ may or may not represent the true conditional causal effect of unit changes in weight change (between baseline and $j = 1$) on end-of-study quality of life.

The problem with naively extending the cross-product modeling strategy to the time-varying setting, as in (2), is that it is not clear what causal effects, if any, the coefficients of D_1 and D_1X_0 in (2) are measuring. The main source of the problem (for causal inference) is that model (2) conditions on X_1 (exercise level between time $j=0$ and $j=1$), which is likely affected by D_1, weight loss or weight gain between time $j=0$ and time $j=1$ (Robins, 1987, 1989, 1994, 1997, 1999a; Bray et al., 2006). This has two undesirable consequences. First, naively conditioning on X_1 cuts off any portion of the effect of weight change (D_1) on Y that is transmitted using X_1; that is, the function $\gamma_2 + \gamma_3 X_0$ does not include the effects (including effect moderation by X_0) of D_1 on Y that are mediated (Baron and Kenny, 1986; Kraemer et al., 2001) by X_1. Second, naively conditioning on X_1 introduces bias in the coefficients (γ_2, γ_3) due to nuisance associations between X_1 and Y that are not on the causal pathway between D_1 and Y. These include nuisance associations due to variables that are related to both X_1 and Y. Thus, while the scientist wishes to condition on the time-varying covariate X because of interest in X's role as a time-varying moderator of the effect of time-varying D on Y, doing so in the traditional way (that is, using standard regression adjustment) is not suitable because of the potential for bias.

Robins' Structural Nested Mean Model (1994) overcomes these problems by clearly specifying the causal and non-causal portions of the conditional mean of Y given the past (the history of weight change and time-varying moderators). The SNMM clarifies the meaning of causal effect moderation when both primary predictors of interest and putative moderators are time varying. The SNMM serves as a guide for properly incorporating potential time-varying moderators in the linear regression.

In Section 10.2 we define, more formally, what is meant by time-varying effect moderation in the context of a causal model for the conditional mean of the outcome given the past (that is, using Robins' SNMM). In Section 10.3 we describe a maximum likelihood (ML) estimator of parameters of the SNMM. In Section 10.4, we demonstrate a SAS PROC NLP implementation of the ML estimator using real data from a weight loss study. In the empirical example, we assess the impact of early versus later weight loss (or gain) on end-of-study vitality (a health-related quality of life measure) as a function of prior weight loss and time-varying covariates (exercise, diet adherence, and prior vitality scores) thought to be moderators of these effects.

10.2 Time-Varying Causal Effect Moderation

10.2.1 Notation

We rely on the potential outcomes notation to define the causal parameters of interest (Rubin, 1974; Holland, 1986, 1990). As described briefly in the introduction, we consider the following general temporal data structure:

$$(X_0, d_1, X_1(d_1), d_2, \ldots, X_{T-1}(d_1, d_2, \ldots, d_{T-1}), \; d_T, \; Y(d_1, d_2, \ldots, d_T)). \tag{3}$$

In this notation, d_j ($j = 1, 2, \ldots, T$) is an index for the primary time-varying predictor variable (for example, time-varying weight change) at time j. In our example, d_j is the change in body weight defined as the difference between weight at the current visit (time j) and the previous visit (at time $j-1$). For instance, $(d_1, d_2) = (-3, 0)$ denotes a loss of 3 pounds in body weight between the first and second visits and no change in body weight between the second and third visits. We use lowercase d_j to distinguish it from the observed data predictors, which are random variables, denoted by uppercase D_j (see Section 10.3). $X_j(d_1, d_2, \ldots, d_j)$ ($j = 1,2,\ldots,T-1$), possibly a vector, denotes the time-varying covariate(s) (the putative time-varying moderator(s) of interest) at time j. X_0 may include assignment to a diet type or structure, baseline patient traits, characteristics, or demographics (such as age, race, gender, and income), as well as baseline measures of the time-varying covariates. We impose no restriction on the type of time-varying covariates considered; $X_j(d_1, d_2, \ldots, d_j)$ and X_0 may be continuous or categorical. Finally, $Y(d_1, d_2, \ldots, d_T)$ denotes the potential outcome at the end of the study (that is, occurring after d_T; for example, end-of-study health-related quality of life). In this chapter, we consider only continuous, unbounded outcomes Y. For example, $Y(d_1, d_2, \ldots, d_T)$ is the outcome a patient would have had had they lost (or gained) weight over the course of the study in increments (decrements) of $(d_1, d_2, \ldots, d_T)$. That is, $Y(d_1, d_2, \ldots, d_T)$ describes the end-of-study outcome under a particular trajectory or course of weight loss or gain. Note that in our notation, $X_j(d_1, d_2, \ldots, d_j)$ ($j = 1,2,\ldots,T-1$) are also indexed by d_j because they are potentially affected by prior levels of d_j. That is, they are also conceived as potential outcomes. Indeed, the vector of time-varying covariates may include prior time-varying instances of the primary outcome variable $Y(d_1, d_2, \ldots, d_T)$. For instance, in the context of our motivating example, prior levels of quality of life may also moderate the future impact of weight loss on end-of-study quality of life.

We use the underscore notation as short-hand to denote the history of a variable or index, as follows:

$$\underline{d}_j = (d_1, d_2, \ldots, d_j);$$
$$\underline{X}_j(\underline{d}_j) = (X_0, X_1(d_1), X_2(\underline{d}_2), \ldots, X_j(\underline{d}_j)); \text{ and}$$
$$Y(\underline{d}_T) = Y(d_1, d_2, \ldots, d_T).$$

In this chapter, we do not consider longitudinal outcomes; we consider only outcomes measured at the end of the study (post-d_T). Therefore, we do not index the outcome $Y(\underline{d}_T)$ by a subscript denoting time. It is possible, however, to extend the methods presented here to handle longitudinal outcomes (Robins, 1994).

10.2.2 Robins' Structural Nested Mean Model

In this subsection, we define our primary causal functions of interest in the context of Robins' SNNM. In general, there are T causal effect functions of interest, one per time point. For simplicity, we present the SNMM in the simple $T = 2$ post-baseline (meaning, post-X_0) time points setting. Thus, we have the following objects to define our causal effects with:

$$(X_0,\ d_1,\ X_1(d_1),\ d_2,\ Y(d_1, d_2)).$$

The first causal effect is denoted by

$$\mu_1(X_0, d_1) = \mathrm{E}(\ Y(d_1,\ 0) - Y(0,\ 0) \mid X_0). \tag{4}$$

$\mu_1(X_0, d_1)$ is the average causal effect of $(d_1, 0)$ versus $(0,0)$ on the outcome conditional on X_0. In the context of our motivating example, $\mu_1(X_0, d_1)$ represents the causal effect on end-of-study health-related quality of life of having lost (or gained) d_1 pounds between the first and second visits to the clinic and no change in weight thereafter ($Y(d_1,\ 0)$) versus no change in weight during the entire study ($Y(0,\ 0)$), as a function of X_0, baseline exercise and/or other demographic characteristics that are a part of X_0.

The second causal effect is defined as

$$\mu_2(\underline{X}_1(d_1), \underline{d}_2) = \mathrm{E}(\ Y(d_1, d_2) - Y(d_1, 0) \mid \underline{X}_1(d_1)), \tag{5}$$

which is the average causal effect of (d_1, d_2) versus $(d_1, 0)$ on the outcome, conditional on both X_0 and $X_1(d_1)$. In the context of our motivating example, $\mu_2(\underline{X}_1(d_1), \underline{d}_2)$ represents the causal effect on end-of-study health-related quality of life of having lost (or gained) d_2 pounds between the second and third visits to the clinic ($Y(d_1, d_2)$) versus no change in weight between the second and third visits to the clinic ($Y(d_1, 0)$) as a function of both X_0 and $X_1(d_1)$, and supposing a change in weight of d_1 between the first and second clinic visits.

In our example, then, $\mu_1(X_0, d_1)$ captures the effect of losing (or gaining) weight early on in the study and not losing any weight thereafter, whereas, $\mu_2(\underline{X}_1(d_1), \underline{d}_2)$ captures the effect of losing (or gaining) weight later on in the study. In addition, by conditioning on the history of time-varying covariates, these functions allow us to model the average effect of losing weight early versus later while taking into account changing patterns in the evolving state of patients in terms of X_j (for example, exercise).

Robins' SNMM is a particular additive decomposition of the conditional mean of $Y(d_1, d_2)$ given $\underline{X}_1(d_1)$ that includes the functions $\mu_1(X_0, d_1)$ and $\mu_2(\underline{X}_1(d_1), \underline{d}_2)$ as part of the decomposition. Specifically, for $T = 2$ the SNMM can be written as follows:

$$\mathrm{E}(\ Y(d_1, d_2) \mid \underline{X}_1(d_1)\ ) = \beta_0 + \varepsilon_1(X_0) + \mu_1(X_0, d_1) + \varepsilon_2(\underline{X}_1(d_1)) + \mu_2(\underline{X}_1(d_1), \underline{d}_2), \tag{6}$$

where β_0 is the intercept equal to $\mathrm{E}(\ Y(0,0)\ )$, which is the mean outcome under no weight gain or loss during the course of the study. The functions $\varepsilon_1(X_0)$ and $\varepsilon_2(\underline{X}_1(d_1))$ are defined to make the right-hand side of (5) equal the conditional mean of $Y(d_1,d_2)$ given $\underline{X}_1(d_1)$. That is, the functions $\varepsilon_1(X_0)$ and $\varepsilon_2(\underline{X}_1(d_1))$ are defined as follows:

$$\varepsilon_1(X_0) = E(\ Y(0,0) \mid X_0) - E(\ Y(0,0)\ ) \qquad (7)$$

$$\varepsilon_2(\underline{X}_1(d_1)) = E(\ Y(d_1,0) \mid \underline{X}_1(d_1)) - E(\ Y(d_1,0) \mid X_0) \qquad (8)$$

We label the functions $\varepsilon_1(X_0)$ and $\varepsilon_2(\underline{X}_1(d_1))$ as *nuisance functions* to distinguish them from our primary causal functions of interest, $\mu_1(X_0, d_1)$ and $\mu_2(\underline{X}_1(d_1), \underline{d}_2)$. They connote both causal and non-causal relationships (associations) between the time-varying moderators and the outcome Y.

The components of the SNMM exhibit two properties, which dictate how we model these quantities:

First, we note that $\mu_j = 0$ whenever $d_j = 0$. (9)

Second, the nuisance functions are mean-zero functions conditional on the past: (10)
$E(\ \varepsilon_j(X_{j-1}(d_{j-1})) \mid X_{j-2}\ ) = 0.$

Thus, in the $T = 2$ *time points setting*, for instance:

a. $E(\ \varepsilon_1(X_0)\ ) = 0$, where the expectation is over the X_0 random variable(s), and
b. $E(\ \varepsilon_2(\underline{X}_1(d_1)) \mid X_0\ ) = 0$,where the expectation is over the $X_1(d_1)$ random variable(s) conditional on X_0.

Property (9) makes sense because causal effects should be 0 when comparing the same course of weight change over time, regardless of covariate history. Property (10) is what makes the SNMM a non-standard regression model because it is a function of conditional mean-zero error terms. Intuitively, $\varepsilon_2(\underline{X}_1(d_1))$ captures the mean association between $Y(d_1,0)$ and having more $(\underline{X}_1(d_1))$ versus less (X_0) covariate information. Property (10) indicates that this information deficit can be expressed as a function of the mean residual information in $X_1(d_1)$ not explained by d_1 and X_0 (which has mean zero). Recognition of the nuisance functions in the model for $E(Y(d_1,d_2) \mid \underline{X}_1(d_1))$ is what makes the SNMM distinct from the standard regression model shown in (2). Further, understanding how to model the nuisance functions properly helps resolve the challenges with the standard regression model (2) that were discussed in the Introduction.

10.3 Estimation

10.3.1 Observed Data and Causal Assumptions

Section 10.2.1 introduced the potential outcomes that were used to define the causal parameters of interest. In this section, we describe the observed data—and their connection to the potential outcomes—which are used to estimate the causal parameters of interest. Let D_j denote the observed value of the primary time-varying predictor of interest at time j; and let $\underline{D}_j = (D_1, D_2, ..., D_j)$ denote the history of the observed time-varying predictor through time j. Let X_j (possibly a vector) denote the observed value of the time-varying covariate (or potential moderator) at time j, and let $\underline{X}_j = (X_1, X_2, ..., X_j)$. Let Y denote the observed end-of-study outcome. The full set of observed data, O, has the following temporal order:

$$O = (X_0,\ D_1,\ X_1,\ D_2, ...,\ X_{T-1},\ D_T,\ Y). \qquad (11)$$

The connection (link) between the potential outcomes in (2) and the observed data in (11) is established by invoking the Consistency Assumption (Robins, 1994) for both the observed time-varying covariates and the observed end-of-study outcome Y. For all subjects in the study, the Consistency Assumption for the end-of-study outcome states that

$$Y = Y(\underline{D}_T), \tag{12}$$

where the right-hand side $Y(\underline{D}_T)$ denotes the potential outcome indexed by values of $\underline{d}_T$ equal to $\underline{D}_T$. Intuitively, this assumption states that the observed outcome Y for a subject that follows the trajectory of observed primary predictor values $\underline{D}_T$ agrees with the potential outcome indexed by the same trajectory of values. Note that the observed potential outcome $Y = Y(\underline{D}_T)$ is just one of many potential outcomes that could have been observed. Similarly, we assume consistency for each of the potential putative time-varying moderators in $\underline{X}_{T-1}(\underline{d}_{T-1})$, to link them up with the observed values $\underline{X}_T$.

In order to estimate the values of μ_j using the observed data, we also assume the No Unmeasured (or Unknown) Confounders Assumption (Robins, 1994):

For every j ($j = 1,2,...,T$), D_j is independent of ($Y(\underline{d}_T)$ for all $\underline{d}_T$) conditional on $\underline{X}_{j-1}$. (13)

Intuitively, this untestable assumption states (for every j) that aside from the history of putative time-varying moderators up to time j, there exist no other variables (measured or unmeasured, known or unknown) that are directly related to both D_j and the potential outcomes. Together with the Consistency Assumption, the No Unmeasured Confounders Assumption allows us to draw causal inferences from observed differences in the data (see Supplementary Web Appendix B in Almirall et al., 2009).

10.3.2 Parametric Models for the Components of the SNMM: Modeling Assumptions

Properties (9) and (10) serve as a guide for parametric models for the causal and non-causal portions of the SNMM. In this chapter, we consider simple linear parametric models for the values of μ_j such as the following:

$$\mu_j(\underline{X}_{j-1}, \underline{D}_j; \beta_j) = D_j(\beta_{j0} + \beta_{j1} X_{j-1}) = \beta_{j0} D_j + \beta_{j1} D_j X_{j-1}, \tag{14}$$

where $\beta_j = (\beta_{j0}, \beta_{j1})$ is an unknown column vector of parameters. This model, for example, implies that the effect of a unit change in D_1 (for example, weight change between baseline and $t = 1$) on the outcome varies linearly in X_{j-1} with slope equal to β_{j1}.

Assume for the moment that X_{j-1} is univariate for all j. For each ε_j, $j = 1, 2,...,T$, we consider parametric models for the nuisance functions such as the following:

$$\varepsilon_j(\underline{X}_{j-1}, \underline{D}_{j-1}; \eta_j, \lambda_j) = \delta_j(\underline{X}_{j-1}, \underline{D}_{j-1}; \lambda_j)\, \eta_j \tag{15}$$

where η_j is an unknown scalar parameter. More complex forms—where the ε_j's are indexed by a row vector of unknown parameters η_j—are discussed in Almirall and colleagues (2009). The residual δ_j is equal to $X_{j-1} - m_j(\underline{X}_{j-2}, \underline{D}_{j-1}; \lambda_j)$, where $m_j(\underline{X}_{j-2}, \underline{D}_{j-1}; \lambda_j) = g_j(F_j\lambda_j)$ is a general linear model (GLM), with link function $g_j()$, for the conditional expectation $E(\underline{X}_{j-1} \mid \underline{X}_{j-2}, \underline{D}_{j-1})$ based on the unknown parameters λ_j. For binary X_{j-1}, $g_j()$ can be either the inverse logit transform or the inverse probit transform. On the other hand, if X_{j-1} were continuous, then $g_j()$ would be the identity function. Note that $E(\delta_j(\underline{X}_{j-1}, \underline{D}_{j-1}; \lambda_j) | \underline{X}_{j-2}, \underline{D}_{j-1}) = 0$ by definition.

As an example, suppose X_j is a binary indicator of exercise measured at time j. In this case, a sample model for ε_j is $\varepsilon_j(\underline{X}_{j-1}, \underline{D}_{j-1}; \eta_j, \lambda_j) = (X_j - p_j(\lambda_j))\, \eta_j$, where $p_j(\lambda_j)$ is the predicted probabilities of a logistic regression of X_j on the past.

The parameterization shown in (15) ensures that models for the nuisance functions satisfy the constraint in (10). Observe that since $E(\delta_j(\underline{X}_{j-1}, \underline{D}_{j-1}; \lambda_j) | \underline{X}_{j-2}, \underline{D}_{j-1}) = 0$, then $E(\varepsilon_j(\underline{X}_{j-1}, \underline{D}_{j-1}; \eta_j, \lambda_j) | \underline{X}_{j-2}, \underline{D}_{j-1}) = E(\delta_j(\underline{X}_{j-1}, \underline{D}_{j-1}; \lambda_j)\, \eta_j | \underline{X}_{j-2}, \underline{D}_{j-1}) = E(\delta_j(\underline{X}_{j-1}, \underline{D}_{j-1}; \lambda_j) | \underline{X}_{j-2}, \underline{D}_{j-1})\, \eta_j = 0$.

The parameterization shown in (15) assumes that each X_j is univariate. For multivariate X_j (say, $X_j = (X_{jk} : k = 1, 2, \ldots, s_j)$, a vector of s_j covariates at time j), we propose modeling the separate ε_{jk}'s for each X_{jk} as in (15) and then summing them together to create a model for j^{th} time-point nuisance function ε_j.

Let β denote the full collection of parameters in the μ_j's, including the SNMM intercept β_0; and let η and λ denote the collection of parameters in the nuisance functions of the SNMM. Note that the parameters λ are shared between the SNMM and the conditional mean models for the time-varying covariates given the past. Next, we describe maximum likelihood estimation of the causal parameters (β) and non-causal (nuisance) parameters (η, λ) of the SNMM.

10.3.3 Maximum Likelihood Estimation

Recall that the full observed data for one person are denoted by O. The probability density function f_O of the observed data O can be written as a product of conditional densities, as follows:

$$f_O(O) = f_Y(Y | \underline{X}_{T-1}, \underline{D}_T) \prod_{j=1}^{T-1} f_j(X_j | \underline{X}_{j-1}, \underline{D}_{j-1}) f_0(X_0) \prod_{j=1}^{T} \pi_j(D_j | \underline{X}_{j-1}, \underline{D}_{j-1}), \qquad (16)$$

where f_Y is the conditional density of Y given $(\underline{X}_{T-1}, \underline{D}_T)$, f_j is the conditional density of X_j given $(\underline{X}_{j-1}, \underline{D}_{j-1})$, $f_0(X_0)$ is the density of X_0, and π_j is the conditional density of D_j given $(\underline{X}_{j-1}, \underline{D}_{j-1})$.

In this chapter we assume that the conditional distribution of Y given $(\underline{X}_{T-1}, \underline{D}_T)$ follows a normal distribution with conditional mean structure following an SNMM with parameters (β, η, λ) and residual square-root variance σ_Y. Thus, f_Y is assumed to be a normal probability density function with parameters (β, η, λ, σ_Y). The form of the conditional densities f_j and f_0 depend on the type of time-varying covariates found in the data. In our data example here, we encounter both continuous and binary random variables in $\underline{X}_{J-1}$; for continuous time-varying covariates, we assume normality, whereas for binary time-varying covariates, we assume a Bernoulli distribution with conditional probability modeled by the logistic transform. In general practice, the quantity $\prod_{j=1}^{T-1} f_j(X_j | \underline{X}_{j-1}, \underline{D}_{j-1}) f_0(X_0)$ may be a mixture of continuous and categorical conditional probability density functions. In any case, $\prod_{j=1}^{T-1} f_j(X_j | \underline{X}_{j-1}, \underline{D}_{j-1}) f_0(X_0)$ is at least a function of λ, the unknown parameters indexing models for the expectation (mean) of X_j given the past. This is important because it means that the parameters λ are shared between the conditional density for Y given the past and other portions of the multivariate distribution of O. This happens because models for the conditional mean of the time-varying covariates are employed in the nuisance functions—that is, the ε_j's—of the SNMM. The densities f_j and f_0 may also be a function of other variance components (for example, σ_j and σ_0, if there are continuous time-varying covariates assumed to follow a normal distribution).

Let θ denote the full collection of unknown parameters in $f_Y(Y \mid \underline{X}_{T-1}, \underline{D}_T) \prod_{j=1}^{T-1} f_j(X_j \mid \underline{X}_{j-1}, \underline{D}_{j-1})$ $f_0(X_0)$. Thus, θ includes $(\beta, \eta, \lambda, \sigma_Y)$ in f_Y, and λ and possibly other variance components (for example, σ_j and σ_0) in $\prod_{j=1}^{T-1} f_j(X_j \mid \underline{X}_{j-1}, \underline{D}_{j-1}) f_0(X_0)$.

To proceed with estimation of θ, we assume we have a data set, $(O_1, O_2, ..., O_N)$, of N independent random variables, each assumed to be drawn from the distribution $f_O(O \mid \theta)$. Therefore, written as a function of the unknown parameters θ, the complete data log-likelihood is

$$\begin{aligned} \text{loglik}_1 &= \textstyle\sum_{i=1}^{N} \log f_O(O_i \mid \theta) \\ &= \textstyle\sum_{i=1}^{N} (\log f_Y(Y_i \mid \underline{X}_{T-1,i}, \underline{D}_{T,i}; \beta, \eta, \lambda, \sigma_Y) + \sum_{j=1}^{T-1} \log f_j(X_{j,i} \mid \underline{X}_{j-1,i}, \underline{D}_{j-1,i}; \\ &\quad \lambda_j, \sigma_j) f_0(X_{0,i}; \lambda_0, \sigma_0) \\ &\quad + \textstyle\sum_{j=1}^{T} \log \pi_j(D_{j,i} \mid \underline{X}_{j-1,i}, \underline{D}_{j-1,i})), \end{aligned} \tag{17}$$

where i denotes subject i in the data set ($i = 1, 2, \ldots, N$). Because the conditional distribution of D_j given $(\underline{X}_{j-1}, \underline{D}_{j-1})$ factorizes and is not a function of any of the parameters in θ, we can obtain a maximum likelihood (ML) estimate of θ by finding the value of θ that maximizes:

$$\begin{aligned} \text{loglik}_2 &= \textstyle\sum_{i=1}^{N} \log f_O(O_i \mid \theta) \\ &= \textstyle\sum_{i=1}^{N} (\log f_Y(Y_i \mid \underline{X}_{T-1,i}, \underline{D}_{T,i}; \beta, \eta, \lambda, \sigma_Y) + \sum_{j=1}^{T-1} \log f_j(X_{j,i} \mid \underline{X}_{j-1,i}, \underline{D}_{j-1,i}; \\ &\quad \lambda_j, \sigma_j) f_0(X_{0,i}; \lambda_0, \sigma_0)). \end{aligned} \tag{18}$$

Denote the ML estimate of θ by $\hat{\theta}$. That is, $\hat{\theta} = \text{argmax}_\theta \, \text{loglik}_2(\theta)$.

The following section demonstrates how to estimate θ using ML with real data.

10.4 Empirical Example: Maximum Likelihood Data Analysis Using SAS PROC NLP

In this section, we demonstrate how to obtain ML estimates of the SNMM using SAS PROC NLP. Data for our illustrative example come from a randomized, controlled clinical trial comparing a low-carbohydrate (LC; $N_{LC} = 59$) diet versus a low-fat diet (LF; $N_{LF} = 60$) for weight loss, hereafter referred to as the LCLF Study (Yancy et al., 2004). Participants in both arms of the LCLF Study had measures of body weight, health-related quality of life (HRQOL), and exercise collected during clinic visits at baseline and every 4 weeks over the course of 16 weeks. In addition, adherence to diet was measured at every clinic visit post-baseline. Our total sample size is $N = 119$.

Using the LCLF Study data, Yancy and colleagues (2004) demonstrated improved weight loss, on average, for patients in the LC diet as compared with those following the LF diet, with most improvements in both arms of the study occurring during the first 12 weeks of study. Yancy and colleagues (2009) examined the effect of the LC diet versus the LF diet on a variety of quality of life measures and found that the LC diet group had greater improvements in the Mental Component Summary score of the Short Form 36 (SF-36), a commonly used and widely validated instrument for assessing HRQOL (McHorney et al., 1992; Ware and Sherbourne, 1992). In ongoing, unpublished research, we have also investigated the marginal impact of weight loss on quality of life using a Marginal Structural Model (MSM) (Robins, 1997, 1999a; Robins et al., 2000) and found some evidence that patients who lose weight faster enjoy a better intermediate and end-of-study health-related quality of life. Given these preliminary findings, we are also interested in better understanding the relationship among diet, weight loss, and quality of life, by studying the impact of weight change (that is, time-varying body weight) on health-related quality of life conditional on (that is, as modified by) the evolving state of the patient with respect to exercise, compliance with the diet, and prior levels of quality of life. While MSMs can be used to study the impact of time-varying weight loss, they cannot be used to study time-varying causal effect moderation (modification) because they do not allow conditioning on time-varying covariates.

10.4.1 Primary Scientific Question of Interest

In this chapter, we apply the SNMM to the LCLF data to study the extent to which assigned diet (LC versus LF), time-varying exercise, time-varying adherence to assigned diet, prior weight change, and prior levels of quality of life moderate the effect of losing (or gaining) weight early versus later over the course of 12 weeks on end-of-study vitality. In other words "do the effects of losing weight early versus later during the course of 12 weeks on end-of-study vitality scores differ depending on diet arm and time-varying covariates such as adherence to diet, exercise, and prior levels of quality of life?"

While our data arise from an experimental study, the causal effect moderation question we are interested in constitutes an observational study of the data because our primary right-hand side (or causal) variable of interest is longitudinal weight (change), which, unlike assignment to diet type (LC versus LF), cannot be manipulated experimentally.

10.4.2 Study Measures and Temporal Ordering

For our illustrative example, we are using LCLF Study data gathered at baseline and at clinic visits occurring every 4 weeks from baseline through week 16. Thus, for our purposes, there are five measurement occasions. In our study, the time-varying covariates of interest—measures of adherence to diet (COMPLY), exercise (EXER), and vitality (VIT)—are self-reported recollections designed to capture these constructs since the last visit or in the past 2 weeks. Thus, the time at which a measure is collected (clinic visits) is not necessarily the time at which the construct being measured actually occurred. In our causal analyses, therefore, we lag our measures appropriately to account for this feature of the data. We also do this acknowledging that in our conception of time-varying causal effect moderation in Section 10.2 we require that time-varying moderators $\underline{X}_{j-1}$ occur prior to, or concurrent with, the primary predictor (or treatments) of interest at time j, D_j. In addition, the primary outcome Y must be measured at the end of the study, meaning after the occurrence of the final measure of the time-varying predictor, D_T.

The first step in our data analysis, therefore, is to identify the primary measures of interest and their temporal ordering both in the data and in terms of the quantities they measure. Figure 10.1 summarizes the relationship among our study measures of interest, their timing in the LCLF Study, and how we use these measures in our data analysis.

Figure 10.1 Temporal Ordering of Study Measurements in LCLF Study

Interval Prior to Baseline	Baseline Visit	Interval Prior to Week 4 Visit	Week 4 Visit	Interval Prior to Week 8 Visit	Week 8 Visit	Interval Prior to Week 12 Visit	Week 12 Visit	Interval Prior to Week 16 Visit	Week 16 Visit
Measurements Collected in LCLF Study†									
	WGT0		WGT4		WGT8		WGT12		WGT16
			COMP4		COMP8		COMP12		COMP16
	EXER0		EXER4		EXER8		EXER12		EXER16
	VIT0		VIT4		VIT8		VIT12		VIT16
	DIET								
Measurements in Real Temporal Order									
	WGT0		WGT4		WGT8		WGT12		WGT16
		COMP4		COMP8		COMP12		COMP16	
EXER0		EXER4		EXER8		EXER12		EXER16	
VIT0		VIT4		VIT8		VIT12		VIT16	
	DIET								
Measurements Used for Data Analysis									
	D1 = WGT4 – WGT0			*D2* = WGT8 – WGT4		*D3* = WGT12 – WGT8			
X_0 =		X_1 =		X_2 =				*Y* =	
		COMP4		COMP8					
EXER0		EXER4		EXER8					
VIT0		VIT4		VIT8				VIT16	
DIET									

†All measurements were collected at the clinic visits, starting at the baseline visit and every 4 weeks thereafter.

Definitions (see also Section 10.2):

DIET = diet type, a binary measure (1=LC diet; 0=LF diet)
WGT = weight, a continuous measure
COMP = adherence to diet, a binary measure
EXER = exercise, a binary measure
VIT = vitality (a quality of life outcome), a continuous measure

10.4.2.1 Primary Predictor of Interest: Successive Changes in Body Weight

Let Z_j be the measure of body weight taken at visit *j*, where $j = 0$ denotes the baseline visit. D_j is defined as the difference in body weight between successive clinic visits: $D_j = Z_j - Z_{j-1}$. For our study, we consider measures of weight change over the course of 12 weeks post-baseline. Because clinic visits were 4 weeks apart, $T = 3$ $(j = 1, 2, 3)$. Thus, we have D_1 = weight change between baseline and the first clinic visit, D_2 = weight change between the second and third clinic visits, and D_3 = weight change between the third and fourth clinic visits.

10.4.2.2 Baseline and Time-Varying Moderators of Interest

The putative time-varying moderators $(X_{j-1}: j = 1, 2, 3)$ include continuous time-varying measures of vitality (VIT0, VIT4, VIT8, respectively) and binary (yes/no = 1/0) time-varying indicators of self-reported exercise (EXER0, EXER4, EXER8, respectively). In addition, (X_1, X_2) include binary (yes/no = 1/0) indicators of compliance to diet between the baseline and the first visit (COMPLY4) and compliance to diet between the first and second visits (COMPLY8), respectively. In addition, X_0 also includes a binary (LC/LF = 1/0) indicator of assigned diet arm (DIET).

We note that X_0 does not include a compliance to diet measure because the diet arm was not assigned until the first clinic visit; therefore, compliance to diet is included only in (X_1, X_2). Technically, the diet arm was assigned immediately after the first body weight measure was taken at the baseline clinic visit. However, we can justify including DIET in X_0 because diet assignment was randomized and, therefore, is unaffected by baseline levels of body weight (Z_0). Further, it is sensible to ask whether the impact of body weight change between the baseline and the first follow-up clinic visit differs according to DIET.

10.4.2.3 Primary Outcome: Vitality

HRQOL is assessed using the Medical Outcomes Study SF-36 instrument (McHorney et al., 1992; Ware and Sherbourne, 1992), which measures HRQOL along eight dimensions of physical and mental health. The primary outcome measure for our analysis, Vitality, is one of the continuous physical HRQOL subscales derived from the SF-36 instrument. We use the Vitality component of the SF-36 for illustrating the SNMM methodology; however, we could have used one or more of the other HRQOL subscales, as well. Let Y = VIT16, a continuous measure of vitality during the interval of time just prior to the week 16 clinic visit. For illustrative purposes, we have restricted the outcome to be an end-of-study outcome, but the methods described in this chapter can be readily extended to handle a longitudinal outcome variable (Robins, 1994).

10.4.3 Parametric Models

For the conditional distribution of VIT16 given the past (that is, for f_Y), we assumed a normal distribution with residual square-root variance σ_Y and conditional mean following a SNMM with this parameterization:

$$E(\text{VIT16} \mid \text{DIET}, \underline{\text{EXER8}}, \underline{\text{VIT8}}, \underline{\text{COMP8}}, \underline{D_3}) \quad (19)$$

$$= \beta_0 \quad \text{[intercept]}$$

$$+ \eta_{14}\delta_{1\text{DIET}} + \eta_{15}\delta_{1\text{EXER0}} + \eta_{16}\delta_{1\text{VIT0}} \quad [\varepsilon_1(X_0; \eta_1)]$$

$$+ \beta_{10} D_1 + \beta_{11} D_1\text{EXER0} + \beta_{12} D_1\text{VIT0} + \beta_{13} D_1\text{DIET} \quad [\mu_1(X_0, D_1; \beta_1)]$$

$$+ \eta_{21}\delta_{2\text{COMPLY4}} + \eta_{22}\delta_{2\text{EXER4}} + \eta_{23}\delta_{2\text{VIT4}} \quad [\varepsilon_2(\underline{X_1}, D_1; \eta_2)]$$

$$+ \beta_{20} D_2 + \beta_{21} D_2\,\text{EXER4} + \beta_{22} D_2\,\text{VIT4} + \beta_{23} D_2\,\text{COMPLY4} \quad [\mu_2(\underline{X_1}, \underline{D_2}; \beta_2)]$$

$$+ \eta_{31}\delta_{3\text{COMPLY8}} + \eta_{32}\delta_{3\text{EXER8}} + \eta_{33}\delta_{3\text{VIT8}} \quad [\varepsilon_3(\underline{X_2}, \underline{D_2}; \eta_3)]$$

$$+ \beta_{30} D_3 + \beta_{31} D_3\,\text{EXER8} + \beta_{32} D_3\,\text{VIT8} + \beta_{33} D_3\,\text{COMPLY8} \quad [\mu_3(\underline{X_2}, \underline{D_3}; \beta_3)]$$

The μ_j models in this SNMM are Markovian in the sense that each model for the effect of D_j on Y is only a function of prior weight change and measures of the time-varying covariates immediately preceding D_j. More complicated models could also be considered—for instance, models that allow the full history of time-varying covariates $\underline{X}_{j-1}$ to moderate the impact of subsequent weight change on vitality.

Because EXER, COMPLY, and DIET are binary, we assume Bernoulli distributions for their conditional distributions given the past (that is, the f_j's), with probabilities modeled using logistic link functions (that is, g = inverse logit link). For example, for COMPLY4, the Bernoulli likelihood takes the form

$$f_{\text{COMPLY4}} = p_{\text{COMPLY4}}\,(\text{COMPLY4}) + (1\text{-}p_{\text{COMPLY4}})\,(1\text{-COMPLY4}),$$

where p_{COMPLY4} denotes the predicted probability that COMPLY4 = 1 from a logistic regression of COMPLY4 on covariates (EXER0, VIT0, DIET, and D1). (See Section 10.4.4.2 for the corresponding SAS PROC NLP code.) For baseline (VIT0) and follow-up (VIT4, VIT8), which are continuous time-varying variables, we assume normal distributions for their conditional distributions with residual square-root variance σ_{VIT0}, σ_{VIT4}, and σ_{VIT8} respectively (with g = identity function). In terms of the specific form of the linear portion of the GLMs (that is, models for the $F_j\lambda_j$), all models for the post-baseline variables included main effects for the history of covariates that preceded it and first-order interactions with prior levels of weight change, whereas for the baseline covariates, we use intercept-only models.

10.4.4 SAS PROC NLP

The NLP procedure in SAS provides a powerful set of optimization tools for minimizing or maximizing multi-parameter non-linear functions with constraints, such as our loglik_2 (Property [18]). Recall from Property (18) that the complete data log-likelihood is a function of f_Y and f_j and the parameters θ. In this parameterization, θ includes (β, η, λ, σ_Y and λ) and possibly other variance components (for example, σ_j and σ_0) depending on the distribution of the time-varying covariates that are used. Here we demonstrate how to use PROC NLP to find the value of the parameters in θ that maximize $\text{loglik}_2(\theta)$. PROC NLP is particularly well-suited for this application because the log-likelihood function loglik_2 is both non-linear in θ, and it includes simple inequality constraints. Specifically, the vector of parameters λ appears in the f_Y portion of the log-likelihood as a multiplicative product with parameters in η, and λ also appears in other portions of the log-likelihood. In addition, we constrain the variance components (for example, σ_Y) in loglik_2 to be positive.

We begin by inputting our data set into SAS and printing the data to ensure they were loaded correctly:

```
libname lib1 '\My Documents\WeightData';

proc print data=lib1.weight_data;
 var subject diet exer0 vit0 d1 comply4 exer4 vit4 d2 comply8 exer8
vit8 d3 vit16;
run;
```

We show the first 12 lines of data here. The outcome is VIT16. DIET, EXER0, and VIT0 are baseline moderators of interest; D1 is weight change between baseline and week 4; COMPLY4, EXER4 and VIT4 are week 4 moderators; D2 is weight change between week 4 and week 8; COMPLY8, EXER8, and VIT8 are week 8 moderators of interest; and D3 is weight change between week 8 and week 12.

Output 10.1 SAS PROC NLP Analysis Data Set

Obs	subject	DIET	exer20	VIT0	D1	comply4	exer24	VIT4	D2	comply8	exer28	VIT8	VIT16
1	1	0	0	75.00	-7.40	0	0	75.00	-4.00	0	0	70.00	80.00
2	2	1	0	60.00	-12.4	1	1	80.00	-6.40	1	1	65.00	65.00
3	3	0	1	80.00	-4.20	0	1	80.00	-3.40	0	1	80.00	87.92
4	4	1	1	53.33	-12.4	1	1	50.00	-4.20	1	1	45.00	65.00
5	5	1	1	65.79	-6.85	0	1	52.65	-4.97	0	1	50.80	83.38
6	6	0	0	70.00	-6.00	1	1	90.00	-0.20	1	0	90.00	65.00
7	7	1	0	55.00	-11.6	1	1	80.00	-5.20	0	1	90.00	75.00
8	8	1	1	70.00	-16.6	1	1	90.00	-1.20	0	1	90.00	100.0
9	9	0	1	55.00	-4.00	1	1	50.00	-5.00	1	1	60.00	75.00
10	10	0	0	55.00	-13.2	1	1	55.00	-6.80	1	1	50.00	80.00
11	11	0	0	70.00	-10.0	1	1	90.00	-7.40	1	0	90.00	100.0
12	12	1	0	45.00	-18.0	1	1	69.53	-3.27	0	1	73.51	74.85

The data set should have only one record per subject with time-varying variables coded appropriately. For example VIT0 represents the vitality measure for baseline, VIT4 is the vitality measure taken at week 4, and so on. If the data set is in person-period format (one record per measurement time period), it should be converted to a wide data set (one record per subject).

10.4.4.1 Initial Model Selection and Starting Values Using a Two-Stage Regression Approach

PROC NLP requires starting values for the numerical optimization routine that maximizes loglik_2 (Property [18]). Appendix 10.A describes the SAS code we used to obtain the starting values for PROC NLP. We employed a moments-based two-stage regression estimator to obtain starting values and to carry out initial model selection for our working models. For more details concerning the two-stage regression estimator, see Almirall and colleagues (2009). For completeness, we briefly describe the two-stage regression estimator here.

The two-stage regression estimator is the moments-based analog of the ML estimator described in Section 10.3.3. In the first stage, the parameters λ_j are estimated, separately for each j, by GLM. In fitting the models $m_j(\underline{X}_{j-2},\underline{D}_{j-1};\lambda_j) = g_j(F_j\lambda_j)$, we performed an ad hoc stepwise model selection procedure to find the best fitting, parsimonious models for the conditional mean $E(\underline{X}_{j-1} \mid \underline{X}_{j-2},\underline{D}_{j-1})$. Details are explained in Appendix 10.A. Then, based on the estimates of λ_j, the residuals δ_j are calculated and subsequently used as covariates in a second regression (that is, the second stage) of the outcome based on the SNMM in Property (19).

10.4.4.2 Explanation of the PROC NLP Code

Once initial model selection for the nuisance models has been performed and starting values based on the initial working models have been calculated using the two-stage approach, we are ready to set up our PROC NLP code to obtain ML estimates that maximize Property (18). The complete program is presented in Appendix 10.B. This section provides a step-by-step explanation of portions of the code.

In the first line of code, we give our SAS data analysis a title; the ODS OUTPUT statements in the second and third lines of code instruct SAS to output the estimated parameters and variance-covariance matrix as SAS data sets.

```
TITLE "MLE of the Weight Data Using PROC NLP -- &sysdate. ";
ods output "Resulting Parameters"=lib1.NLPestimates;
ods output "Covariances"=lib1.NLProbustvarcov;
```

Next, we call the NLP procedure and specify the name of the data set using the DATA= option:

```
PROC NLP data=lib1.all_weight_data vardef=n covariance=1 pcov;
```

Here, we also specify the type of standard errors we want calculated using the VARDEF= and COVARIANCE= options. SAS PROC NLP uses standard asymptotic results from ML theory (for example, Section 5.5 in Vaart, 1998) to compute an estimate of the so-called robust (or sandwich) variance-covariance matrix of $\hat{\theta}$, which we denote by $\hat{\Delta}(\hat{\theta})$. We can obtain $\hat{\Delta}(\hat{\theta})$ by specifying **vardef=n covariance=1**. Estimated standard errors are computed as the square roots of the diagonal elements of $\hat{\Delta}(\hat{\theta})$. The PCOV option instructs PROC NLP to print the estimated variance-covariance matrix in the output. As mentioned previously, the ODS OUTPUT statement shown earlier allows us to retrieve $\hat{\Delta}(\hat{\theta})$ as a SAS data set for later computations. In Section 10.4.4.3, the variance-covariance matrix is used to calculate standard errors (and, thus, confidence intervals) for particular linear combinations of the estimated parameters.

The next statement specifies the numerical optimization to be carried out. In our case, we are interested in carrying out ML estimation; therefore, we instruct SAS PROC NLP to maximize loglik, which we define for PROC NLP in subsequent programming statements:

```
MAX loglik;
```

The next statement needed is the PARMS statement. The PARMS statement identifies the parameters to be estimated and sets starting values for the numerical optimization routine. It is easier to set up the PARMS statement after one has written out the programming statements for the likelihood. The syntax for the PARMS statement, which we shorten here for reasons of space, is as follows:

```
PARMS sig2= 17.18, sig2_vit4= 15.99,sig2_vit8= 11.96, sig2_vit0=
18.23, beta0= 65.45, /*...etc...*/;
```

The complete PARMS statement for our data analysis is shown in Appendix 10.B.

The BOUNDS statement, which follows next, is where we specify parameter constraints. In our analysis, we bound the residual square-root variances to be positive, as follows:

```
BOUNDS sig2 > 1e-12, sig2_vit0 > 1e-12, sig2_vit4 > 1e-12, sig2_vit8
> 1e-12;
```

No other parameters in loglik_2 have constraints.

Next we move to the programming statements used to set up the log-likelihood to be maximized. The goal here is to work toward defining loglik. Recall that the log-likelihood is a function of the distribution of the moderators given the past, the f_j's, as well as a function of the distribution of VIT16 given the past, f_Y, which includes our primary SNMM of interest. For clarity, pedagogical purposes, and ease of debugging later, we found it better to set up the likelihood using multiple programming statements rather than writing out the likelihood in one line of code. PROC NLP allows one to do this immediately after the BOUNDS statement.

First, we calculate portions of the log-likelihood corresponding to the baseline nuisance conditional density functions, the f_0's. In addition, we calculate the relevant portions of the f_0's that will be used in the SNMM conditional likelihood. Here we show the code for DIET, a binary baseline moderator:

```
dietlin1=gamma11_0;       /* intercept only logistic regression model  */
dietp=exp(dietlin1)/(1+exp(dietlin1));
                          /* probability using inverse-logit transform */
fdiet=diet*dietp+(1-diet)*(1-dietp);
                          /* used in Bernoulli likelihood for DIET*/
ddiet=diet-dietp;         /* residual to be used in the SNMM for VIT16 */
```

The residual ddiet is $\delta_{l\text{DIET}}$ in Property (19) (see Section 10.3.2 for details concerning parametric models for the nuisance functions). To maintain consistency, we apply the inverse-logit transformation on the sole parameter gamma11_0 (the odds that **DIET=1**) to calculate the probability that **DIET=1**, but we also could have set up PROC NLP to estimate the probability dietp directly. Either method works fine, but if you want to calculate dietp directly, you should be sure to include **dietp>0** in the BOUNDS statement. We use similar coding for the other dichotomous baseline moderator EXER0 (see Appendix 10.B).

For the continuous baseline moderator VIT0, the code is much simpler. One line of code creates the residual $\delta_{l\text{VIT0}}$ used in the SNMM for VIT16 [see Property (19)]. Again, here we use an intercept-only model because there is no history preceding the baseline moderator VIT0:

```
dvit0=VIT0-(gamma13_0); /* residual to be used in the SNMM for VIT16 */
```

Next, we calculate portions of the log-likelihood corresponding to the post-baseline nuisance conditional density functions, the f_j's. Here we show the code for COMPLY4, a week 4 binary moderator:

```
comply4lin1= gamma21_0 + gamma21_1*DIET + gamma21_2*EXER0 +
gamma21_3*D1;   /* logit model */
comply4p=exp(comply4lin1)/(1+exp(comply4lin1));
            /* probability */
fcomply4=comply4*comply4p+(1-comply4)*(1-comply4p);
   /* used in the Bernoulli likelihood */
dcomply4=comply4-comply4p;
   /* residual to be used in the SNMM for VIT16 */
```

The residual dcomply4 is $\delta_{2\text{COMPLY4}}$ in Property (19). The covariates chosen for the logistic regression model for COMPLY4—that is, DIET, EXER0, and D1—were chosen based on initial model selection (see Section 10.4.4.1 and Appendix 10.A). Note that the initial model selection suggested removing VIT0 from the logistic regression for COMPLY4. Similar code was used for EXER4.

For the continuous moderator VIT4 at week 4, we need only the following programming statement to create the residual, $\delta_{2\text{COMPLY4}}$:

```
dvit4=VIT4-(gamma23_0 + gamma23_1*VIT0 + gamma23_2*D1 +
gamma23_3*VIT0*D1);
```

Again, here the covariates in the final model were chosen based on initial model selection (see Section 10.4.4.1 and Appendix 10.A). We use similar code for the dichotomous or continuous moderator variables at week 8.

The penultimate step in our programming statements is to calculate the conditional mean (that is, the SNMM), and the residuals to be used in the log-likelihood corresponding to the conditional distribution of VIT16 given (DIET, <u>EXER8</u>, <u>VIT8</u>, <u>COMP8</u>, $\underline{D}_3$), f_Y:

```
snmmVIT16=beta0 + eta14_res14_DIET*ddiet + eta15_res15_EXER0*dexer0
         + eta16_res16_VIT0*dvit0
         + beta10_D1*D1
         + beta14_D1DIET*D1*DIET + beta15_D1EXER0*D1*EXER0 +
beta16_D1VIT0*D1*VIT0
         + eta21_res21_COMPLY4*dCOMPLY4 + eta22_res22_EXER4*dEXER4
         + eta23_res23_VIT4*dVIT4
         + beta20_D2*D2 + beta21_D2COMPLY4*D2*COMPLY4 +
beta22_D2EXER4*D2*EXER4
         + beta23_D2VIT4*D2*VIT4
         + eta31_res31_COMPLY8*dCOMPLY8 + eta32_res32_EXER8*dEXER8
         + eta33_res33_VIT8*dVIT8
         + beta30_D3*D3 + beta31_D3COMPLY8*D3*COMPLY8 +
beta32_D3EXER8*D3*EXER8
         + beta33_D3VIT8*D3*VIT8;
epsilon=VIT16-snmmVIT16;
```

The object snmmVIT16 is precisely Property (19) (that is, our SNMM of interest). The primary parameters of interest—that is, those in the μ_j's—are those labeled beta.

The final step is to program the complete data log-likelihood (see Property [18]). At each of the three time points, we have two dichotomous moderators and one continuous moderator. Therefore, the complete data log-likelihood is a function of 10 conditional density functions (nine for the time-varying moderators, plus one corresponding to the conditional distribution of VIT16 given the past). As in Section 10.3.3, we assume normal distributions for all of the continuous variables:

```
loglik =   log(fdiet)                                    /* [DIET] ~ bernoulli          */
           +  log(fexer0)                                /* [EXER0] ~ bernoulli         */
           log(sig2_vit0) - (dvit0**2/(2*sig2_vit0**2))  /* [VIT0] ~ normal             */
           +  log(fcomply4)                              /* [COMPLY4 | past]~bernoulli */
           +  log(fexer4)                                /* [EXER4 | past] ~ bernoulli */
           log(sig2_vit4) - (dvit4**2/(2*sig2_vit4**2))  /* [VIT4 | past] ~ normal     */
           +  log(fcomply8)                              /* [COMPLY8 | past]~bernoulli */
           +  log(fexer8)                                /* [EXER8 | past]~bernoulli   */
           -  log(sig2_vit8) - (dvit8**2/(2*sig2_vit8**2)) /* [VIT8 | past]~normal     */
           log(sig2) - (epsilon**2/(2*sig2**2))          /* [VIT16 | past]~normal      */
;
```

10.4.5 PROC NLP Output, Model Results, and Interpretation

PROC NLP produces many sections of output based on the options that are specified. The first section of output describes how the gradient and Hessian matrix are calculated (that is, based on analytic formulas and finite difference approximations). The second section, titled Optimization Start, lists all of the parameters to be estimated, the starting values that were used, and the constraints placed on the parameters. The third section of the output provides information about the optimization procedure, including the type of optimization procedure employed by PROC NLP, a summary of the number of parameters being estimated, and the number of subjects (*N*). This section also shows details concerning the number of iterations, the improvement in the log-likelihood at each iteration (that is, the objective function), and the final value of log-likelihood and slope at the solution. It is essential to review these sections first to ensure that the correct parameters are being estimated, to check starting values, to ensure that the correct constraints were placed on the parameters, and to ensure convergence of the numerical optimization routine.

The next section of output, titled "Optimization Results," produces the ML estimates, $\hat{\theta}$, and their corresponding standard errors, and *p*-values. PROC NLP automatically produces a column for the standard errors whenever the COVARIANCE= option has been set.

Output 10.2 SAS PROC NLP: Optimization Results

Optimization Results						
Parameter Estimates						
N	Parameter	Estimate	Approx Std Err	t Value	Approx Pr > |t|	Gradient Objective Function
1	sig2	11.529426	0.757505	15.220273	8.590079E-30	-0.008322
2	sig2_vit4	15.653134	1.237725	12.646695	8.080688E-24	0.075107
3	sig2_vit8	11.755608	1.050688	11.188491	2.429932E-20	0.183281
4	sig2_vit0	18.149850	1.084132	16.741372	3.521951E-33	0.002445
5	gamma11_0	0.013609	0.182551	0.074547	0.940699	-0.340098
6	gamma12_0	0.408751	0.186436	2.192447	0.030277	-0.077163
7	gamma13_0	59.835944	1.657568	36.098645	2.733837E-66	-0.009119
8	gamma21_0	-0.159239	0.435969	-0.365254	0.715565	0.134506
9	gamma21_1	0.862473	0.464470	1.856899	0.065778	-0.025547
10	gamma21_2	-0.842582	0.453436	-1.858214	0.065589	0.528869
11	gamma21_3	-0.089199	0.039831	-2.239417	0.026971	0.044023
12	gamma22_0	1.213170	0.343850	3.528196	0.000594	-0.010149
13	gamma22_1	1.185886	0.548098	2.163638	0.032474	-0.007180
14	gamma23_0	20.256117	9.185571	2.205210	0.029345	-0.003342
15	gamma23_1	0.780218	0.146865	5.312483	0.000000505	-0.002393
16	gamma23_2	-2.210745	0.619396	-3.569195	0.000516	0.041969
17	gamma23_3	0.034491	0.010694	3.225275	0.001622	-0.153887

Optimization Results						
Parameter Estimates						
N	**Parameter**	**Estimate**	**Approx Std Err**	**t Value**	**Approx Pr > |t|**	**Gradient Objective Function**
18	**gamma31_0**	-2.427822	0.663753	-3.657718	0.000379	0.003286
19	**gamma31_1**	2.376449	0.493118	4.819234	0.000004260	-0.001026
20	**gamma31_2**	-0.296078	0.088441	-3.347735	0.001089	-0.000436
21	**gamma32_0**	0.124178	0.486114	0.255450	0.798813	-0.001161
22	**gamma32_1**	1.809607	0.565670	3.199051	0.001764	0.005892
23	**gamma33_0**	21.943562	3.944913	5.562496	0.000000164	-0.000270
24	**gamma33_1**	0.719654	0.052663	13.665289	3.247824E-26	-0.000962
25	**eta14_res14_DIET**	-6.151747	5.501784	-1.118137	0.265742	-0.021217
26	**eta15_res15_EXER20**	-1.641192	4.546778	-0.360957	0.718766	-0.003707
27	**eta16_res16_VIT0**	0.518775	0.162683	3.188863	0.001822	-0.067273
28	**Beta0**	65.523505	3.697128	17.722810	2.66664E-35	0.044318
29	**Beta10_D1**	-0.597441	0.758160	-0.788014	0.432242	-0.071963
30	**Beta14_D1Diet**	-0.261892	0.490731	-0.533678	0.594552	0.239752
31	**Beta15_D1exer20**	-0.593875	0.406696	-1.460243	0.146837	0.043617
32	**Beta16_D1VIT0**	0.012537	0.010124	1.238343	0.218006	0.193041
33	**eta21_res21_COMPLY4**	-12.810076	4.621290	-2.771970	0.006461	0.009694
34	**eta22_res22_EXER24**	0.454148	5.481000	0.082859	0.934102	-0.147914
35	**eta23_res23_VIT4**	0.507970	0.162578	3.124476	0.002234	-0.009587
36	**Beta20_D2**	-0.650131	1.979927	-0.328361	0.743211	-0.176000
37	**Beta21_D2comply4**	-1.819338	0.711255	-2.557928	0.011775	0.420162
38	**Beta22_D2exer24**	-1.222696	0.759832	-1.609166	0.110208	0.026772
39	**Beta23_D2VIT4**	0.030631	0.023828	1.285507	0.201090	0.324085
40	**eta31_res31_COMPLY8**	-2.525218	3.484324	-0.724737	0.470024	0.284945
41	**eta32_res32_EXER28**	-0.519705	3.714897	-0.139898	0.888975	0.042493
42	**eta33_res33_VIT8**	0.146175	0.108052	1.352819	0.178657	-0.004925
43	**Beta30_D3**	1.596084	0.970481	1.644632	0.102663	0.126292
44	**Beta31_D3comply8**	-0.425010	0.360160	-1.180061	0.240310	-0.103302
45	**Beta32_D3exer28**	0.017113	0.329711	0.051903	0.958692	0.026872
46	**Beta33_D3VIT8**	-0.019246	0.012146	-1.584584	0.115693	-0.374166

The ML estimate of the intercept β_0 is 65.5 (95%CI = [59, 72]). Therefore, the data suggest that in the absence of any weight change over the course of 12 weeks (that is, $D_1=D_2=D_3=0$), the (population) mean vitality score at week 16 is estimated at 66 (95%CI = [58.3, 72.8]). This is an estimate of the mean vitality score at week 16 had the entire sample experienced no weight change over the course of 12 weeks. As expected—since the majority of people in the study lost weight—β_0 is statistically significantly lower than the observed mean vitality score at week 16 of 74 (median = 77).

The estimates $\hat{\beta}_j$ of the causal effects of interest seem to suggest that the impact of weight change between baseline and week 4 has a negligible impact on mean vitality scores at week 16, whereas COMPLY4 and VIT8 are possibly significant moderators of the impact of D_2 and D_3 on week 16 vitality scores, respectively.

The causal parameter estimates $\hat{\beta}_j$ by themselves, however, are not as useful for making inferences as it is to consider particular linear combinations of interest. That is, since we have estimated conditional causal effects at each time point, it is more interesting to consider the causal effect of increases or decreases in weight change at different levels of the time-varying covariates (that is, the putative moderators of interest). For example, consider the characteristics defining the most common patient in the data set (the median value for each variable):

a) exercised throughout the entire study (EXER0=EXER4=EXER8=1),
b) always adhered to their assigned diet (COMPLY4=COMPLY8=1),
c) had a baseline vitality score of 60 (VIT0=60),
d) had a week 4 vitality score of 70 (VIT4=70), and
e) had a week 8 vitality score of 75 (VIT8=75).

For patients exhibiting these characteristics, we consider the average impact at each time point j ($j = 1, 2, 3$) of a 5-pound negative change in weight (that is, $D_j = -5$ = 5 pound weight loss) versus no change in weight ($D_j = 0$). The results of our SNMM analysis estimate this impact to be 3.5 (95%CI = [-0.2, 7.2]) at time $j = 1$ for patients in the LC group and 2.2 (95%CI = [-1.6, 6.0]) for patients in the LF group, 7.61 (95%CI = [3.0, 12.5]) at time $j = 2$, and 2.2 (95%CI = [-1.6, 6.0]) at time $j = 3$. Because higher values of vitality indicate better quality of life, the direction of the effects at each time point is intuitive—that is, weight loss results in higher values of vitality at the end of the study. Keeping everything else fixed, the effect of weight loss between weeks 4 and 8 disappears for patients who do not comply with their assigned diet during the first four weeks of study (effect = -1.4 ; 95%CI = [-6.9, 4.2]); therefore, this is evidence that compliance with diet moderates the impact of weight loss between weeks 4 and 8 on end-of-study vitality scores. Patients who comply with diet (either diet) during the first four weeks of the study see more benefits resulting from their weight loss between weeks 4 and 8 in terms of improved quality of life at the end of the study.

To see how we calculated the specified conditional effects described here, observe, for example, that the conditional causal effect of weight change between weeks 4 and 8 given prior levels of exercise, vitality, and compliance with assigned diet is estimated as

$$\hat{\mu}_2(\underline{X}_1, \underline{D}_2; \hat{\beta}_2) = (-0.650)\, D_2 + (-1.223)\, D_2\, \text{EXER4} + (0.031)\, D_2\, \text{VIT4} + (-1.819)\, D_2\, \text{COMPLY4}.$$

Therefore, the average effect of 5 pounds of weight loss between weeks 4 and 8 among patients who exercise (EXER4=1), adhere to their assigned diet (COMPLY4=1), and have a median week-4 vitality score (VIT4=70) is estimated as

$$7.61 = -5 \times ((-0.650) + (-1.223) + (0.031) \times 70 + (-1.819)).$$

In order to calculate the standard errors (and, thus, the 95% confidence intervals) for this estimate, we used the estimated variance-covariance matrix of $\hat{\beta}$ and standard formulas for the variance of linear combinations. Appendix 10.C shows a simple SAS script written in PROC IML that calculates the 95%CI.

10.5 Discussion

In this chapter, we have reviewed Robins' Structural Nested Mean Model for studying the time-varying causal effect moderation and demonstrated a maximum likelihood implementation using SAS PROC NLP with real data. This work was motivated by an interest in the impact of weight loss or gain (where weight is measured repeatedly over time) on health-related quality of life.

This work builds on work by Almirall and colleagues (2009) on the use of the SNMM to examine time-varying causal effect moderation. In particular, the conceptualization and use of linear models for the nuisance functions presented in Almirall and colleagues (2009) was used in this chapter to facilitate an MLE implementation. Further, in Section 10.4.4.1, we briefly described the use of the two-stage regression estimator Almirall and colleagues (2009) proposed both to obtain starting values for the ML estimator and for initial model selection. The main difference between the two-stage estimator and the MLE is that the two-stage estimator does not require distributional assumptions (for example, normality); that is, the two-stage estimator is a moments-based estimator. It remains to be seen how these two estimators compare.

Having an adequate model selection procedure is important for the successful implementation of the ML estimator. We know that fitting an MLE with misspecified models for the nuisance functions results in biased estimates of the primary causal parameters of interest. Performing initial model selection for the working models (the f_j's) used in the ML procedure based on the separate model fits in stage one of the two-stage regression estimator, as we suggest in Section 10.4.4.1, is intuitive and useful. Indeed, had we not done this initial model selection first, PROC NLP would have been required to find the MLE for over 90 parameters using just $N = 119$ subjects! (In contrast, our final log-likelihood was a function of 46 parameters.) It is not clear, however, that this is the most optimal strategy for model selection for the SNMM, nor what is the impact of our ad hoc model selection procedure on the distribution of our ML estimator. In addition, even if our general approach of performing model selection on working models first before doing model selection on the SNMM is adopted, it is not clear that ad hoc piecewise model selection based on *p*-value cut offs, which we employed in our empirical example, will ensure that we arrive at the true model. In future work, we will explore and compare different model selection procedures for the SNMM, including likelihood-based selection procedures such as Akaike and Bayes information criterion methods.

Our illustrative data analysis has a number of limitations. First, it is possible that we do not meet the untestable sequential ignorability (no unmeasured confounders) assumption in our analysis. That is, there may be other (time-varying) covariates that were not a part of our model that may impact both weight loss and HRQOL directly. For example, we do not include the amount or type of food consumed between clinic visits. Future studies of the impact of weight loss on HRQOL, or any other outcome, should include nutrient intake data (as measured by self-reported food diaries, for example). Further, even plausible confounders that we measured in this study (and included in the data analysis)—for example, time-varying exercise—could be measured more carefully (for example, amount of exercise in minutes since the last clinic visit) in future studies in order to further reduce the possibility of time-varying confounding bias. Sensitivity analyses, such as those discussed in Robins (1997, 1999a) will be useful for exploring the consequences of selection bias due to violations of the sequential ignorability (no unmeasured confounders) assumption. Secondly, an important concern that we do not address in this chapter has to do with missing data. The ML method we propose is a complete case estimator. Therefore, patients with missing weight values at any time point are excluded from the analysis. Two options for dealing with missing data in this context include inverse-probability weighting methods that can handle missing covariate data (Robins et al., 1994) or multiple imputation (Schafer, 1997). Third, in this chapter we focus solely on an end-of-study quality of life measure. The methods discussed in this chapter, however, can be extended to handle a longitudinal outcome as well, as in Robins (1994). The longitudinal approach would involve specifying an SNMM for each occasion of the longitudinal outcome—that is, for each Y_t, say—and estimating the parameters simultaneously. A final limitation of the ML method as proposed in this chapter is that we did not allow for residual correlation between the conditional models for the vector of X_j's (and Y). Assuming correct model specification, we conjecture that the use of this conditional independence assumption will not lead to bias in the estimates of the causal parameters, although it may have consequences in terms of inference (that is, variance estimation and therefore *p*-values). To guard against improper inference, therefore, we have suggested the use of so-called robust (or sandwich) standard errors via the `covariance=1` option in PROC NLP (White, 1980). Future methodological work will explore the full impact of the working conditional independence assumption and its consequence both in terms of bias and standard error estimation.

The version of the SNMM shown in Property (6) defines the nuisance function at the first time point as

$$\varepsilon_1(X_0) = E(\ Y(0,0) \mid X_0) - E(\ Y(0,0)\ ).$$

This definition for $\varepsilon_1(X_0)$ was chosen so that intercept, $\beta_0 = E(\ Y(0,0)\ )$, has the interpretation as the population mean outcome supposing that all subjects had $d_1 = d_2 = 0$ (averaged over all covariate values). An alternate specification of the SNMM is to set $\varepsilon_1(X_0) = E(Y(0,0) \mid X_0)$, and to define the intercept as $\beta_0 = E(Y(0,0) \mid X_0 = 0)$. With this specification, the intercept can be interpreted as the mean outcome among all patients with $X_0 = 0$ supposing that all subjects had $d_1 = d_2 = 0$. Using the alternate specification requires maximizing over fewer parameters as λ_0, indexing the distribution of the baseline variables f_0, would not appear as part of $\varepsilon_1(X_0)$ in the SNMM. The drawback, of course, is that having the intercept defined as $\beta_0 = E(Y(0,0) \mid X_0 = 0)$ may not be meaningful because the value zero may not lie in the range of plausible values for X_0. Despite this, scientists implementing the likelihood method in the future may wish to use the alternate specification. This may be an important consideration when the set of baseline covariates is much larger than the corresponding set of time-varying covariates or there is little interest in $\beta_0 = E(Y(0,0))$. Importantly, the definition (and therefore interpretation) of the causal functions $\mu_1(X_0, d_1)$ and $\mu_2(\underline{X}_1(d_1), \underline{d}_2)$ remain unchanged with either set of definitions for (β_0, $\varepsilon_1(X_0)$). However, $\varepsilon_2(\underline{X}_1(d_1))$ must remain as defined in Property (6) in order for $\mu_1(X_0, d_1)$ to keep its interpretation as the conditional causal effect at time 1.

In the absence of time-varying causal effect moderation, the SNMM identifies marginal time-varying causal effects, such as those indexing the Marginal Structural Model (Robins, 1997, 1999a, 1999b; Robins et al., 2000). This is true because the absence of time-varying causal effect moderation at time *j* means that the effect of D_j on the outcome is constant across levels of time-varying $\underline{X}_{j-1}$. In other words, the causal parameters $\mu_j(\underline{X}_{j-1}, \underline{D}_j; \beta_j)$ are independent of $\underline{X}_{j-1}$. In this special (testable) case, therefore, the MLE method presented here can be used to estimate marginal causal effects.

Appendix 10.A

SAS code for obtaining starting values for maximizing $loglik_2$ [Property (18)]. Starting values are obtained using a two-stage regression estimator.

This appendix describes how we obtained starting values for the data analysis using PROC NLP, using a moments-based, two-stage regression estimator. The two-stage regression estimator is described briefly in Section 10.4.4.1 and in more detail elsewhere (Almirall et al., 2009).

The first step in the two-stage regression analysis is to define models for our nuisance functions, f_j. In our example data set, we have six nuisance models, three at the 4-week time point (COMPLY4, EXER4, and VIT4) and three at the 8-week time point (COMPLY8, EXER8, and VIT8). At each time point, we have two dichotomous outcomes (COMPLY and EXER) that we will model using logistic regression models and one continuous outcome (VIT) that we will model with linear regression. Due to our limited sample size ($N = 119$), we performed variable selection in these models using hierarchical stepwise variable selection. For the nuisance models for the second time point (week 4), we fit the main effects (DIET, EXER0, VIT0, and D1) and then all interaction variables with D1. For the nuisance models for the third time point (week 8), we fit the main effects (DIET, D1, D2, VIT4, EXER4, and COMPLY4) and then all interaction variables of the second time point variables with D2.

Our first step in the hierarchical stepwise variable selection was to examine the interactions; if *p*-values for the interactions were > 0.10, they were removed from the model. The second step was to fit the models based on interaction selection and then remove main effect variables with *p*-values > 0.10. As a note, if an interaction was significant we did not remove the main effect of the interaction. Once the final model was determined, we output the predicted probabilities in the data set defined by the OUT statement here (**`out=predCOMPLY4`**) to create the residuals needed for the second stage of the SNMM model. In the following example code, *pCOMPLY4* is the variable for the predicted probabilities from this model.

For the 4-week time point for COMPLY4, a dichotomous variable, the following SAS code was used:

```
proc logistic data=lib1.all_weight_data;
      model COMPLY4(event='1')=DIET EXER0 VIT0 D1
                                D1*DIET D1*EXER0 D1*VIT0;
      output out=predCOMPLY4 pred=pCOMPLY4;
run;
```

In this case, none of the interaction terms were kept in the model (all *p*-values > 0.10) and based on the main effects only model, the variables selected for COMPLY4 were DIET, EXER0, and DIET. We followed the same steps for EXER4 and VIT4. However, for VIT4 we used PROC GLM to fit a linear model using the following SAS code. For continuous variables, we output the residuals directly to a file (**`out=predVIT4`**) to be used for the second stage of the SNMM model. In the following example code, rVIT4 is the variable for the residuals from this model:

```
proc GLM data=lib1.all_weight_data;
      model VIT4=DIET EXER0 VIT0 D1
                 D1*DIET D1*EXER0 D1*VIT0;
      output out=predVIT4 r=rVIT4;
run;
```

For the 8-week time point for COMPLY8, the following SAS code was used:

```
proc logistic data=lib1.all_weight_data;
      model COMPLY8(event='1')=DIET D1
                              D2 VIT4 EXER4 COMPLY4
                              D2*EXER4 D2*VIT4 D2*COMPLY4;
      output out=predCOMPLY8 pred=pCOMPLY8;
run;
```

We followed similar steps for EXER8 and VIT8 (except fit the model using PROC GLM). The following table shows the variables selected using hierarchical stepwise variable selection:

Outcome	Final Model Variables
COMPY4	DIET EXER0 D1
EXER4	EXER0
VIT4	VIT0 D1 D1*VIT0
COMPLY8	COMPLY4 D2
EXER8	EXER4
VIT8	VIT4

Once the final models are set for the nuisance models, we need the parameter estimates from each of the models as well as from the second-stage SNMM model to use as starting values for the likelihood model (Property [18]) that we will run in PROC NLP. Running the models first as a two-stage process is also a good check that everything is set up properly in PROC NLP. As shown here, from each of the nuisance models, we will use either the residuals (from PROC GLM) or predicted values from PROC LOGISTIC to create residuals to be used in the second-stage SNMM model. For the second-stage SNMM, we need to create one file that includes the residuals created from the logistic models as well as the residuals from the linear regression models.

For each dichotomous nuisance model, the following DATA step should be executed using the appropriate file names:

```
data predcomply4;
  set predcomply4;
  res21_comply4=COMPLY4-pCOMPLY4;
  keep subject res21_comply4;
 run;
```

For each continuous nuisance model, the following DATA step should be executed using the appropriate file names:

```
data predvit4;
  set predvit4;
  res21_comply4=pVIT4;
  keep subject res21_VIT4;
 run;
```

Once all the models have been run and the DATA steps have been run for each model, the files with the residuals should be merged with the main data set as follows:

```
proc sort data=lib1.weight_data;
by subject;

data lib1.all_weight_data;
 merge lib1.weight_data predcomply4 predexer4 predvit4 predcomply8
predexer8 predvit8;
 by subject;
run;
```

Macros can also be written to streamline these separate model fits and data merges. Sample macros that do this are available from the second author (Coffman) upon request.

The last step that we need to perform is to create baseline residual variables for inclusion in the second-stage SNMM model. We can do this with intercept only models in either PROC LOGISTIC for dichotomous outcomes or PROC GLM for continuous outcomes and follow the same steps described previously. Or we can find the means and create residuals in the DATA step as shown:

```
data temp;
 set lib1.weight_data;
run;

/* Get means of baseline variables */
proc means data=temp_data mean n print;
 var DIET EXER0 VIT0;
 output out=varmeans;
run;

/* rename mean variables and keep only MEANs */
data varmeans;
 set varmeans (rename=( diet=mean_diet exer0=mean_exer0
vit0=mean_vit0));
 keep mean_diet mean_exer0 mean_vit0;
 if _STAT_="MEAN";
run;

/* Trick for merging data sets, set "dummy" id */
data temp;
 set temp;
 dummy=1;
run;

data varmeans;
 set varmeans;
 dummy=1;
run;
```

```
proc sort data=temp;  by dummy;
proc sort data=varmeans;  by dummy;
run;

data lib1.all_weight_data;
 merge temp varmeans;
 by dummy;
  res14_DIET=DIET-mean_diet;
  res15_EXER0=EXER0-mean_exer0;
  res16_VIT0=VIT0-mean_vit0;
  drop dummy mean_diet mean_exer0 mean_vit0;
run;
```

Now we are ready to run the second-stage SNMM model to get the starting values for the PROC NLP. Because our outcome, VIT16, is continuous, we will run a regression model using PROC GLM as follows:

```
Title "Second stage of model, &sysdate.";
proc glm data=lib1.all weight data;
model vit16=res14_DIET res15_EXER0 res16_VIT0
            D1 D1*DIET D1*EXER0 D1*VIT0
            res21_COMPLY4 res22_EXER4 res23_VIT4
            D2 D2*COMPLY4 D2*EXER4 D2*VIT4
            res31_COMPLY8 res32_EXER8 res33_VIT8
            D3 D3*COMPLY8 D3*EXER8 D3*VIT8;
run;
```

Appendix 10.B

Complete SAS PROC NLP code for the data analysis in Section 10.4; see subsection 10.4.4 for a step-by-step explanation of this code.

The following is the full set of code for PROC NLP for maximizing $loglik_2$ (Property [18]). This code includes the use of starting values from the two-stage regression estimator (see Appendix 10.A):

```
*************************************;
* Use ODS output statements to store ;
* parameter estimates and covariance ;
* matrix from PROC NLP in a data set ;
*************************************;
ods output "Resulting Parameters"= lib1.NLPestimates;
ods output "Covariances"=lib1.NLProbustvarcov;
title "NLP Analysis, data=coffman.all_weight_data, covariance=2
&sysdate. ";

proc nlp data=Coffman.all_weight_data vardef=n covariance=2 sigsq=1;
max loglik;

************************************;
* Starting values for parameters    ;
*  from 2 stage models              ;
************************************;
  PARMS sig2=17.18,sig2_vit4=15.99,sig2_vit8=11.96, sig2_vit0=18.23,

  gamma11_0=         0.0,
  gamma12_0=         0.405,
  gamma13_0=         59.87,
  gamma21_0=         -0.2502     ,
```

```
  gamma21_1=         0.8204      ,
  gamma21_2=         -0.736      ,
  gamma21_3=         -0.0929     ,
  gamma22_0=         1.213 ,
  gamma22_1=         1.1849      ,
  gamma23_0=         20.26176227 ,
  gamma23_1=         0.78232267  ,
  gamma23_2=         -2.20983446 ,
  gamma23_3=         0.03465106  ,
  gamma31_0=         -2.4376     ,
  gamma31_1=         2.3763      ,
  gamma31_2=         -0.2975     ,
  gamma32_0=         0.1178      ,
  gamma32_1=         1.8171      ,
  gamma33_0=         21.94588492 ,
  gamma33_1=         0.7197243   ,
  eta14_res14_DIET=  -6.14788684,
  eta15_res15_EXER20=      -1.62651224,
  eta16_res16_VIT0=  0.55882648,
  Beta0=             65.44918016 ,
  Beta10_D1=         -0.65772698 ,
  Beta14_D1Diet=           -0.2536632  ,
  Beta15_D1exer20=   -0.53823094 ,
  Beta16_D1VIT0=           0.0129085   ,
  eta21_res21_COMPLY4=     -12.87304274      ,
  eta22_res22_EXER24=      0.58517074,
  eta23_res23_VIT4=  0.4379589   ,
  Beta20_D2=         -0.30852128 ,
  Beta21_D2comply4=  -1.71415978 ,
  Beta22_D2exer24=   -1.24239297 ,
  Beta23_D2VIT4=           0.02440274,
  eta31_res31_COMPLY8=     -2.75818127,
  eta32_res32_EXER28=      -0.55345255 ,
  eta33_res33_VIT8=  0.11863987  ,
  Beta30_D3=         1.73649321  ,
  Beta31_D3comply8=  -0.48168742,
  Beta32_D3exer28=   0.03547696,
  Beta33_D3VIT8=           -0.02095646
  ;
    bounds sig2 > 1e-12, sig2_vit0 > 1e-12, sig2_vit4 > 1e-12,
sig2_vit8 > 1e-12;

***********************************;
*  Baseline DIET - Intercept only   ;
***********************************;
    dietlin1=gamma11_0;
    dietp=exp(dietlin1)/(1+exp(dietlin1));
    fdiet=diet*dietp+(1-diet)*(1-dietp);
    ddiet=diet-dietp;

***********************************;
*  Baseline EXER20 - Intercept only ;
***********************************;
    exer20lin1=gamma12_0;
    exer20p=exp(exer20lin1)/(1+exp(exer20lin1));
    fexer20=exer20*exer20p+(1-exer20)*(1-exer20p);
    dexer20=exer20-exer20p;
```

```
*************************************;
*  Baseline VIT0 - Intercept only    ;
*************************************;
    dvit0=VIT0-(gamma13_0);

************;
*  COMPLY4  ;
************;
    comply4lin1=gamma21_0 + gamma21_1*DIET + gamma21_2*EXER20 +
gamma21_3*D1;
    comply4p=exp(comply4lin1)/(1+exp(comply4lin1));
    fcomply4=comply4*comply4p+(1-comply4)*(1-comply4p);
    dcomply4=comply4-comply4p;

************;
*  EXER24   ;
************;
    exer24lin1=gamma22_0 + gamma22_1*EXER20;
    exer24p=exp(exer24lin1)/(1+exp(exer24lin1));
    fexer24=exer24*exer24p+(1-exer24)*(1-exer24p);
    dexer24=exer24-exer24p;

**********;
*  VIT4   ;
**********;
    dvit4=VIT4-(gamma23_0 + gamma23_1*VIT0 + gamma23_2*D1 +
gamma23_3*VIT0*D1);

*************;
*  COMPLY8   ;
*************;
       comply8lin1=gamma31_0 + gamma31_1*COMPLY4+ gamma31_2*D2;
    comply8p=exp(comply8lin1)/(1+exp(comply8lin1));
    fcomply8=comply8*comply8p+(1-comply8)*(1-comply8p);
    dcomply8=comply8-comply8p;

************;
*  EXER28   ;
************;
    exer28lin1=gamma32_0 + gamma32_1*EXER24;
    exer28p=exp(exer28lin1)/(1+exp(exer28lin1));
    fexer28=exer28*exer28p+(1-exer28)*(1-exer28p);
    dexer28=exer28-exer28p;

**********;
*  VIT8   ;
**********;
    dvit8=VIT8-(gamma33_0 + gamma33_1*VIT4);

********************;
*  Outcome - VIT16  ;
********************;
    epsilon= VIT16 -( beta0 + eta14_res14_DIET*ddiet +
eta15_res15_EXER20*dexer20
         + eta16_res16_VIT0*dvit0
         + beta10_D1*D1
         + beta14_D1DIET*D1*DIET + beta15_D1EXER20*D1*EXER20 +
beta16_D1VIT0*D1*VIT0
         + eta21_res21_COMPLY4*dCOMPLY4 + eta22_res22_EXER24*dEXER24
         + eta23_res23_VIT4*dVIT4
         + beta20_D2*D2 + beta21_D2COMPLY4*D2*COMPLY4 +
```

```
beta22_D2EXER24*D2*EXER24
         + beta23_D2VIT4*D2*VIT4
         + eta31_res31_COMPLY8*dCOMPLY8 + eta32_res32_EXER28*dEXER28
         + eta33_res33_VIT8*dVIT8
         + beta30_D3*D3 + beta31_D3COMPLY8*D3*COMPLY8 +
beta32_D3EXER28*D3*EXER28
         + beta33_D3VIT8*D3*VIT8);

*********************;
*  SNMM - Likelihood  ;
*********************;
    loglik =  log(fdiet)+log(fexer20)-log(sig2_vit0)-
(dvit0**2/(2*sig2_vit0**2))
        + log(fcomply4) + log(fexer24)- log(sig2_vit4)-
(dvit4**2/(2*sig2_vit4**2))
        + log(fcomply8)+ +log(fexer28)- log(sig2_vit8)-
(dvit8**2/(2*sig2_vit8**2))
        - log(sig2)-(epsilon**2/(2*sig2**2));

run;
```

Appendix 10.C

Sample PROC IML code used to calculate 95% confidence intervals for linear combinations of interest.

The following code, written in PROC IML, can be used to calculate the 95% confidence intervals for different linear combinations of $\hat{\beta}$ of interest. The sample code shown here shows how to do this for one of the linear combinations described in the results at the end of Section 10.4.5. Namely, this code shows how to calculate a 95% confidence interval for the average impact on the end-of-study vitality of a 5-pound weight loss between weeks 4 and 8, for patients that exercised, adhered to their assigned diet, and have a median week-4 vitality score.

This code relies on two SAS data sets—one holding the parameter estimates (lib1.NLPestimates) and the other holding the variance-covariance matrix (lib1.NLProbustvarcov)—both of which were created during the PROC NLP analyses described previously. The code also requires the user to know the location of the β parameters in the PROC NLP output. For example, from the output shown in Section 10.4.5, it is easy to see that the intercept β_0 is the 28th parameter.

```
proc iml;
   /* define an indexing vector for the beta (causal) estimates */
   /* for example, the 28th parameter was the intercept = beta0 */
   beta0ind = 28; beta1ind = 29:32; beta2ind = 36:39; beta3ind =
43:46;
   betaind = beta0ind || beta1ind || beta2ind || beta3ind;

   /* read in the parameter estimates into a vector called
'estimates'*/
   use lib1.NLPestimates;
   read all var {estimate} into estimates;

   /* using betaind, index only the betas (the causal parameters)*/
   betaestimates = estimates[betaind];
```

```
    /* read in variance-covariance matrix into matrix called 'varcov'*/
    use lib1.NLProbustvarcov;
    read all into varcov;

    /* using betaind, index only the betas portion of varcov*/
    betavarcov = varcov[betaind,betaind];

    /* set the linear combinations of interest */
    /* here we show the combination for a 5lbs */
    /* weight loss between weeks 4 and 8 for   */
    /* patients who comply with their assigned   */
    /* diet, exercise, and have a median week */
    /* 4 vitality score equal to 70.            */
    linearcombo1 = {
          /* set to zero intercept and time 1 betas */
          0,0,0,0,0,
          /* contrasts for beta 2 */
          -5,                /* -5 = D2                  */
          -5,                /* -5*1 = D2*COMPLY4        */
          -5,                /* -5*1 = D2*EXER28         */
          -350,              /* -5*70 = D2*VIT4          */
          /* set to zero intercept and time 3 betas */
          0,0,0,0
          };

    /* calculate the impact on end-of-study vitality */
    effect1 = t(betaestimates) * linearcombo1;
    /* calculate the standard error for effect1 */
    se1 = sqrt( ( t(linearcombo1) * betavarcov ) * linearcombo1 ) ;
    /* calculate the confidence interval for effect1 */
    ci95perct = effect1 + se1*1.96*{-1,1};

    /* print the results */
    print effect1 se1 ci95perct;
quit;
```

References

Almirall, D., T. Ten Have, et al. 2009. “Structural nested mean models for assessing time-varying effect moderation.” *Biometrics* in press.

Baron, R. M., and D. A. Kenny. 1986. “The moderator-mediator variable distinction in social psychological-research: conceptual, strategic, and statistical considerations.” *Journal of Personality and Social Psychology* 51(6): 1173–1182.

Bray, B. C., D. Almirall, R. S. Zimmerman, D. Lynam, and S. A. Murphy. 2006. “Assessing the total effect of time-varying predictors in prevention research.” *Prevention Science* 7(1): 1–17.

Holland, P. W. 1986. “Statistics and causal inference.” *Journal of the American Statistical Association* 81(396): 945–960.

Holland, P. W. 1990. “Rubin's model and its application to causal inference in experiments and observational studies.” *American Journal of Epidemiology* 132(4): 825–826.

Kraemer, H. C., E. Stice, et al. 2001. “How do risk factors work together? Mediators, moderators, and independent, overlapping, and proxy risk factors.” The *American Journal of Psychiatry* 158(6): 848–856.

McHorney, C. A., J. E. Ware, et al. 1992. "The validity and relative precision of MOS short- and long-form health status scales and Dartmouth COOP charts—results from the medical outcomes study." *Medical Care* 30(5): MS253–MS265.

Petersen, M. L., S. G. Deeks, J. N. Martin, and M. J. van der Laan. 2007. "History-adjusted marginal structural models for estimating time-varying effect modification." *American Journal of Epidemiology* 166(9): 985–993.

Robins, J. 1987. "A graphical approach to the identification and estimation of causal parameters in mortality studies with sustained exposure periods." *Journal of Chronic Diseases* 40(Supp 2): S139–S161.

Robins, J. 1989. "The control of confounding by intermediate variables." *Statistics in Medicine* 8(6): 679–701.

Robins, J. M. 1994. "Correcting for non-compliance in randomized trials using structural nested mean models." *Communications in Statistics—Theory and Methods* 23(8): 2379–2412.

Robins, J. M. 1997. "Estimating the causal effects of time varying endogeneous treatments by G-estimation of structural nested models. " *Latent Variable Modeling and Applications to Causality*. Maia Berkane. New York: Springer-Verlag**:** 69–117.

Robins, J. M. 1999a. "Association, causation, and marginal structural models." *Synthese* 121(1–2): 151–179.

Robins, J. M. 1999b. "Marginal structural models versus structural nested models as tools for causal inference." *Statistical Models in Epidemiology: The Environment and Clinical Trials*. Edited by M. E. Halloran and D. Berry. IMA Volume 116. New York: Springer-Verlag, 95–134.

Robins, J. M., A. Rotnitzky, et al. 1994. "Estimation of regression coefficients when some regressors are not always observed." *Journal of the American Statistical Association* 89(427): 846–866.

Robins, J. M., M. A. Hernán, et al. 2000. "Marginal structural models and causal inference in epidemiology." *Epidemiology* 11(5): 550–560.

Rubin, D. B. 1974. "Estimating causal effects of treatments in randomized and nonrandomized studies." *Journal of Educational Psychology* 66(5): 688–701.

Schafer, J. L. 1997. *Analysis of Incomplete Multivariate Data*. London: Chapman and Hall/CRC.

van der Vaart, A. W. 1998. *Asymptotic Statistics*. Cambridge, UK: Cambridge University Press.

Ware, J. E. and C. D. Sherbourne 1992. "The MOS 36-item short-form health survey (SF-36). 1. Conceptual framework and item selection." *Medical Care* 30(6): 473–483.

White, H. 1980. "A heteroskedasticity-consistent covariance-matrix estimator and a direct test for heteroskedasticity." *Econometrica* 48(4): 817–838.

Yancy, W. S., D. Almirall, et al. 2009. "Effects of two weight- loss diets on health-related quality of life." *Quality of Life Research* 18(3): 281–289.

Yancy, W. S., M. K. Olsen, J. R. Guyton, R. P. Bakst, and E. C. Westman. 2004. "A low-carbohydrate, ketogenic diet versus a low-fat diet to treat obesity and hyperlipidemia—A randomized, controlled trial." *Annals of Internal Medicine* 140(10): 769–777.

Chapter 11

Regression Models on Longitudinal Propensity Scores

Aristide Achy-Brou
Michael Griswold
Constantine Frangakis

Abstract

Estimating causal treatment effect in longitudinal, observational data can be complex due to the need to control for selection bias in the full history of covariates used in the treatment assignment. Having a robust approach to deal with the lack of randomization between treatment groups is critical because the history of covariates used in the treatment assignment grows rapidly with the length of the observation period.

We present regression estimators that can compare longitudinal treatments using only the longitudinal propensity scores as regressors. These estimators, which assume knowledge of the variables used in the treatment assignment, are important for reducing the large dimension of covariates for two reasons. First, if the regression models on the longitudinal propensity scores are correct, then these estimators share advantages of correctly specified likelihood-based estimators, a benefit not shared by estimators based on weights alone. Second, if the models are incorrect, the misspecification can be more easily limited through model checking than with models based on the full covariates. Thus, the proposed estimators can also be used in place of the regression on the full covariates.

We analyze data from a naturalistic schizophrenia study using Regression Models on Longitudinal Propensity Scores (RMLPS). SAS code for performing the analysis is provided, and output using data from the schizophrenia study is examined.

11.1 Introduction

Our goal is to estimate the effects of longitudinal treatments in observational studies in the presence of treatment-assignment confounding using Regression Models on Longitudinal

Propensity Scores (RMLPS) (Achy-Brou et al., 2009; Segal et al., 2007). In such studies, there is a need to control the growing dimension of history variables that predict the assignment of treatments. The longer the observation period, the more acute the problem of dealing with this common treatment-assignment confounding issue becomes.

One method for estimating these effects is through Robins's G-computation formula (1987). This method has rarely been used because it generally needs to adjust for the entire history of the longitudinal covariates. This adjustment is subject to model misspecification as the numerous models are difficult to check and fix. For this reason, the most widely used methods for estimating the effect of sustained longitudinal treatments are derived from the Horvitz-Thompson (1952) inverse propensity score weighting approach using marginal structural models (Robins et al., 2000). These methods are quite useful for providing generally consistent estimators when the propensity scores are correct. However, they can be inefficient because they do not directly use the available covariate information except through augmentations of the estimators (Tsiatis, 2006). The augmentation methods, though, do not compete but rather can be used in combination with RMLPS.

Using RMLPS to estimate causal effects is a generalization of the widely used approach based on regression models on the propensity scores introduced by Rosenbaum and Rubin (1983, 1984) for single time treatment. To better appreciate the more fundamental role of the propensity score, consider the setting where the scores are known and only those scores are kept as summaries of the patients' histories. The optimal statistical methods for using the propensity scores should use only the subclassification of patients that these scores define, not the actual values.

We now provide the essential notation and steps of the RMLPS approach. The times where a treatment can change are denoted by $t = 1, 2, \ldots T$. At each time, let $z_t = 1, 2, \ldots K$ indicate the levels of the treatment. If patient i would have taken some longitudinal treatment of interest, $z = (z_1, z_2, \ldots, z_T)$, we let $Y_i(z) = Y_i(z_1, z_2, \ldots, z_T)$ be the potential outcome that is observed at the evaluation time period (Neyman, 1928; Rubin, 1974, 1978). Note that the treatment regime of interest, z, may be different from the treatment regime actually observed for given patients. For a particular longitudinal treatment, we are interested in estimating outcome quantities such as $E\{Y_i(z)\}$, which is the expectation we would observe if all patients received a particular longitudinal treatment. For the ith patient, let $X_{i,t}^{obs}$ be the vector of variables observed after the patient received a specific treatment at time $t-1$ but before taking a specific treatment at time t. Let the actual treatment received be denoted by $Z_{i,t}$, and let Z_i be the vector of these treatment assignments. Let the patient history, $H_{i,t}$, be the cumulative information observed before the patient received treatment at time t, that is:

$$H_{i,t} = \{ (X_{i,1}^{obs}, Z_{i,1}), \ldots (X_{i,t-1}^{obs}, Z_{i,t-1}), X_{i,t}^{obs} \}.$$

Let Y_i^{obs} denote the observed outcome at the end of the last period, which, based on the potential outcomes notation, is equal to $Y_i(Z_i)$. Finally, let the conditional probability for the ith subject at time point t to receive treatment k, $Z_{i,t} = z$, given the history $H_{i,t}$, be denoted by:

$$e_{i,t,z} = \Pr(Z_{i,t} = z \mid H_{i,t}),$$

which is the propensity score.

We wish to compare outcomes among such possible longitudinal treatments. Note that this comparison is not the same as the comparison between the observed distribution of outcome in each longitudinal treatment group versus its observed control (everyone not in that specific longitudinal treatment group) or the comparison between observed distributions of outcome in each longitudinal treatment group.

Given that only one treatment assignment is actually made for each patient at each time point, and that the treatment assignment, or adherence to original treatment assignment, can change over the observation period, this contrast of interest is not directly observable. We need the three usual assumptions underpinning any estimation of the causal effects of longitudinal treatment in observational studies. The first assumption is that the patients are a random sample drawn from the appropriate reference population. The second assumption, already implicit in the notation $Y_i(\mathbf{z})$, is that the treatment assignment for one patient does not affect the outcome of a different patient (stable unit treatment values [SUTVA]) (Rubin, 1978). The third assumption is that all variables related to treatment assignment have been measured, in the sense that, conditional on the observed variables up to a particular time, the assignment to the treatment at the next time is random (sequential ignorability) (Robins, 1987).

11.2 Estimation Using Regression on Longitudinal Propensity Scores

Under these three stated assumptions, Achy-Brou and colleagues (2009) showed that an evaluation of $E\{Y(z)\}$ may be done using the g-computation formula (Robins, 1987) where the history of the full covariates is replaced by the history of propensity scores:

$$E\{Y(z)\} = \sum_{e1, z1, \ldots, eT, zT} \Pr(Y^{obs} \mid e_{1,z1}, Z_1^{obs} = z1, \ldots e_{T,zT}, Z_T^{obs} = z_T) \,.$$

$$\Pr(e_{1,z1}) \ldots \Pr(e_{1,z1}, Z_1^{obs} = z1, \ldots e_{T-1,zT-1}, Z_{T-1}^{obs} = z_{T-1})$$

Thus, given models for $\sum_{e1, z1, \ldots, eT, zT} \Pr(Y^{obs} \mid e_{1,z1}, Z_1^{obs} = z1, \ldots e_{T,zT}, Z_T^{obs} = z_T)$, $\Pr(e_{1,z1})$, … and $\Pr(e_{1,z1}, Z_1^{obs} = z1, \ldots e_{T-1,zT-1}, Z_{T-1}^{obs} = z_{T-1})$, we can estimate the causal effects of the longitudinal treatments in an observational study. The key advantage of the formula used in Achy-Brou and colleagues (2009) over the g-computation formula is that the dimension of the covariates in the models is dramatically reduced. This is useful because models for the regressions on the propensity scores can be built and checked more easily. Here we illustrate how the estimation algorithm works in practice. We also include the steps needed to check and improve the accuracy of the models used in the estimation. First, using a greedy stepwise selection algorithm based on the Akaike Information Criterion (AIC), we select the best performing transition and outcome models among the class of models with various interaction terms. Then, for each treatment, we rerun the estimation of the outcome models' coefficients using only patients who received that specific treatment. Using only patients who received the specific treatment is desirable when we have a good sample size and we want to minimize any of the side effects associated with borrowing strength across different treatment groups. The important point is that the proposed approach allows you to easily try different models and to understand what parts of the data carry more information.

11.3 Example

11.3.1 Study Description

Simulated data based on a schizophrenia study (Tunis et al., 2006) utilized to demonstrate a marginal structural model analysis in Chapter 9 are also used here to illustrate the RMLPS approach. Refer to Chapter 9 or Tunis and colleagues (2006) for details. In brief, we compare the effectiveness of two groups of medications (labeled treatments 1 and 2) at the end of the 1-year treatment period as assessed by the total score from the Brief Psychiatric Rating Scale (BPRS), a measure of schizophrenia symptom severity where lower scores indicate lesser symptom severity. The follow-up period was naturalistic, thus patients were allowed to switch or discontinue as in usual care.

11.3.2 Data Analysis

The analysis follows the 6-step algorithm presented by Segal and colleagues (2007):

- form a multinomial
- propensity model
- classify propensity scores into strata
- estimate transition probabilities of the longitudinal propensity strata
- estimate expected outcomes for the longitudinal treatment patterns of interest
- estimate the average potential outcome over all patients for the longitudinal treatment patterns of interest
- obtain uncertainty estimates using bootstrapping

The analysis data set was structured based on one observation per patient per visit, with all potential confounder variables and outcome measures. For simplicity of presentation, our analysis focused only on the outcome at the final visit for all patients who continued in the study through the final visit. The treatment comparison of interest was between continuous use of treatment 1 and continuous use of treatment 2. Table 11.1 summarizes the medication switching patterns over time during the study. There was more switching from treatment 2 to treatment 1 and few patients with the reverse pattern.

Table 11.1 also includes a summary of the outcome variable (change from baseline to endpoint in BPRS total score) by treatment pattern. Mean reductions in symptoms were largest for the group that started and stayed on treatment 1.

Table 11.1 Numbers of Patients Following Each Medication Treatment Pattern and Unadjusted Mean Changes in Outcome Scores (BPRS Total) at the Final Visit

		Time 3	
Time 1	Time 2	Trt 1	Trt 2
Trt 1	Trt 1	N = 273 Mean(SD): -13.2 (13.8)	N = 3 Mean(SD): -5.4 (15.0)
	Trt 2	N = 0	N = 6 Mean(SD): -7.7 (11.4)
Trt 2	Trt 1	N = 6 Mean(SD): -6.4 (14.4)	N = 0
	Trt 2	N = 10 Mean(SD): -9.4 (14.2)	N = 54 Mean(SD): -11.4 (14.9)

Analysis Steps 1 and 2

The first step of the analysis involves estimating the propensity scores and classifying propensity scores into five strata for each of the three time periods (visits) assessed in this analysis. Program 11.1 demonstrates the SAS code to perform these steps. PROC LOGISITIC is used to estimate the probability of receiving treatment 1. The model includes as covariates a set of a priori selected variables—designed to cover demographic variables and the domains of symptom severity, functioning, tolerability, and major medical resource utilization. The output data set (Predtrt) containing the estimated propensity scores is created for later analysis. In Step 2, the propensity scores are ranked by visit, and five strata for each visit are created using quintile cutoff scores. This is accomplished using PROC RANK.

An assessment of the overlap in propensity score distributions and the balance created using the propensity score should be conducted at this step. There are several approaches to assessing the overlap and the quality of the propensity model, as discussed by Austin (2008). In this example, we provide simple evaluations of the distribution of the propensity scores by treatment group for visit 7 (because the final visit was the key visit for this analysis) and an assessment of treatment imbalance in key covariates before and after propensity score adjustment.

The propensity score distributions had adequate overlap. Propensity score adjustment generally reduced the imbalance in covariate scores between the groups. However, there is no strong indication of selection bias in these data prior to adjustment because none of the variables were statistically different.

Program 11.1 Estimation of Longitudinal Propensity Models

```
*********************************************************************;
*  STEP 1: Estimate the Propensity Models                          *;
*     PROC LOGISTIC is used to estimate propensity scores and output *;
*     to a data set where they are ranked and formed into quintile   *;
*     subgroups in the next step.  PREDTRT1 is the propensity score  *;
*     (probability of receiving treatment 1)                         *;
*********************************************************************;

ODS LISTING CLOSE;
PROC LOGISTIC DATA = INPDS;
  CLASS VIS THERAPY GENDER RACE B_HOSP B_EVNT P_HOSP P_EVNT;
  MODEL TRT = VIS AGEYRS GENDER RACE B_HOSP B_EVNT B_GAF B_BPRS P_EVNT
              P_HOSP P_BPRS P_GAF;
  OUTPUT OUT = PREDTRT PRED = PREDTRT1;
  run;
ODS LISTING;
```

Program 11.2 Stratification of Longitudinal Propensity Scores

```
*********************************************************************;
*  STEP 2: Categorize propensity scores into 5 strata              *;
*     PROC RANK is used for form quintile subgroups. BIN_PS is the   *;
*     variable denoting the subgroup (propensity score bin). At this *;
*     step one should assess the propensity score distributions to   *;
*     confirm sufficient overlap in scores between treatment groups  *;
*     and check the balance in covariates achieved between treatment *;
*     groups before and after adjustment. Simple output is used here *;
*     but histograms, boxplots and other graphics could be of value. *;
*********************************************************************;

PROC SORT DATA = PREDTRT;
  BY VIS; RUN;

PROC RANK DATA = PREDTRT GROUPS = 5 OUT = RANKPS;
  BY VIS;
  RANKS RNK_PREDTRT1;
  VAR PREDTRT1 ;
run;

DATA RANKPS;
  SET RANKPS;
  BIN_PS = RNK_PREDTRT1 + 1;
run;

    * THERE ARE 3 POSTBASELINE VISITS IN THIS ANALYSIS DATA SET *;
DATA V5 V6 V7;
  SET RANKPS;
  IF VIS = 5 THEN OUTPUT V5;
  IF VIS = 6 THEN OUTPUT V6;
  IF VIS = 7 THEN OUTPUT V7;
run;

    * A BRIEF EVALUATION OF PROPENSITY BALANCE IS HERE *;

PROC SORT DATA = RANKPS;
  BY VIS TRT; RUN;
```

```
PROC UNIVARIATE DATA = RANKPS;
  BY VIS TRT;
  VAR PREDTRT1;
  TITLE 'Distribution of propensity scores'; RUN;
PROC FREQ DATA = RANKPS;
  TABLES VIS*BIN_PS*TRT;
  TITLE 'Therapy distribution among bins by visit'; RUN;
```

Output from Program 11.2

```
                    Distribution of propensity scores

  ---------------------------------- VIS=7 TRT=T_1 ---------------------------------

                           The UNIVARIATE Procedure
                    Variable:  PREDTRT1  (Estimated Probability)

                                   Moments

            N                          324    Sum Weights                324
            Mean                 0.8057059    Sum Observations    261.048713
            Std Deviation       0.03392898    Variance            0.00115118
            Skewness            -0.0941572    Kurtosis            0.27851063
            Uncorrected SS      210.700319    Corrected SS        0.37182968
            Coeff Variation     4.21108704    Std Error Mean      0.00188494

                            Quantiles (Definition 5)

                            Quantile          Estimate

                            100% Max          0.905350
                            99%               0.885617
                            95%               0.866251
                            90%               0.844593
                            75% Q3            0.827277
                            50% Median        0.806746
                            25% Q1            0.782808
                            10%               0.765259
                            5%                0.748839
                            1%                0.720833
                            0% Min            0.708961

  ---------------------------------- VIS=7 TRT=T_2 ---------------------------------

The UNIVARIATE Procedure
                    Variable:  PREDTRT1  (Estimated Probability)

                                   Moments

            N                           79    Sum Weights                 79
            Mean                0.79685171    Sum Observations    62.9512849
            Std Deviation       0.03829261    Variance            0.00146632
            Skewness            -0.2814442    Kurtosis            0.13622492
            Uncorrected SS      50.2772121    Corrected SS        0.11437325
            Coeff Variation     4.80548728    Std Error Mean      0.00430825

                            Quantiles (Definition 5)

                            Quantile          Estimate

                            100% Max          0.883209
                            99%               0.883209
                            95%               0.853460
```

(continued)

Output *(continued)*

```
                    90%              0.844921
                    75% Q3           0.825901
                    50% Median       0.794077
                    25% Q1           0.774749
                    10%              0.752936
                    5%               0.720296
                    1%               0.694857
                    0% Min           0.694857


Therapy distribution among bins by visit
                  Controlling for VIS=7

                BIN_PS
                          TRT(TREATMENT PRESCRIBED AT THIS VISIT
                            (A_C,_B_,__C,A__,___) /TRT/)
```

Frequency / Percent / Row Pct / Col Pct	T_1	T_2	Total
1	58 14.39 72.50 17.90	22 5.46 27.50 27.85	80 19.85
2	63 15.63 77.78 19.44	18 4.47 22.22 22.78	81 20.10
3	69 17.12 85.19 21.30	12 2.98 14.81 15.19	81 20.10
4	66 16.38 81.48 20.37	15 3.72 18.52 18.99	81 20.10
5	68 16.87 85.00 20.99	12 2.98 15.00 15.19	80 19.85
Total	324 80.40	79 19.60	403 100.00

Table 11.2 Summary of Covariate Balance before and after Propensity Score Strata Adjustment (Visit 7)

	Before Subclassification		After Subclassification	
Covariate	*F*-Statistic	*P*-value	*F*-Statistic	*P*-value
Age	.09	.767	.03	.871
Baseline GAF	.42	.517	.02	.895
Baseline BPRS	.18	.669	.10	.748
Previous GAF	1.23	.268	.86	.354
Previous BPRS	2.58	.109	.47	.492
	Chi-Square Statistics	*P*-value	Chi-Square Statistic	*P*-value
Previous Event	.66	.416	.05	.820
Previous Hosp	.02	.879	.04	.840

Analysis Step 3

In Step 3, estimated probabilities of transitioning between the longitudinal propensity score strata are computed. PROC LOGISTIC in the macro EST (see Program 11.3) conducts the initial calculations for the transition probabilities. A proportional odds logistic model is run, with the propensity score bin as the dependent variable (five possible values) and a simple model with the previous visit's treatment and propensity bins as covariates. Data manipulation of the output data set is required in order to modify the output cumulative values into the transition values necessary for later analysis steps. At the end of this section, we have included data sets with the transition probabilities for visit 5 to visit 6 and from visit 6 to visit 7 (TRPR_V6 and TRPR_V7).

Program 11.3 Estimation of Transition Probabilities

```
**********************************************************************;
*  STEP 3: Estimate transitional probabilities of the longitudinal   *;
*  propensity score strata. The first part of this section creates   *;
*  an analysis data set with variables to denote the propensity      *;
*  score bin and treatment at each visit (data set UPD which is then *;
*  merged with visitwise analysis data sets). Summary statistics on  *;
*  the propensity score bins and treatments over time can be easily  *;
*  summarized using PROC FREQ. The EST macro runs a proportional     *;
*  odds logistic regression model to assess the transitional         *;
*  probabilities for each possible combination of propensity bin     *;
*  over time. The steps following the macro compute the transition   *;
*  probabilities from the parameter estimates of the logistic model  *;
**********************************************************************;

    * Input for macro denotes the visit number *;
%MACRO PM(VN);

  DATA F1_&VN;
    SET &VN;
    BIN_PS_&VN = BIN_PS;
    TRT_&VN = TRT;
    KEEP PATSC BIN_PS_&VN TRT_&VN;
  RUN;
```

Program 11.3 *(continued)*

```
%PM(V5); RUN;
%PM(V6); RUN;
%PM(V7); RUN;

PROC SORT DATA = F1_V5; BY PATSC; RUN;
PROC SORT DATA = F1_V6; BY PATSC; RUN;
PROC SORT DATA = F1_V7; BY PATSC; RUN;

DATA UPD;
  MERGE F1_V5 F1_V6 F1_V7;
  BY PATSC;

PROC FREQ DATA = UPD;
        TABLES BIN_PS_V5*BIN_PS_V6*BIN_PS_V7;
        TITLE 'PATTERN OF BINS OVER TIME'; RUN;
PROC FREQ DATA = UPD;
        TABLES TRT_V5 TRT_V6 TRT_V7 TRT_V5*TRT_V6*TRT_V7;
        TITLE 'PATTERN OF TRTS OVER TIME'; RUN;

PROC SORT DATA = UPD; BY PATSC; RUN;
PROC SORT DATA = V5; BY PATSC; RUN;
PROC SORT DATA = V6; BY PATSC; RUN;
PROC SORT DATA = V7; BY PATSC; RUN;

DATA V5;
  MERGE V5 UPD;
  BY PATSC;
DATA V6;
  MERGE V6 UPD;
  BY PATSC;
DATA V7;
  MERGE V7 UPD;
  BY PATSC;

ODS LISTING CLOSE;

 /* Input for macro includes the analysis data set for a specific visit (INDAT), name
for the output data set containing the parameter estimates (PARM_EST), list of
variables for the CLASS statement (CLASSVARS), and list of variables in the MODEL
statement (MODELVARS).  Run macro for the 2nd and 3rd time points to assess
transitions.             */

%MACRO EST(INDAT, PARM_EST, CLASSVARS, MODELVARS);

  PROC LOGISTIC DATA = &INDAT OUTEST = &PARM_EST;
    CLASS &CLASSVARS;
    MODEL BIN_PS =  &MODELVARS;
   RUN;

%MEND EST;

%EST(V6, PARM_V6, TRT_V5 BIN_PS_V5, TRT_V5 BIN_PS_V5); RUN;
%EST(V7, PARM_V7, TRT_V5 BIN_PS_V5 TRT_V6 BIN_PS_V6, TRT_V5 BIN_PS_V5 TRT_V6
BIN_PS_V6); RUN;

ODS LISTING;

 /* Data trpr_v7 uses the parameter estimates output from the EST macro to compute
the actual transition probabilities for time period 2 to 3. Arrays are used in order
to more efficiently calculate the 250 different transition probabilities (5x5x5x2:  5
propensity bins at each of 3 time points for each of two treatment patterns of
interest).    */
```

Program 11.3 *(continued)*

```
   DATA TRPR_V7;
     SET PARM_V7;
     IF _TYPE_ = 'PARMS';

   * parameters are set to zero automatically in SAS modeling and are
     specifically set to zero here for clarity.                        *;

     INTERCEPT_5 = 0;
     BIN_PS_V55 = - BIN_PS_V51 - BIN_PS_V52 - BIN_PS_V53 - BIN_PS_V54;
     BIN_PS_V65 = - BIN_PS_V61 - BIN_PS_V62 - BIN_PS_V63 - BIN_PS_V64 ;
     TRT_V5T_2 = - TRT_V5T_1;
     TRT_V6T_2 = - TRT_V6T_1;

      X1 = INTERCEPT_1;
      X2 = INTERCEPT_2;
      X3 = INTERCEPT_3;
      X4 = INTERCEPT_4;
      X5 = INTERCEPT_5;

      Y1= BIN_PS_V51;
      Y2= BIN_PS_V52;
      Y3= BIN_PS_V53;
      Y4= BIN_PS_V54;
      Y5= BIN_PS_V55;

      Z1= BIN_PS_V61;
      Z2= BIN_PS_V62;
      Z3= BIN_PS_V63;
      Z4= BIN_PS_V64;
      Z5= BIN_PS_V65;

      W1= TRT_v5T_1;
      W2= TRT_v5T_2;
      V1= TRT_v6T_1;
      V2= TRT_v6T_2;
   run;

 DATA TRPR_V7;
   SET TRPR_V7;
    ARRAY X[5] X1 - X5;
    ARRAY Y[5] Y1 - Y5;
    ARRAY Z[5] Z1 - Z5;
    ARRAY W[2] W1 - W2;
    ARRAY V[2] V1 - V2;
    ARRAY PRE[5, 5, 5, 2 ];

    DO A = 1 TO 2;             * LOOP FOR 2 TREATMENT GROUPS    *;
      DO I = 1 TO 5;           * LOOP FOR BINS AT TIME PERIOD 3 *;
        DO J = 1 TO 5;         * LOOP FOR BINS AT TIME PERIOD 1 *;
          DO K = 1 TO 5;       * LOOP FOR BINS AT TIME PERIOD 2 *;

   * Computation of probabilities using logistic model. Initial (pre)
     probabilites are cumulative as they are from proportional odds
     model - and are adjusted to individual outcome probabilities here*;
         PRE[I, J, K, A ]= EXP(X[I] + W[A] + V[A] + Y[J] + Z[K]) / (1 +
                           EXP(X[I] + W[A] + V[A] + Y[J] + Z[K]));
         TRPR7 = PRE[I, J, K, A ];

         IF 2 LE I LE 4 THEN DO;
           TRPR7 = PRE[I, J, K, A ] - (EXP(X[I-1] + W[A] + V[A] + Y[J] +
                   Z[K]) / (1 + EXP(X[I-1] + W[A] + V[A] + Y[J] +
                   Z[K])));
        END;
```

Program 11.3 (*continued*)

```
        IF I = 5 THEN DO;
          TRPR7 = 1 - (EXP(X[I-1] + W[A] + V[A] + Y[J] + Z[K]) / (1 +
                  EXP(X[I-1] + W[A] + V[A] + Y[J] + Z[K])));
        END;
        OUTPUT;

        END;
       END;
      END;
    END;;
  KEEP A I J K TRPR7;


* Repeat the same process for trpr_v6 as for trpr_v7.  Here there are 50 transitional
probabilities to compute.          *;

  DATA TRPR_V6;
    SET PARM_V6;
    IF _TYPE_ = 'PARMS';

     INTERCEPT_5 = 0;
     BIN_PS_V55 = - BIN_PS_V51 - BIN_PS_V52 - BIN_PS_V53 - BIN_PS_V54;
     TRT_V5T_2 = - TRT_V5T_1;

     X1 = INTERCEPT_1;
     X2 = INTERCEPT_2;
     X3 = INTERCEPT_3;
     X4 = INTERCEPT_4;
     X5 = INTERCEPT_5;

     y1= BIN_PS_V51;
     y2= BIN_PS_V52;
     y3= BIN_PS_V53;
     y4= BIN_PS_V54;
     y5= BIN_PS_V55;

     z1= TRT_V5T_1;
     z2= TRT_V5T_2;
run;

 DATA TRPR_V6;
   SET TRPR_V6;
   ARRAY X[5] X1 - X5;
   ARRAY Y[5] Y1 - Y5;
   ARRAY Z[2] Z1 - Z2;
   ARRAY PRE[5, 5, 3 ];     /* it is a three-dimensional array */

   DO A = 1 TO 2;
     DO K = 1 TO 5;
       DO J= 1 TO 5;

         PRE[K, J, A]= EXP(X[K] + Y[J] + Z[A]) / (1 + EXP(X[K] + Y[J] +
                       Z[A]));
         TRPR6 = PRE[K, J, A];

         IF 2 LE k LE 4 THEN DO;
           TRPR6 = PRE[K, J, A]  -  (EXP(X[K-1] + Y[J] + Z[A]) / (1 +
                   EXP(X[K-1] + Y[J] + Z[A])));
         END;
```

Program 11.3 *(continued)*

```
        IF K = 5 THEN DO;
          TRPR6 = 1 - (EXP(X[K-1] + Y[J] + Z[A]) / (1 + EXP(X[K-1] +
                  Y[J] + Z[A])));
       END;
       OUTPUT;

       END;
    END;
  END;
 KEEP A J K TRPR6 SECTION6; RUN;
```

Analysis Step 4

In this step, we estimate the expected outcomes for the longitudinal treatment patterns of interest. Specifically, we are interested in the expected outcomes for treatment 1 at all time periods and treatment 2 at all time points. PROC GENMOD (with the NORMAL distribution for our continuous outcome measure) was used to estimate the expected values. The model, with the change in outcome measure at endpoint as the dependent measure, included the previous treatments and previous propensity score strata as dependent measures. The final result of this step is an analysis data set containing the predicted values for each treatment and propensity bin combination over time (2*5*5*5 = 250 combinations: two treatment patterns of interest and 125 propensity bin combinations) —along with the probabilities of those transitions from Step 3. An example listing of this data set (ALL) is provided after Program 11.4.

The listing shows that a patient on treatment 1 at time point 1 in propensity strata 1 had a 56% chance of being in strata 1 at time 2. Furthermore, a patient in strata 1 at time 2 had a 69% chance of remaining in strata 1 at time 3. The expected outcome of a patient on treatment 1 at each time point and in propensity strata 1 at each time point was -8.6.

Program 11.4 Estimation of Expected Outcomes for each Transition Path

```
*********************************************************************;
*  STEP 4: Estimate longitudinal treatment expected outcomes in      *;
*    groups of interest (AAA and BBB). This code runs a simple model *;
*    with only the treatment and propensity score bins at each time- *;
*    point included as covariates and the outcome measure as the     *;
*    dependent variable. This macro can be used to assess sensitivity*;
*    via comparisons with other models.  After the macro call, the   *;
*    parameter estimates are output to a data set to allow for       *;
*    calculation of the expected outcome for all possible transition *;
*    paths (all treatment and propensity bin options over time).     *;
*********************************************************************;

DATA V7;
  SET V7;
  TRT_V5_  = TRT_V5;
  TRT_V6_  = TRT_V6;
  TRT_V7_  = TRT_V7;

DATA OUTCV7;
  SET RANKPS;
  IF VIS = 7;
  KEEP PATSC BAVAR AVAR CAVAR;

PROC SORT DATA = V7; BY PATSC; RUN;
```

```
PROC SORT DATA = OUTCV7; BY PATSC; RUN;

DATA ADAT7;
  MERGE V7 (IN=A) OUTCV7 (IN=B);
  BY PATSC;
  IF A AND B;

          * Summary statistics on analysis data set *;
PROC MEANS DATA = ADAT7;
  CLASS TRT_V5_ TRT_V6_ TRT_V7_;
  VAR CAVAR;
  TITLE2 'SUMMARY STATS FROM ADAT7'; run;

PROC TABULATE DATA = ADAT7;
  CLASS TRT_V5_ TRT_V6_ TRT_V7_;
  VAR BAVAR CAVAR;
  TABLES (TRT_V5_*TRT_V6_*TRT_V7_)*(N MEAN STD),(BAVAR CAVAR);
  TITLE2 'SUMMARY STATS FROM ADAT7'; run;

/* Input for macro includes the analysis data set for a specific visit
(DATA_2), name for the output data set containing the parameter estimates
(DATA_1), list of variables for the CLASS statement (CLASSVAR2), and list
of variables in the MODEL statement (MODELVAR2).  */


%MACRO G_ESTS(DATA_2, DATA_1, CLASSVAR2, MODELVAR2);

 ODS OUTPUT ParameterEstimates= &data_1 ;
 PROC GENMOD DATA = &DATA_2;
   CLASS &CLASSVAR2;
   MODEL CAVAR = &MODELVAR2 / DIST = NOR LINK = ID;
   run;

%MEND G_ESTS;

%g_ests(ADAT7, vis7_OUTCESTS, TRT_V5_ TRT_V6_ TRT_V7_ BIN_PS_V5
   BIN_PS_V6 BIN_PS_V7, TRT_V5_ TRT_V6_ TRT_V7_ BIN_PS_V5 BIN_PS_V6
   BIN_PS_V7);
run;

    * get parameter estimates from model to allow computation *;
    * of expected values for all transition paths            *;

DATA VIS7_OUTCESTS;
  SET VIS7_OUTCESTS;
  KEEP PARAMETER LEVEL1 ESTIMATE;

PROC TRANSPOSE DATA = VIS7_OUTCESTS OUT=TR_OUTCESTS;
  RUN;

DATA TR_OUTCESTS;
  SET TR_OUTCESTS;
   INTERCEPT = COL1;
    X1 = COL2;  * TRT AT V5 *;
    X2 = COL3;
    Y1 = COL4;  * TRT AT V6 *;
    Y2 = COL5;
    Z1 = COL6;  * TRT AT V7 *;
    Z2 = COL7;
```

```
    B1=COL8; B2=COL9; B3=COL10; B4=COL11; B5=COL12;   * BIN AT V5 *;
    C1=COL13; C2=COL14; C3=COL15; C4=COL16; C5=COL17; * BIN AT V6 *;
    L1=COL18; L2=COL19; L3=COL20; L4=COL21; L5=COL22; * BIN AT V7 *;
run;

 DATA OUTC;
   SET TR_OUTCESTS;
   ARRAY X[2] X1 - X2;
   ARRAY Y[2] Y1 - Y2;
   ARRAY Z[2] Z1 - Z2;
   ARRAY B[5] B1 - B5;
   ARRAY C[5] C1 - C5;
   ARRAY L[5] L1 - L5;
   ARRAY PRE[2, 5, 5, 5 ];

   DO A = 1 TO 2;
    DO J = 1 TO 5;
      DO K = 1 TO 5;
          DO I = 1 TO 5;

   PRE[A, J, K, I ]= COL1 + X[A] + Y[A] + Z[A] + B[J] + C[K] + L[i];
               EOUT = PRE[A, J, K, I ];
               OUTPUT;

         END;
       END;
      END;
    END;
  run;


 DATA OUTC;
   SET OUTC;
   KEEP A J K I EOUT;
     run;

PROC SORT DATA = TRPR_V7; BY A J K I; RUN;
PROC SORT DATA = OUTC; BY A J K I; RUN;
PROC SORT DATA = TRPR_V6; BY A J K; RUN;

DATA ALL1;
  MERGE TRPR_V7 OUTC;
  BY A J K I;

DATA ALL;
  MERGE ALL1 TRPR_V6;
  BY A J K;
  SUM_EO = EOUT*(.2)*TRPR6*TRPR7;
  IF A = 1 THEN TRTPTTRN = 'AAA';
  IF A = 2 THEN TRTPTTRN = 'BBB';

PROC PRINT DATA = ALL;
  VAR TRTPTTRN J K I TRPR6 TRPR7 EOUT;
  TITLE 'LISTING OF DATASET ALL (TRANSITION PROBS AND EXPECTED OUTCOMES)';
RUN;
```

Output from Program 11.4

LISTING OF DATASET ALL (TRANSITION PROBS AND EXPECTED OUTCOMES

Obs	TRTPTTRN	J	K	I	TRPR6	TRPR7	EOUT
1	AAA	1	1	1	0.56184	0.68756	-8.5755
2	AAA	1	1	2	0.56184	0.23807	-10.9945
3	AAA	1	1	3	0.56184	0.05502	-13.0868
4	AAA	1	1	4	0.56184	0.01634	-17.8012
5	AAA	1	1	5	0.56184	0.00301	-20.6457
6	AAA	1	2	1	0.28214	0.48647	-11.0129
7	AAA	1	2	2	0.28214	0.35624	-13.4318
8	AAA	1	2	3	0.28214	0.11345	-15.5242
9	AAA	1	2	4	0.28214	0.03687	-20.2385
10	AAA	1	2	5	0.28214	0.00697	-23.0830
11	AAA	1	3	1	0.11399	0.22977	-12.3396
12	AAA	1	3	2	0.11399	0.39809	-14.7585
13	AAA	1	3	3	0.11399	0.24504	-16.8509
14	AAA	1	3	4	0.11399	0.10530	-21.5652
15	AAA	1	3	5	0.11399	0.02180	-24.4097
. . . .							
125	AAA	5	5	5	0.62377	0.75457	-17.1169
. . . .							

Analysis Step 5

This step utilizes the output of Steps 3 and 4 (contained in data set ALL) to estimate the average of the potential outcomes for the longitudinal treatment patterns of interest (treatment 1 at all time points [denoted AAA] and treatment 2 at all time points [denoted BBB]). This is accomplished using simple summations of the appropriate probabilities in data set ALL. The summation produces an estimated treatment difference favoring treatment 1 of 2.5 points on the BPRS scale (see Output from Program 11.5).

Program 11.5 Estimation of Outcomes in Treatment Patterns of Interest

```
******************************************************************;
*  STEP 5: Estimate the average, over all patients, of the potential *;
*    outcomes for longitudinal treatment groups of interest (AAA vs  *;
*    BBB).  This code uses the expected values for all patterns      *;
*    created in step 4 and sums the values across the corresponding  *;
*    patterns of interest.  The final estimates are then printed.    *;
******************************************************************;

PROC SORT DATA = ALL;
  BY A; RUN;

DATA ALL;
  SET ALL;
  IF A = 1 THEN DO; * COUNTERS FOR TREATMENT 1 *;
    WTEST_AAA + SUM_EO;
    SUM_TRPR6A + TRPR6;
    SUM_TRPR7A + TRPR7;
  END;
  IF A = 2 THEN DO; * COUNTERS FOR TREATMENT 2 *;
    WTEST_BBB + SUM_EO;
    SUM_TRPR6B + TRPR6;
    SUM_TRPR7B + TRPR7;
  END;
  DUM = 1;
```

```
PROC SORT DATA = ALL;
  BY DUM; RUN;

DATA ALL;
  SET ALL;
  BY DUM;
  IF LAST.DUM;
  DIFF = WTEST_AAA - WTEST_BBB;
  KEEP WTEST_AAA WTEST_BBB DIFF;

PROC PRINT DATA = ALL;
  TITLE 'FINAL ESTIMATE DATASET';
  TITLE2 'WTEST_AAA: ESTIMATED RESPONSE FOR LONGITUDINAL TREATMENT PATTERN
AAA';
  TITLE3 'WTEST_BBB: ESTIMATED RESPONSE FOR LONGITUDINAL TREATMENT PATTERN
BBB';
  TITLE4 'DIFF: ESTIMATED DIFFERENCE IN RESPONSE BETWEEN TWO TREATMENT
PATTERNS';
RUN;
```

Output from Program 11.5

```
                         FINAL ESTIMATE DATASET
     WTEST_AAA: ESTIMATED RESPONSE FOR LONGITUDINAL TREATMENT PATTERN AAA
     WTEST_BBB: ESTIMATED RESPONSE FOR LONGITUDINAL TREATMENT PATTERN BBB
    DIFF: ESTIMATED DIFFERENCE IN RESPONSE BETWEEN TWO TREATMENT PATTERNS

                              WTEST_       WTEST_
                     Obs        AAA          BBB          DIFF

                      1      -13.0024     -10.1465     -2.85589
```

Analysis Step 6

In this step, Steps 3 through 5 are repeated using a bootstrap algorithm (5,000 replications used here) in order to estimate the variability of our propensity score sub-classification treatment difference estimate. The specific code is not shown, but simply creates a loop to repeat the process 5,000 times and output the resulting treatment difference estimate. The distribution of treatment difference estimates is summarized by PROC UNIVARIATE. Using the percentile method, the 95% 2-sided confidence interval was found to be (-6.91, 1.30) with a corresponding *p*-value of 0.185.

Output from Analysis Step 6

```
               SUMMARY STATS ON BOOTSTRAP DIFFERENCES: AAA - BBB

                          The UNIVARIATE Procedure
                              Variable:  DIFF

                                  Moments

      N                        5000    Sum Weights               5000
      Mean               -2.7978146    Sum Observations    -13989.073
      Std Deviation      2.09761783    Variance            4.40000058
      Skewness           0.02795663    Kurtosis            -0.1326878
      Uncorrected SS     61134.4344    Corrected SS        21995.6029
      Coeff Variation    -74.973441    Std Error Mean       0.0296648
```

(*continued*)

Output from Analysis Step 6 *(continued)*

```
                Basic Statistical Measures

       Location                    Variability

   Mean      -2.79781     Std Deviation            2.09762
   Median    -2.79368     Variance                 4.40000
   Mode       .           Range                   14.18360
                          Interquartile Range      2.87671


                 Tests for Location: Mu0=0

      Test           -Statistic-     -----p Value------

      Student's t    t  -94.3143     Pr > |t|    <.0001
      Sign           M     -2028     Pr >= |M|   <.0001
      Signed Rank    S  -5878113     Pr >= |S|   <.0001


                  Quantiles (Definition 5)

                  Quantile         Estimate

                  100% Max        4.8827501
                  99%             1.9440237
                  95%             0.6811120
                  90%            -0.0688069
                  75% Q3         -1.3916694
                  50% Median     -2.7936758
                  25% Q1         -4.2683819
                  10%            -5.4915107
                  5%             -6.2668682
                  1%             -7.6076745
                  0% Min         -9.3008516

                Frequency Counts
                           Percents
           Value Count  Cell   Cum
              . . .
   -6.908590145030     1   0.0   2.5
              . . .
    1.295190177818     1   0.0  97.5
```

Sensitivity / Model Checks

As mentioned previously, a key feature of using regression on the longitudinal propensity score is that we can more easily check the relative validity of the models. Here we present SAS code (Program 11.6) to graphically depict the predictive accuracy of the outcome model. The code produces a scatterplot of the predicted and actual means for each bin and treatment combination—with the area of each plotted circle representing the sample size in each longitudinal subclass. From the output, there are noted outliers, though all subclasses of reasonable sample sizes were well predicted by the model.

To further assess the validity of the models, we also followed the two approaches presented in Section 11.2. First, we assessed model improvement for both the transition and outcome models using the AIC criteria. Second, we re-ran the outcome model using only the subset of patients who did not switch treatments during the study. The AIC criteria can be assessed by modifying the MODEL (transition and outcome) statements in the EST (Program 11.3) and G_ESTS (Program 11.4) macros (not shown). For these data, the AIC was slightly improved by the inclusion of the treatment interactions (for example, visit 5 by visit 6 and visit 6 by visit 7 interactions) and the treatment by propensity bin interactions (for example, visit 5 treatment by visit 5 bin). However, the inferences from this model were the same and the model was less stable—with a much larger variance from the bootstrap evaluation. Thus, the simple model results are retained here. The same SAS code was also used to assess the outcome using the subset of patients not switching treatments during the study. This was accomplished by modifying the data set entering the analysis macros. Once again, inferences from this approach were similar.

Program 11.6 Graphical Assessment of Analysis Models

```
*******************************************************;
** Graph of observed and expected outcomes to assist  **;
** in model assessment                                 **;
*******************************************************;

PROC MEANS DATA = ADAT7 NOPRINT;
  CLASS TRT_V5_ TRT_V6_ TRT_V7_ BIN_PS_V5 BIN_PS_V6 BIN_PS_V7;
  VAR CAVAR;
  OUTPUT OUT = MEANOUT N = NPT MEAN = AVGVAL; RUN;

DATA OUTC;
  SET OUTC;
  BIN_PS_V5 = J;
  BIN_PS_V6 = K;
  BIN_PS_V7 = I;
DATA MEANOUT;
  SET MEANOUT;
  IF (TRT_V5_ = 'T_1' AND TRT_V6_ = 'T_1' AND TRT_V7_ ='T_1' AND
        BIN_PS_V5 NE . AND BIN_PS_V6 NE . AND BIN_PS_V7 NE .) OR
     (TRT_V5_ = 'T_2' AND TRT_V6_ = 'T_2' AND TRT_V7_ ='T_2' AND
        BIN_PS_V5 NE . AND BIN_PS_V6 NE . AND BIN_PS_V7 NE .);
  IF TRT_V5_ = 'T_1' AND TRT_V6_ = 'T_1' AND TRT_V7_ ='T_1' THEN A = 1;
  IF TRT_V5_ = 'T_2' AND TRT_V6_ = 'T_2' AND TRT_V7_ ='T_2' THEN A = 2;

PROC SORT DATA = OUTC; BY A BIN_PS_V5 BIN_PS_V6 BIN_PS_V7; RUN;
PROC SORT DATA = MEANOUT; BY A BIN_PS_V5 BIN_PS_V6 BIN_PS_V7; RUN;

DATA GRPH;
  MERGE OUTC (IN=X) MEANOUT (IN=Y);
  BY A BIN_PS_V5 BIN_PS_V6 BIN_PS_V7;
  IF X AND Y;

TITLE 'Scatterplot of Expected and Actual Outcomes by Bin/Treatment
Trajectory';

SYMBOL1 C=RED V=CIRCLE;
AXIS1 LABEL = (ANGLE=90 "OBSERVED OUTCOME")  ORDER = (-70 TO 20 BY 10);
AXIS2 LABEL = (ANGLE=0 "EXPECTED OUTCOME")  ORDER = (-70 TO 20 BY 10);

PROC GPLOT DATA=GRPH;
 BUBBLE AVGVAL*EOUT = NPT / vaxis = axis1 haxis = axis2;
 PLOT AVGVAL*EOUT = 1 / vaxis = axis1 haxis = axis2;
RUN;
```

Output from Program 11.6

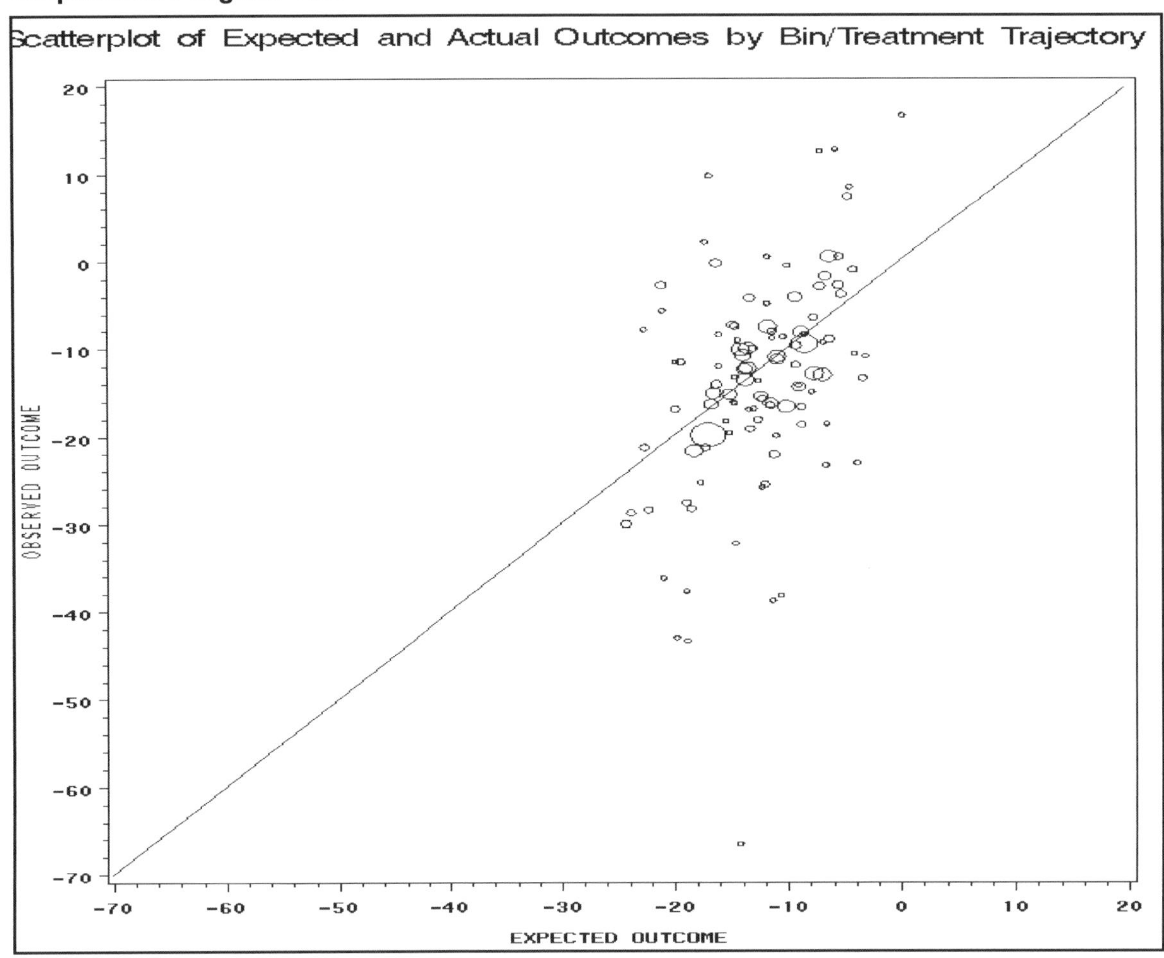

11.4 Summary

The method presented in this chapter can be viewed first as an extension of the propensity score regression adjustment methods to a longitudinal setting. It can also be seen as a robust, yet easier, way of applying and extending g-computation-based methods by replacing the full covariate history with the longitudinal propensity scores. In the chapter, we gave a quick and practical overview of the methodology and presented a detailed illustration of the steps needed to evaluate longitudinal treatment using regression models on the propensity scores.

References

Achy-Brou, A. C., C. E. Frangakis, and M. Griswold. "Estimating treatment effects of longitudinal designs using regression models on propensity scores." *Biometrics*. Published online October 10, 2009. DOI: 10.1111/j.1541-0420.2009.01334.x.

Austin, P. C. 2008. "Goodness-of-fit diagnostics for the propensity score model when estimating treatment effects using covariate adjustment with the propensity score." *Pharmacoepidemiology and Drug Safety* 17(12): 1202–1217.

Horvitz, D. G., and D. J. Thompson. 1952. "A generalization of sampling without replacement from a finite universe." *Journal of the American Statistical Association* 47: 663–685.

Neyman, J. 1928. "On the application of probability theory to agricultural experiments. Essay on principles." Section 9, translated. 1990. *Statistical Science* 5: 465–80.

Robins, J. M. 1987. "A graphical approach to the identification and estimation of causal parameters in mortality studies with sustained exposure periods." *Journal of Chronic Diseases* 40, Supplement 2: 139S–161S.

Robins, J. M., M. A. Hernán, and B. Brumback. 2000. "Marginal structural models and causal inference in epidemiology." *Epidemiology* 11: 550–560.

Rosenbaum, P. R, and D. B. Rubin. 1983. "The central role of the propensity score in observational studies for causal effects." *Biometrika* 70: 41–55.

Rosenbaum, P. R., and D. B. Rubin. 1984. "Reducing bias in observational studies using subclassification on the propensity score." *Journal of the American Statistical Association* 79: 516–24.

Rubin, D. B. 1974. "Estimating causal effects of treatments in randomized and nonrandomized studies." *Journal of Educational Psychology* 66(5): 688–701.

Rubin, D. B. 1978. "Bayesian inference for causal effects: the role of randomization." *Annals of Statistics* 6: 34–58.

Segal, J. B., M. Griswold, A. C. Achy-Brou, and R. Herbert. 2007. "Using propensity scores subclassification to estimate effects of longitudinal treatments: an example using a new diabetes medication." *Medical Care* 45: S149–157.

Tsiatis, A. A. 2006. *Semiparametric Theory and Missing Data* (page 336). New York: Springer-Verlag.

Tunis, S. L., D. E. Faries, A. W. Nyhuis, B. J. Kinon, H. Ascher-Svanum, and R. Aquila. 2006. "Cost-effectiveness of olanzapine as first-line treatment for schizophrenia: results from a randomized, open-label, 1-year trial. *Value in Health* 9(2): 77–89.

Part 4

Claims Database Research

Chapter 12

Good Research Practices for the Conduct of Observational Database Studies

Bradley C. Martin
Brenda Motheral
John Brooks
Bill Crown
Peter Davey
Dave Hutchins
Paul Stang

Abstract

Retrospective databases describing health information have become a common source of data for investigators to explore a wide range of economic, epidemiologic, safety, and effectiveness studies. This chapter describes an abridged checklist containing 10 of the most important points to consider when evaluating or designing a retrospective database study. As a quick guide, the 10 points are described summarily in table form followed by a more detailed discussion of each point. This checklist can be viewed as a guide to assess the nuances commonly encountered in retrospective observational studies in the health care arena. Some familiarity with general research principles is assumed and, in order to adequately assess some questions, relevant research training or additional reading will be required.

12.1 Introduction

Retrospective databases describing health information have become a common source of data for investigators to explore a wide range of economic, epidemiologic, safety, and effectiveness studies. An important strength of most retrospective databases is that they allow researchers to examine medical care utilization as it occurs in routine clinical care. They often provide large study populations and longer observation periods, allowing for examination of specific subpopulations. In addition, retrospective databases provide a relatively inexpensive and expedient approach for answering the time-sensitive questions posed by decision makers. Two recent studies have suggested that adequately controlled observational studies produce results similar to randomized controlled trials (Concato et al., 2000; Benson and Hartz, 2000). Analyses derived from retrospective observational sources also present an array of limitations and factors that must be considered when conducting an investigation. Because treatment patterns and outcome measures are only observed and never randomized, investigators must overcome selection bias, or endogeneity, that influences treatment selection and the propensity to have some outcome of interest. In addition to the issues of selection bias, researchers using retrospective data sources, particularly those derived from paid claims not collected for research purposes, must address other factors such as data quality including missing data, HIPAA, timeliness, developing appropriate operational definitions, and local coding conventions and practice patterns.

In 2000, the International Society for Pharmacoeconomics and Outcomes Research (ISPOR) convened an expert panel to develop good research practice guidelines for retrospective database studies. The panel members met and developed several drafts and presented prior versions of the checklist to the ISPOR membership at their U.S. and European meetings to solicit feedback resulting in a checklist accepted by the ISPOR Board of Directors in 2002. The complete checklist has been published (Motheral et al., 2003) and is available on the Internet (http://www.ispor.org/workpaper/healthscience/ret_dbTFR0203.asp). In 2008–2009, ISPOR as well as the U.S. Food and Drug Administration (FDA) were developing additional guidelines on the conduct of observational studies to estimate treatment effects derived from retrospective data sources. Interested readers should follow up with these organizations to identify the latest guidance. The guidelines that are being developed at the time of this writing will offer readers more clarity and detail regarding specific research design and statistical issues common in these types of studies.

The checklist presented in this chapter represents an abridged checklist containing 10 of the most important points to consider when evaluating a retrospective database study. The complete checklist contains 27 points or questions and should be used when designing a retrospective study or when a more thorough and detailed review of a retrospective database study is warranted, such as when one is serving as a journal referee.

Numerous databases are available for use by researchers, particularly within the U.S. Because the databases have varying purposes, their content can vary dramatically. Accordingly, the unique advantages and disadvantages of a particular database must be considered. In conducting or reviewing a database study, it is important to assess whether the database is suitable for addressing the research question and whether the investigators have used an appropriate methodology in reaching the study conclusions. While the checklist was written in the form of 10 questions to guide readers and decision-makers as they consider a database study, it can also serve as a guide to researchers designing, analyzing, or reporting retrospective studies. This checklist is intended to raise general issues, not to offer detailed prescriptive recommendations. Some familiarity with general research principles is assumed and, in order to adequately assess some questions, relevant research training or additional reading will be required. This is particularly true for assessing questions relating to statistics. Other important issues in the use of retrospective databases, including patient confidentiality, credibility, and study sponsorship, are not addressed in this checklist. Readers should consult with their own professional society's guides and their own institutional guidelines on conflicts of interest, research involving human subjects, or other guidelines to inform them on these important issues. Other chapters in this text describe the statistical techniques and the SAS programming steps that can be used to implement some of the issues covered in this chapter; however, this checklist does not offer specific SAS programming steps.

12.1.1 How Should the Checklist Be Used?

This checklist was developed primarily for the commonly used medical claims or encounter-based databases but could potentially be used to assess retrospective studies that employ other types of databases, such as disease registries and national survey data. The checklist is meant to serve as a supplement to already available checklists for economic evaluations (Clemens et al., 1995; Weinstein et al., 1996). Only those issues that are unique to database studies or are particularly problematic in database research were included in the checklist. Not every question will be applicable to every study, but the checklist should prompt researchers to at least consider important factors affecting the quality of the study.

12.2 Checklist and Discussion

CHECKLIST

Topic	Question
1. **Database Relevance**	Has the database content and study population been described in sufficient detail to determine the rationale for using the database to answer the research question and to assess how the findings can be interpreted in the context of other organizations?
2. **Database Quality**	Have the reliability and validity of the data been described, including any data quality checks and handling of missing data?
3. **Research Plan**	Has an a priori research plan been developed, including a rationale for selecting the particular research design, and have the potential limitations of that design been acknowledged?
4. **Sample Selection**	Have inclusion and exclusion criteria been used to derive the final sample from the initial population, has the rationale for their use been described, and has the impact of these criteria on sample representativeness been discussed?
5. **Variable Definitions**	Has a rationale and/or supporting literature for the selection criteria and variable definitions been provided and were sensitivity analyses performed for definitions or criteria that are controversial, uncertain, or novel?
6. **Resource Valuation**	For studies that examine costs, has a method and rationale for valuing resources (costs, charges, payments, fee schedules) been described, and is it consistent with the study perspective?
7. **Confounding**	If the goal of the study is to examine treatment effects, have the authors adequately controlled for confounding variables through use of a comparison group *and* i) multivariate statistical techniques or ii) stratification of the sample by different levels of the confounding variables to compare outcomes?
8. **Statistical Analysis**	Have the appropriate statistical techniques been used, taking into account the particular nuances of utilization and cost data, such as skewness and correlations within and among population subgroups?

Topic	Question
9. Practical Significance	Has the practical significance of the findings been explained by discussing the statistical versus clinical or economic significance of the results and the variance explained/goodness of fit of the statistical models?
10. Theoretical Basis	Has a theory for the findings been provided and have alternative explanations for the observed findings been discussed?

1. *Relevance:* Has the database content and study population been described in sufficient detail to determine the rationale for using the database to answer the research question and to assess how the findings can be interpreted in the context of other organizations?

   Each database represents a particular situation in terms of study population, benefit coverage, and service organization. To appropriately interpret a study, key attributes should be described, including the sociodemographic and health care profile of the population, limitations on available services, such as those imposed by socialized medicine, plan characteristics, and benefit design (for example, physician reimbursement approach, cost-sharing for office visits, drug exclusions, mental health carve outs). For example, in an economic evaluation that compares two drugs, it would be important to know the formulary status of the drugs as well as any other pharmacy benefit characteristics that could affect the use of the drugs, such as step therapy, compliance programs, and drug utilization review programs.

2. *Data Quality:* Have the reliability and validity of the data been described, including any data quality checks and handling of missing data?

   With any research data set, quality assurance checks are necessary to determine the reliability and validity of the data, keeping in mind that reliability and validity are not static attributes of a database but can vary dramatically depending on the questions asked and the analyses performed. Quality checks are particularly important with administrative databases from health care payers and providers because the data were originally collected for purposes other than research, most often for claims processing and payment. This fact creates a number of potential challenges for conducting research.

   First, services may not be captured in the claims database because the particular service is not covered by the plan sponsor or because the service is carved out and not captured in the data set (for example, mental health). Second, data fields that are not required for reimbursement may be particularly unreliable. Similarly, data from providers who are paid on a capitated basis often have limited utility because providers may not be required to report detailed utilization information. Third, changes in reporting/coding over time or differences across study groups can result in unreliable data as well. It is common for procedure codes and drug codes, among others, to change over time, and the frequency with which particular codes are used can change over time as well, often in response to changes in health plan reimbursement policies.

   For all these reasons, investigators should describe the quality assurance checks performed and any steps taken to normalize the data or otherwise eliminate data suspected to be unreliable or invalid, particularly when there is the potential to bias results to favor one study group over another (for example, outliers). The authors should describe any relevant changes in reporting/coding that may have occurred over time and how such variation affects the study findings. Data quality should be addressed even when the data have been pre-processed (for example, grouped into episodes) prior to use by the researcher. Examples of important quality checks include missing and out-of-range values, consistency of data (for example, patient age), claim duplicates, and comparison of data figures to established norms (for example, rates of asthma diagnosis compared with prevalence figures). Some studies cite previous literature in which the database's reliability and validity have been examined.

3. *A Priori Research Plan:* Has an a priori research plan been developed, including a rationale for selecting the particular research design, and have the potential limitations of that design been acknowledged?

   One of the easiest ways to drive results in a certain direction would be to impose post hoc changes in the research plan or design. A research plan describing sample inclusion criteria, variable definitions, model specifications, and statistical approaches should be developed prior to initiating the research and the results based on the a priori plan should be described. Naturally, investigators acquire new knowledge through the conduct of a study, and it is often important to implement post hoc design changes. The research report, however, should clearly describe any post hoc decisions and, when relevant, report the results of both the a priori plan and after applying any post hoc decisions.

   Many research designs (for example, pre-post with control group) are available to the investigator, each with particular strengths and weaknesses, depending on setting, research question, and data. The investigator should provide a clear rationale for the selection of the design and describe the salient strengths and weaknesses of the design, including how potential biases will be addressed.

4. *Sample Selection:* Have inclusion and exclusion criteria been used to derive the final sample from the initial population, has the rationale for their use been described, and has the impact of these criteria on sample representativeness been discussed?

   The inclusion/exclusion criteria are the minimum rules that are applied to each potential subject's data in an effort to define a study group(s). Regardless of the database used, the inclusion/exclusion criteria can dramatically change the composition of the study group(s). Has a description been provided of the subject number for the total population, sample and after application of each inclusion and exclusion criterion? In other words, is it clear who and how many individuals were excluded and why?

   Second, was there a discussion of the impact of study inclusion and exclusion criteria on study findings, because the inclusion/exclusion criteria can bias the selection of the population and distort the applicability of the study findings? For example, continuous eligibility during the study period is a common inclusion criterion for database studies. However, in government entitlement programs where eligibility is determined monthly, limiting the study population to only those with continuous eligibility would tend to include the sickest patients because they would most likely remain in conditions that make them eligible for coverage. The extent to which this would affect the applicability of study findings depends upon the study question.

5. *Variable Definitions:* Has a rationale and/or supporting literature for the selection criteria and variable definitions been provided and were sensitivity analyses performed for definitions or criteria that are controversial, uncertain, or novel?

   Operational definitions are required to identify cases (subjects) and endpoints (outcomes), often using diagnoses codes, medication uses, and/or procedure codes to indicate the presence or absence of a disease or treatment. The operational definition(s) for all variables should be provided because different definitions can potentially lead to different results and interpretations. For example, investigators attempting to identify group(s) of persons with a particular disorder (Alzheimer's disease) should provide a rationale and, when possible, cite evidence that a particular set of coding (ICD-9-CM, CPT-4, Drug Intervention) criteria is valid. Ideally, this evidence would take the form of validation against a primary source but more often will involve the citation of previous research.

When there is controversial evidence or uncertainty about such definitions, the investigator should perform a sensitivity analysis using alternative definitions to examine the impact of these different ways of defining events. Sensitivity analysis tests different values or combinations of factors that define a critical measure in an effort to determine how those differences in definition affect the results and interpretation. Databases allow investigators to perform sensitivity analyses in a hierarchical fashion, or *caseness*, where the analysis is conducted using different definitions or levels of certainty (for example, definite, probable, and possible cases).

For economic evaluations, a particularly challenging issue is the identification of disease-related costs in a claims database. For example, when studying depression, does one include only services with a depression diagnosis, those with a depression-related code (for example, anxiety), or all services regardless of the accompanying diagnosis code? As mentioned earlier, sensitivity analyses of varying operational definitions are important in these situations.

6. *Resource Valuation:* For studies that examine costs, has a method and rationale for valuing resources (costs, charges, payments, fee schedules) been described, and is it consistent with the study perspective?

   As with any economic evaluation, reviewers should ensure that the resource costs included in the analysis match the responsibilities of the decision-maker whose perspective is taken in the research. For example, if the study is from the perspective of the insurer, the resource list should include only those resources that will be paid for by the insurer, which would exclude member co-pays and noncovered services (for example, over-the-counter medications).

   Likewise, the resource should be valued in a manner that is consistent with the perspective. For a variety of reasons, the resource price information available within retrospective databases may provide an imperfect measure of the actual resource price. Typically, claims data provide a number of cost figures, including the submitted charge, eligible charge, amount paid, and member co-pay. The perspective of the study determines which cost figure to use. Rarely would charge be used as few, if any, actually pay this price. When the perspective is the insurer or plan sponsor, one typically expects the amount paid to be used to value the resource consumed. However, if trying to generalize findings beyond a specific plan, an investigator may use an average discount off charge minus an average member co-pay to arrive at an amount paid. This standardized amount is then applied to actual utilization.

   That said, reported costs may not always reflect additional discounts, rebates, and other negotiated arrangements. These additional price considerations can be particularly important for economic evaluations of drug therapies, where rebates can represent a significant portion of the drug cost. In addition, prices will vary over time with inflation and across geographic areas with differences in the cost of living. In most cases, prices should be adjusted to a reference year and place using relevant price indexes.

7. *Confounding:* If the goal of the study is to examine treatment effects, have the authors adequately controlled for confounding variables through use of a comparison group *and* i) multivariate statistical techniques or ii) stratification of the sample by different levels of the confounding variables to compare outcomes?

One of the greatest dangers in retrospective database studies is incorrectly attributing an effect to a treatment that is actually due, at least partly, to some other variable. If the investigation attempts to make inferences about a particular intervention, a design in which there is no control group is rarely adequate. Without a control group (persons not exposed to an intervention) or comparison group (persons exposed to a different intervention), there often exist too many potential biases that could otherwise account for an observed treatment effect. Even with a control group, failure to account for the effects of all variables that have an important influence on the outcome of interest can lead to biased estimates of treatment effects. Two common approaches for addressing this problem include using regression modeling techniques and stratifying the sample by different levels of the confounding variables, comparing treatments within strata/potential confounders (for example, age, gender). Each of these approaches has strengths and weaknesses.

8. *Statistical Analysis:* Have the appropriate statistical techniques been used, taking into account the particular nuances of utilization and cost data, such as skewness and correlations within and among population subgroups?

   Statistical methods are based upon a variety of underlying assumptions. Often these stem from the distributional characteristics of the data being analyzed. As a result, in any given retrospective analysis, some statistical methods will be more appropriate than others. Authors should explain the reasons why they chose the statistical methods that were used in the analysis. There is rarely, if ever, a statistical estimation approach that is singularly the most appropriate. When there is uncertainty in selecting various statistical or modeling approaches, sensitivity analyses should ideally be conducted to explore the impact the modeling approach has on study findings. There are instances when the modeling approach can have profound impacts on the study results, particularly when contrasting instrumental variable approaches with traditional regression-based approaches (Stukel et al., 2007).

9. *Practical Significance:* Has the practical significance of the findings been explained by discussing the statistical versus clinical or economic significance of the results and the variance explained/goodness of fit of the statistical models?

   In retrospective database studies, the sample sizes are often extremely large, which can render potentially unmeaningful differences to be statistically significantly different. Furthermore, in studies with relatively small sample sizes, the large variance in cost data can render meaningful differences statistically insignificant. Accordingly, it is imperative that both the statistical and the clinical or economic relevance of the findings be discussed.

   In addition, authors should provide the reader with information about how well the model predicts what it is intended to predict. Numerous approaches, such as goodness of fit or split samples, can be used. For example, in ordinary least squares regression models, the adjusted R-square, which measures the proportion of the variance in the dependent variable explained by the model, is a useful measure. Nonlinear models have less intuitive goodness-of-fit measures. Models based on micro-level data (for example, patient episodes) can be good fits even if the proportion of the variance in the outcome variable that they explain is 10% or less. In fact, models based on micro-level data that explain more than 50% of the variation in the dependent variable should be viewed with suspicion.

10. *Theoretical Basis:* Has a theory for the findings been provided and have alternative explanations for the observed findings been discussed?

    Because large sample sizes render many statistically significant findings of questionable meaning, it is essential that the investigator provide a theory (economic, clinical, behavioral, and so on) that explains the observed findings. The examination of causal relationships is a particular challenge with retrospective database studies because subjects are not randomized to treatments. Accordingly, the burden is on the author to rule out plausible alternative explanations to the findings when examining relationships between two variables.

Acknowledgments

We would like to recognize the efforts of Fredrik Berggren, James Chan, Mary Ann Clark, Sueellen Curkendall, Bill Edell, Shelah Leader, Marianne McCollum, Newell McElwee, and John Walt, who are reference group members that provided comments on earlier drafts.

References

Benson, K., and A. J. Hartz. 2000. "A comparison of observational studies and randomized, controlled trials." *The New England Journal of Medicine* 342(25): 1878–1886.

Clemens, K., R. Townsend, F. Luscombe, et al. 1995. "Methodological and conduct principles for pharmacoeconomic research." *PharmacoEconomics* 8(2):1 69–174.

Concato, J., N. Shah, and R. I. Horwitz. 2000. "Randomized, controlled trials, observational studies, and the hierarchy of research designs." *The New England Journal of Medicine* 342(25): 1887–1892.

Motheral, B., J. Brooks, M. A. Clark, et al. 2003. "A checklist for retrospective database studies—report of the ISPOR task force on retrospective databases." *Value in Health* 6(2): 90–97.

Stukel, T. A., E. S. Fisher, D. E. Wennberg, et al. 2007. "Analysis of observational studies in the presence of treatment selection bias: effects of invasive cardiac management on AMI survival using propensity score and instrumental variable methods." The *Journal of the American Medical Association* 297 (3): 278–285.

Weinstein, M. C., J. E. Siegel, M. R. Gold, S. Mark, et al. 1996. "Recommendations of the panel on cost-effectiveness in health and medicine." The *Journal of the American Medical Association* 276(15): 1253–1258.

Chapter 13

Dose-Response Safety Analyses Using Large Health Care Databases

Ouhong Wang
Xiang Ling

Abstract

The marginal structural models (MSM) method has been introduced in Chapter 9 in a traditional two-group comparison setting. In this chapter, the application of MSM is demonstrated using a large observational database to assess dose response of a single treatment that's dynamic over time. The endpoint is mortality, which frequently is the focus of analyses performed using such databases.

13.1 Introduction

13.1.1 Overview

While clinical trials in a controlled environment provide the basis for regulatory approval, large-scale observational databases are usually the means for long-term safety assessment. Statistical methods are critical in dealing with such databases because the data almost without exception suffer from confounding, sometimes even time-dependent confounding. In this chapter the marginal structural models (MSMs) approach is illustrated in analyzing safety information using such a database. It uses inverse probability of treatment weights to create a pseudo-randomized population to facilitate causal inferences. The association between treatments and safety signals is less confounded and, under the assumption of no model misspecification, may even have a causal interpretation. The approach is demonstrated using a dialysis claims database to study the Epoetin alfa dose relationship with mortality. This large-scale database contains additional variables that are not often found in smaller databases, and through the MSM analysis, these additional variables enabled us to reduce the impact of confounding and to more precisely estimate the hazard ratios associated with treatment dosage.

We first introduce some background information on the complex and dynamic interactions among end-stage renal disease (ESRD), anemia, and dialysis treatment, together with some conventional analyses that attempt to assess the dose-mortality relationship. The fact that these analyses suffer from apparent confounding makes it clear that more sophisticated causal inference methods should be applied. Next, we describe in detail the database used and its structure that facilitates the MSM analysis. Following the technical details presented in Chapter 9, we then describe the setup of the treatment model, the censoring model, and the structural model that we used to carry out the MSM analysis. SAS code and the main SAS output are included. Results are interpreted based on these outputs, and some discussions are provided on the caveats in performing analysis using MSM.

13.1.2 Disease, Treatment, and Analysis Background

Patients who suffer from kidney failure almost always experience anemia as a co-morbid condition. This is because erythropoietin, a protein that regulates red blood cell production, is produced in the kidney. End-stage renal disease results in decreased production of erythropoietin by the kidneys, which then causes low levels of hemoglobin, or anemia. Dialysis treatment helps maintain the body's internal equilibrium of water and minerals, but it does not compensate for the lost erythropoietin function. Therefore, an important aspect of dialysis treatment is anemia management. Over the years, the standard of care in the dialysis setting has evolved to routinely include erythropoiesis-stimulating agents, or ESAs. ESAs are proteins that function as endogenous erythropoietin but are manufactured using recombinant DNA technology. The clinical benefit of ESAs is to increase the red blood cell level, measured by hemoglobin (Hb, in g/dL). An ESA that has been used since the early 1990's is Epoetin alfa (Epogen, Amgen Inc., Thousand Oaks, CA).

Some analyses based on observational data have attempted to assess the safety outcomes of Epoetin alfa. The most noticeable analysis involved association between Epoetin alfa dose and mortality using conventional Cox model, with dose as a baseline or time-dependent variable. For example, the analysis conducted by Zhang and colleagues (2004) seemed to show a clear trend of higher mortality associated with higher dose. This finding was replicated using the same statistical method by Bradbury and colleagues (2008) (Figure 13.1). Using a more granular data set, Bradbury and colleagues (2008) showed that the hazard ratio (HR) was approximately 1.22 using dose at baseline, and it dropped to around 1.0 when dose was used as a time-dependent variable.

Figure 13.1 Conventional Cox Regression Results

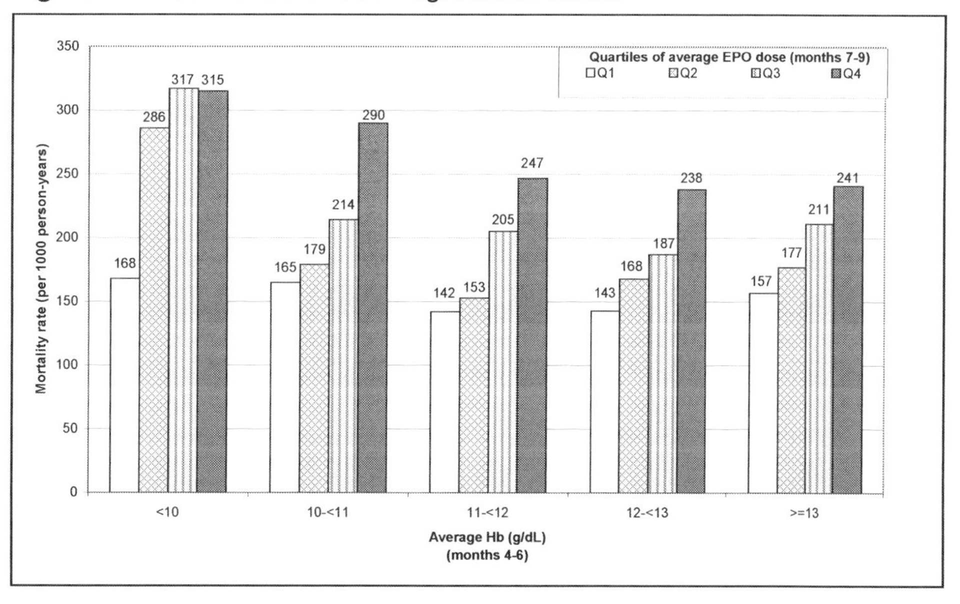

However, it is well recognized that sicker patients have lower Hb levels and are likely to be prescribed higher doses of Epoetin alfa. The sicker patients also are more likely to die. This is a classic confounding problem for point treatment cases. Moreover, observed Hb levels affect subsequent Epoetin alfa dose prescription, which in turn impacts the following Hb level. In order to maintain a certain Hb level, Epoetin alfa doses need to be adjusted periodically. Therefore, it's a typical time-dependent confounding problem. As mentioned in Chapter 9, traditional inferences in this situation, including Cox proportional hazard models with time-dependent treatment, do not have a causal interpretation. This is because the assumptions required for a causal interpretation do not hold due to the presence of confounding. In order to assess the causal relationship between Epoetin alfa doses and mortality, more sophisticated statistical methods are called for, and we used a marginal structural model as an alternative (Robins et al., 2000; Hernán et al., 2000).

We have obtained medical records data from one of the dialysis chains. A subset of patient data collected by this dialysis chain is available to us under private utilization agreements. These data include patient demographics, ESA doses, Hb levels, and co-morbid conditions. Numerous analyses have been done using data from dialysis chains to understand treatment effects and improve patient care.

Note that another example demonstrating the MSM application is discussed in Chapter 9. However, this chapter is different because the outcome here is survival. We discuss a single treatment at different doses instead of two treatment groups, and dose response is our focus rather than a comparison between two treatment groups.

13.2 Data Structure

Before we dive into the MSM analysis details, let's first understand the database at hand. This dialysis chain provides hemodialysis to more than 100,000 patients in the United States and collects information on laboratory parameters, medications, demographic characteristics, dialysis care, and clinical outcomes, including hospitalization and death. For this analysis, data were available for a random sample of 60,000 hemodialysis patients who were at least 18 years of age with no history of peritoneal dialysis and who received hemodialysis for at least 1 month between July 2000 and June 2002. We restricted our study population to patients whose first appearance in the database was before January 2001 and who had a 6-month baseline period to allow for patient characterization. Patients were followed up for 12 months.

Most laboratory parameters (for example, albumin, ferritin, transferrin saturation [TSAT]) were collected monthly; hemoglobin values were collected more frequently (about two times per month) in most facilities. Data were available for Epoetin alfa (EPO) and iron doses (recorded at each administration), demographic characteristics (captured when patients began receiving dialysis), and dialysis care information, including urea reduction ratio (URR), number of missed dialysis visits, and vascular access (VA) information. Hospitalization data were collected on an ongoing basis and included admission and discharge dates and diagnoses based on *International Classification of Disease—9th Revision* (ICD-9) codes. Mortality information was routinely collected, as were reasons for loss to follow up, which included renal transplantation, facility transfer, withdrawal, and modality change.

We assessed Epoetin alfa dosing at 2-week intervals, to be consistent with the Hb assessment frequency in usual care. In each interval, we calculated the cumulative outpatient Epoetin alfa dose (sum of all available doses recorded in the dialysis facility). Epoetin alfa dosing information is not captured in the inpatient setting and, therefore, was unavailable to us. For the purpose of this analysis, we imputed the inpatient portion of the Epoetin alfa treatment using the last dose before hospitalization.

The reason that this database was selected for this analysis, as opposed to other choices (for example, the United States Renal Data System [USRDS] data collected through Medicare), is that Epoetin alfa dose information is available for every administration, and all assessed Hb values are available in the database. In other words, the critical data are much more granular than databases used in other analyses; that is, the data include more observations of more variables and, in general, provide a more complete view of the patient condition, treatment factors, and variables used by doctors in making dosing decisions. This should be an important consideration when applying the MSM analysis because the assumption of no unmeasured confounders is a critical assumption for causal inferences.

The actual SAS database used in this analysis has one record per patient-time point. Patient characteristics were assessed through a corresponding demographics database (with one record per patient) using Program 13.1 to provide a general idea of the patient population. The SAS output is quite long and, instead of the SAS output display, the results are summarized in Table 13.1 as a more concise alternative. Continuous variables are presented as mean (standard deviation) and categorical variables as count (frequency). Note that the summaries are presented per dose categories (bldosequartile, or baseline dose quartiles, plus the zero dose group), which is explained in more detail later.

Program 13.1 Patient Characteristics Summary

```
*** Compute means for continuous variables;
proc means data=demog mean;
  var AGE HEMODIALYRS BMI BLFER BLSAT BLALB BLHGB;
  by bldosequartile;
  OUTPUT OUT=mean MEAN=AGE HEMODIALYRS BMI BLFER BLSAT BLALB BLHGB;
run;

*** Compute standard deviations for continuous variables;

proc means data=demog stddev;
  var age HEMODIALYRS BMI BLFER BLSAT BLALB BLHGB;
  by bldosequartile;
  OUTPUT out=stddev stddev=AGE HEMODIALYRS BMI BLFER BLSAT BLALB
BLHGB;
run;

*** Compute count and frequency for categorical variables;

proc freq data=demog;
  table AGEGROUP/out=a;
  table ETH/out=b;
  table SEX/out=c;
  table REGION/out=d;
  table BLHYPERTENSN/out=e;
  table GLE/out=f;
  by bldosequartile;
run;
```

Similar code was run for the overall patient population.

Table 13.1 Patient Demographics and Baseline Characteristics

	Dose group 0	Dose group 1	Dose group 2	Dose group 3	Dose group 4	All
N	304	5544	7904	8336	5703	27791
Age (years)	54.77 (13.99)	61.01 (15.01)	61.8 (15.08)	60.51 (14.73)	58.13 (14.74)	60.43 (14.74)
Dialysis Vintage (years)	4.95 (4.77)	3.44 (3.81)	2.66 (3.28)	2.49 (3.36)	2.83 (3.6)	2.82 (3.6)
Baseline BMI (kg/m^2)	27.98 (8.07)	26.17 (6.69)	26.37 (6.65)	27.17 (7.15)	28.27 (7.9)	26.98 (7.9)
Baseline Ferritin (ng/ml)	500.8 (322.9)	591.8 (360.7)	527.4 (341.5)	478.7 (343.6)	473.3 (351.8)	514.2 (351.8)
Baseline TSAT (%)	31.54 (10.44)	32.08 (9.66)	29.12 (9.17)	26.49 (8.88)	24.32 (9.33)	27.97 (9.33)
Baseline Albumin (g/dl)	3.88 (0.32)	3.89 (0.28)	3.83 (0.3)	3.76 (0.33)	3.66 (0.36)	3.79 (0.36)
Baseline Hb (g/dl)	12.9 (1.31)	12.11 (0.78)	11.89 (0.76)	11.63 (0.88)	11.01 (1.07)	11.69 (1.07)
Age < 45 years	83 (27.3)	831 (15)	1159 (14.7)	1304 (15.6)	1103 (19.3)	4480 (16.1)
Age >= 45 to < 65 years	138 (45.4)	2181 (39.3)	2869 (36.3)	3304 (39.6)	2482 (43.5)	10974 (39.5)
Age >= 65 years	83 (27.3)	2532 (45.7)	3876 (49)	3728 (44.7)	2118 (37.1)	12337 (44.4)
Female	83 (27.3)	2252 (40.6)	3835 (48.5)	4197 (50.3)	2908 (51)	13275 (47.8)
Black	128 (42.1)	2060 (37.2)	3030 (38.3)	3548 (42.6)	2778 (48.7)	11544 (41.5)
Region=MIDWEST	39 (12.8)	488 (8.8)	758 (9.6)	841 (10.1)	568 (10)	2694 (9.7)
Region=NORTHEAST	50 (16.4)	927 (16.7)	1277 (16.2)	1450 (17.4)	1111 (19.5)	4815 (17.3)
Region=SOUTH	184 (60.5)	3226 (58.2)	4847 (61.3)	5265 (63.2)	3595 (63)	17117 (61.6)
Region=WEST	31 (10.2)	903 (16.3)	1022 (12.9)	780 (9.4)	429 (7.5)	3165 (11.4)
Hypertension	42 (13.8)	729 (13.1)	1170 (14.8)	1343 (16.1)	997 (17.5)	4281 (15.4)
Diabetic	116 (38.2)	2630 (47.4)	4087 (51.7)	4446 (53.3)	2875 (50.4)	14154 (50.9)

13.3 Treatment Model and Censoring Model Setup

We estimated the mortality hazard ratio using marginal structural models (MSMs), where the inverse probability of treatment weighting (IPTW) was used to adjust for confounding by indication. This two-step approach calculates the weights first as the inverse of the predicted Epoetin alfa doses using a treatment model and then assesses the HRs using a weighted structural model. Specifically, IPTW down-weights patients who receive doses close to what was predicted and up-weights patients who receive doses that vary appreciably from what was predicted. This weighting creates a pseudo-population in which confounding between factors influencing treatment and the actual treatment received is mitigated. Consequently, HRs based on this pseudo-population can have a causal interpretation, provided that the weights are modeled accurately and other assumptions are met (Robins, 2000). One important assumption is the ETA assumption—namely, the probability of observing a specific treatment regimen is >0 and <1. In other words, the treatment decision is not a deterministic function of the past. Therefore, each treatment decision is not independent and random (otherwise there is no confounding) and yet cannot be fixed given the past either.

We calculated treatment weights, which were related to predicted EPO doses, for each patient in 2-week intervals using ordinal regression. Our goal was to construct a model that reflects the physician decision-making process in deciding what the next Epoetin alfa dose is for a particular patient. The model is constructed using the entire patient population, and both statistical and clinical considerations are put to work. A simple approach is to recognize the role of observed Hb values and the inertia/momentum of previous doses. This results in a "simple" model with Hb and dose in the previous four time intervals. Some clinicians argue that they also take into consideration a patient's hospitalization status, iron indices, vascular access, and other co-morbid conditions. That led to an "expanded" model, which added days in hospital, number of non-hospital doses, albumin, ferritin, TSAT, vascular access type, hypertension status, and dialysis adequacy in the previous time interval to the simple model. Finally, a "full" model was constructed by adding the interaction between Hb and dose to the "expanded" model, recognizing the dynamics between the two factors, which makes good clinical sense.

The calculations are implemented in SAS using PROC GENMOD. The three models are implemented similarly, and only the full model is illustrated here. Note that the treatment weights are ratios, with the time-dependent confounders included in the denominator only. See Program 13.2. The numerator and the denominator, both predicted dose quartiles, are calculated separately. Weights calculated this way are called *stabilized weights*, denoted as "sw".

Program 13.2 Treatment Weights Calculation

```
*** Compute the treatment part of the IPTW weights;

*** Numerator part, including baseline covariates and time-dependent
intercept;

proc genmod data=infile rorder=formatted order=formatted;
      class ETH SEX REGION VITDFLAG GLU BLVAC CDAYSINHOSP BLHYPERTENSN
            BLHXADEQUACY bldosequartile lag1dosequartile lag2dosequartile
            lag3dosequartile lag4dosequartile
            lag1HYPERTENSION lag1HXADEQUACY lag1VASCULAR;
      model dosequartile = ETH SEX REGION VITDFLAG GLU BLVAC
            CDAYSINHOSP BLHYPERTENSN BLHXADEQUACY AGE BMI HEMODIALYRS
            NOCHGDOSES NOHLDDOSES PERLESS11 BLHGB BLIRON BLALB BLFER BLSAT
            BLPTH bldosequartile lag1dosequartile lag2dosequartile
            lag3dosequartile lag4dosequartile
            hmthno hmthno1 hmthno2 hmthno3
```

```
          / dist=multinomial link=clogit;
      output out=preds pred=pred;
run;

proc sort data=preds;
      by patient biweekno dosequartile _order_;
run;

proc transpose data=preds out=predst(keep=patient theta1 theta2 theta3
           theta4  biweekno dosequartile) prefix=theta;
      by patient biweekno dosequartile;
      id _order_;
      var pred;
run;

data model1;
      set predst;
      prob1=theta1;
      prob2=theta2-theta1;
      prob3=theta3-theta2;
      prob4=theta4-theta3;
      prob5=1-theta4;
      if dosequartile=1 then treat_top=prob1;
        else if dosequartile=2 then treat_top=prob2;
        else if dosequartile=3 then treat_top=prob3;
        else if dosequartile=4 then treat_top=prob4;
        else if dosequartile=5 then treat_top=prob5;
    keep patient biweekno dosequartile treat_top;
run;

*** Denominator part, including baseline covariates, time-dependent
intercept, and also any time-dependent covariates;

proc genmod data=infile rorder=formatted order=formatted;
      class ETH SEX REGION VITDFLAG GLU BLVAC CDAYSINHOSP BLHYPERTENSN
            BLHXADEQUACY bldosequartile lag1dosequartile lag2dosequartile
            lag3dosequartile lag4dosequartile
            lag1HYPERTENSION lag1HXADEQUACY lag1VASCULAR;
      model dosequartile = ETH SEX REGION VITDFLAG GLU BLVAC
            CDAYSINHOSP BLHYPERTENSN BLHXADEQUACY AGE BMI HEMODIALYRS
            NOCHGDOSES NOHLDDOSES PERLESS11 BLHGB BLIRON BLALB BLFER BLSAT
            BLPTH bldosequartile lag1dosequartile lag2dosequartile
            lag3dosequartile lag4dosequartile
            lag1hb lag2hb lag3hb lag4hb
            lag1HYPERTENSION lag1HXADEQUACY lag1VASCULAR lag1NHSPDNUM
            lag1hospitaldays lag1iron lag1sat lag1alb lag1fer
            lag1hbdose0 lag1hbdose1 lag1hbdose2 lag1hbdose3 lag1hbdose4
            hmthno hmthno1 hmthno2 hmthno3
            / dist=multinomial link=clogit;
      output out=preds pred=pred;
run;

proc sort data=preds;
      by patient biweekno dosequartile _order_;
run;

proc transpose data=preds out=predst(keep=patient theta1 theta2 theta3
         theta4  biweekno dosequartile) prefix=theta;
      by patient biweekno dosequartile;
      id _order_;
      var pred;
run;
```

```
data model2;
      set predst;
      prob1=theta1;
      prob2=theta2-theta1;
      prob3=theta3-theta2;
      prob4=theta4-theta3;
      prob5=1-theta4;
      if dosequartile=1 then treat_bottom=prob1;
        else if dosequartile=2 then treat_bottom=prob2;
        else if dosequartile=3 then treat_bottom=prob3;
        else if dosequartile=4 then treat_bottom=prob4;
        else if dosequartile=5 then treat_bottom=prob5;
    keep patient biweekno dosequartile treat_top;
run;

data trtmodels;
      merge model1 (keep=patient biweekno treat_top)
            model2 (keep=patient biweekno treat_bottom)
      by patient biweekno;
      if nmiss(treat_top, treat_bottom)>0 then treat_sw=1;
      if nmiss(treat_top, treat_bottom)=0 then
            treat_sw=treat_top/treat_bottom;
run;
```

In a usual MSM implementation, weights at each time point are aggregated by multiplying all the weights in the study prior to the particular time point. As can be imagined, the variability associated with weights at later time points gets bigger and bigger. These weights are summarized and illustrated in Figure 13.2.

Figure 13.2 MSM Weights

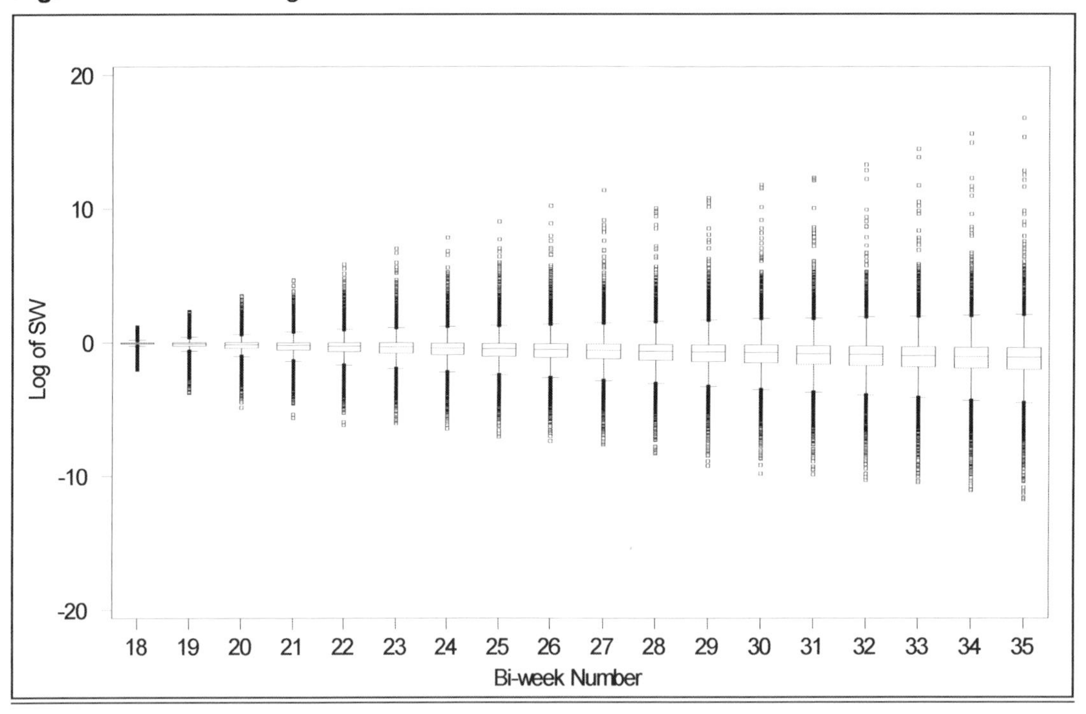

In complicated treatment scenarios with a titratable drug, some of the calculated IPTWs could get very large due to unusual patient characteristics, unconventional treatment decisions, large variability in data assessment, or even data recording errors. Model inadequacy early on may cause the inaccurate weights to be multiplied again and again for later time points because weights are cumulative. In order to prevent the analysis from being dominated by a handful of patients with large weights, in our implementation of MSM the aggregated weights were calculated based on only the previous four time intervals, instead of all previous time points. This variation has the effect of stabilizing the weights, as shown in Figure 13.3. Note the smaller range and the uniformity of the range over the bi-weekly periods. We also truncated the highest weight to either the 98th or 99th percentile values (weights of 82 and 471, respectively, in the full treatment model case). By excluding relatively few outliers that would otherwise greatly influence the model, we were able to improve the performance of the hazard ratio estimates using MSM.

Figure 13.3 Modified MSM Weights

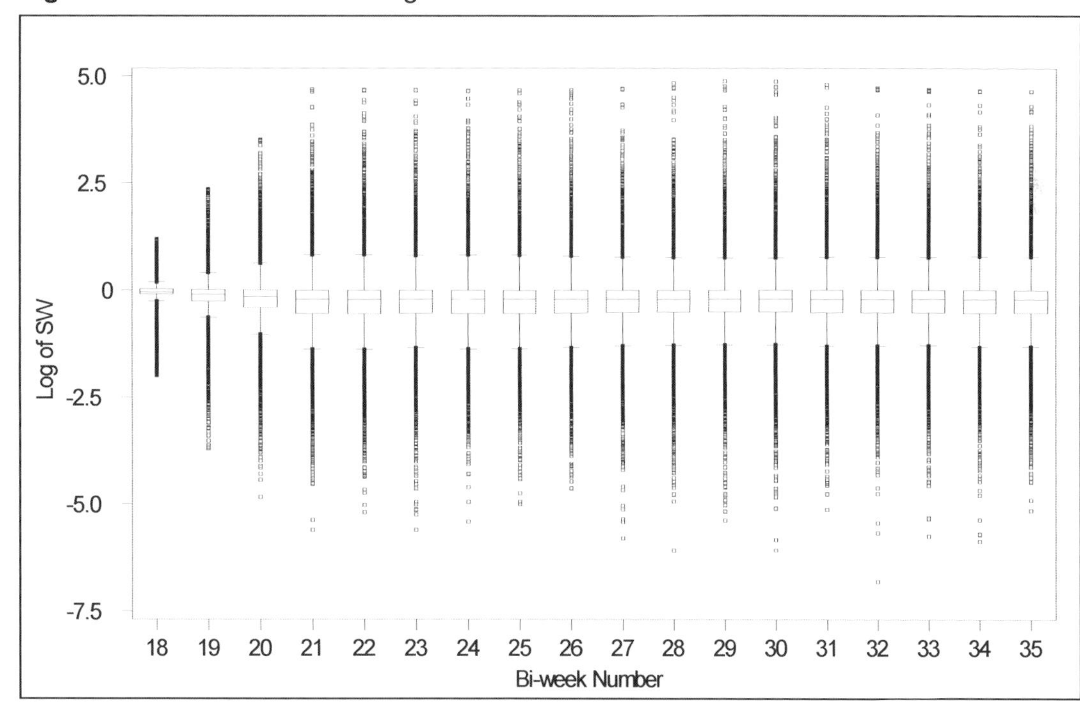

Patient censoring was considered in a similar way to the treatment information, predicted at each time point (given the observed past), and incorporated into the weighting. Censoring events included loss to follow up for various reasons. Censoring weights are calculated using Program 13.3, which is similar to Program 13.2. The censoring weights are not summarized here.

Program 13.3 Censoring Weights Calculation

```
*** Compute the censoring part of the IPTW weights;
*** Numerator part, including baseline covariates and time-dependent
intercept;

proc logistic data=infile;
      class lag1dosequartile lag2dosequartile lag3dosequartile
            lag4dosequartile bldosequartile ETH SEX REGION VITDFLAG GLU BLVAC
            CDAYSINHOSP BLHYPERTENSN BLHXADEQUACY;
      model censored = lag1dosequartile lag2dosequartile
            lag3dosequartile lag4dosequartile bldosequartile ETH SEX REGION
            VITDFLAG GLU BLVAC CDAYSINHOSP BLHYPERTENSN BLHXADEQUACY AGE BMI
```

```
            HEMODIALYRS NOCHGDOSES NOHLDDOSES PERLESS11 BLHGB BLIRON BLALB
            BLFER BLSAT BLPTH hmthno hmthno1 hmthno2 hmthno3;
      output out=model3 p=censored_top;
run;

*** Denominator part, including baseline covariates, time-dependent intercept,
and also any time-dependent covariates;

proc logistic data=infile;
      class ETH SEX REGION VITDFLAG GLU BLVAC CDAYSINHOSP BLHYPERTENSN
            BLHXADEQUACY bldosequartile lag1dosequartile lag2dosequartile
            lag3dosequartile lag4dosequartile
            lag1HYPERTENSION lag1HXADEQUACY lag1VASCULAR;
      model censored = ETH SEX REGION VITDFLAG GLU BLVAC CDAYSINHOSP
            BLHYPERTENSN BLHXADEQUACY AGE BMI HEMODIALYRS NOCHGDOSES
            NOHLDDOSES PERLESS11 BLHGB BLIRON BLALB BLFER BLSAT BLPTH
            bldosequartile lag1dosequartile lag2dosequartile lag3dosequartile
            lag4dosequartile
            lag1hb lag2hb lag3hb lag4hb
            lag1HYPERTENSION lag1HXADEQUACY lag1VASCULAR lag1NHSPDNUM
            lag1hospitaldays lag1iron lag1sat lag1alb lag1fer
            lag1hbdose0 lag1hbdose1 lag1hbdose2 lag1hbdose3 lag1hbdose4 hmthno
            hmthno1 hmthno2 hmthno3;
      output out=model4 p=censored_bottom;
run;

data censormodels;
      merge model3 (keep=patient biweekno censored_top)
            model4 (keep=patient biweekno censored_bottom) ;
      by patient biweekno;
      if nmiss(censored_top, censored_bottom)>0 then censored_sw=1;
      if nmiss(censored_top, censored_bottom)=0 then
            censored_sw=censored_top/censored_bottom;
run;
```

13.4 Structural Model Implementation

The structural model is step two in the MSM method implementation. This is where the causal inferences are made using weighted observations. In our database, the clinical outcome we are assessing is mortality, and survival analysis is needed to estimate its relationship with dose. The actual implementation in SAS, however, is through PROC GENMOD because PROC PHREG does not handle weighted analyses. The generalized estimating equations (GEE) approach using PROC GENMOD is used for hazard ratio point estimates. The confidence intervals associated with these point estimates must be derived from bootstrapping instead of directly utilizing intervals produced by PROC GENMOD. This is discussed in detail later.

The GEE model includes dose and baseline covariates to estimate mortality hazard ratios, with weighting on the Epoetin alfa doses. Mortality was assessed during a 1-year period following the patient's index date and aggregated into bi-weekly intervals. Epoetin alfa doses were grouped into a zero dose category and dose quartiles (1st quartile: ≤ 14000 IU/2 weeks; 2nd quartile: 14000–27000 IU/2 weeks; 3rd quartile: 27000–49000 IU/2 weeks; 4th quartile: > 49000 IU/2 weeks). The lowest non-zero dose quartile was used as the reference group in the structural model. The exposure variable, Epoetin alfa dose category, was lagged by 8 weeks (four time intervals) to allow for the fact that severely ill patients are often hospitalized approximately 4 to 8 weeks prior to death, and their in-hospital Epoetin alfa doses, if any, were not available in our database, which was collected through the dialysis chain. For patients with missed Epoetin alfa doses or patients who did not receive a dose during a dialysis session, a zero dose was recorded. For patients who survived hospitalization, an in-hospital Epoetin alfa dose was imputed using the most recent dose prior to hospitalization.

Program 13.4 implements the structural model using GEE.

Program 13.4 Analysis Model

```
proc genmod data=allmodels descending;
      class patient ETH SEX REGION VITDFLAG GLU BLVAC CDAYSINHOSP
            BLHYPERTENSN BLHXADEQUACY bldosequartile;
      model die = ETH SEX REGION VITDFLAG GLU BLVAC CDAYSINHOSP
            BLHYPERTENSN BLHXADEQUACY AGE BMI HEMODIALYRS NOCHGDOSES
            NOHLDDOSES PERLESS11 BLHGB BLIRON BLALB BLFER BLSAT BLPTH
            bldosequartile epoq0 epoq2 epoq3 epoq4
            hmthno hmthno1 hmthno2 hmthno3
            /link=logit dist=bin;
      scwgt wgt;
      repeated subject=patient/type=ind;
run;
```

Output from Program 13.4

Analysis Of GEE Parameter Estimates
Empirical Standard Error Estimates

Parameter		Estimate	Standard Error	95% Confidence Limits		Z	Pr > |Z|
Intercept		0.7441	2.1078	-3.3871	4.8753	0.35	0.7241
Eth	0	0.3070	0.0853	0.1398	0.4743	3.60	0.0003
Eth	1	0.0000	0.0000	0.0000	0.0000	.	.
Sex	0	-0.1429	0.0625	-0.2653	-0.0205	-2.29	0.0221
Sex	1	0.0000	0.0000	0.0000	0.0000	.	.
region	MIDWEST	0.2399	0.1608	-0.0753	0.5551	1.49	0.1358
region	NORTHEST	0.0680	0.1530	-0.2318	0.3678	0.44	0.6564
region	SOUTH	0.3213	0.1427	0.0416	0.6011	2.25	0.0244
region	WEST	0.0000	0.0000	0.0000	0.0000	.	.
vitdflag	0	-0.0684	0.0711	-0.2077	0.0709	-0.96	0.3359
vitdflag	1	0.0000	0.0000	0.0000	0.0000	.	.
glu	0	-0.3425	0.0686	-0.4769	-0.2080	-4.99	<.0001
glu	1	0.0000	0.0000	0.0000	0.0000	.	.
blvac	cath	0.1182	0.0738	-0.0264	0.2628	1.60	0.1090
blvac	fistula	-0.2181	0.0957	-0.4057	-0.0305	-2.28	0.0227
blvac	graft	0.0000	0.0000	0.0000	0.0000	.	.
cdaysinhosp	0	-0.4154	0.0933	-0.5982	-0.2326	-4.45	<.0001
cdaysinhosp	1	-0.3525	0.1199	-0.5876	-0.1174	-2.94	0.0033
cdaysinhosp	2	0.0858	0.1402	-0.1890	0.3606	0.61	0.5405
cdaysinhosp	3	0.0000	0.0000	0.0000	0.0000	.	.
BLHYPERTENSN	0	-0.0023	0.1156	-0.2289	0.2242	-0.02	0.9838
BLHYPERTENSN	1	0.0000	0.0000	0.0000	0.0000	.	.
BLHXADEQUACY	0	0.0998	0.0895	-0.0757	0.2753	1.11	0.2650
BLHXADEQUACY	1	0.0000	0.0000	0.0000	0.0000	.	.
Age		0.0303	0.0027	0.0249	0.0357	11.02	<.0001
bmi		-0.0294	0.0061	-0.0413	-0.0176	-4.87	<.0001
hemodialyrs		0.0374	0.0067	0.0242	0.0506	5.55	<.0001
nochgdoses		-0.0110	0.0102	-0.0311	0.0090	-1.08	0.2806
nohlddoses		0.0009	0.0135	-0.0255	0.0273	0.07	0.9449
perless11		-0.0035	0.0028	-0.0091	0.0020	-1.25	0.2131
blhgb		-0.1621	0.0834	-0.3255	0.0013	-1.94	0.0519
bliron		-0.0007	0.0003	-0.0013	-0.0001	-2.12	0.0337
blalb		-0.9552	0.0907	-1.1330	-0.7775	-10.53	<.0001

(*continued*)

Output from Program 13.4 *(continued)*

```
  blfer                      0.0002   0.0001   0.0000   0.0004    2.42   0.0155
  blsat                     -0.0052   0.0063  -0.0176   0.0071   -0.83   0.4050
  blpth                      0.0004   0.0001   0.0002   0.0007    3.75   0.0002
  bldosequartile 0           0.5692   0.5130  -0.4362   1.5746    1.11   0.2671
  bldosequartile 1          -0.2165   0.1729  -0.5554   0.1225   -1.25   0.2106
  bldosequartile 2          -0.2756   0.1196  -0.5100  -0.0412   -2.30   0.0212
  bldosequartile 3          -0.2755   0.0908  -0.4533  -0.0976   -3.03   0.0024
  bldosequartile 4           0.0000   0.0000   0.0000   0.0000     .       .
  epoq2                      0.0678   0.0941  -0.1167   0.2522    0.72   0.4714
  epoq3                      0.1923   0.1087  -0.0208   0.4054    1.77   0.0770
  epoq4                      0.3292   0.1378   0.0590   0.5994    2.39   0.0169
  epoq0                      0.4433   0.1920   0.0669   0.8197    2.31   0.0210
  hmthno                    -0.0924   0.0991  -0.2866   0.1019   -0.93   0.3515
  hmthno1                    0.5253   0.4379  -0.3330   1.3837    1.20   0.2303
  hmthno2                   -1.4398   1.1266  -3.6479   0.7682   -1.28   0.2012
  hmthno3                    1.5701   1.1024  -0.5906   3.7308    1.42   0.1544
```

Results are summarized in Table 13.2 for easy examination. Note that the Estimate column in the Output from Program 13.4 is exponentiated to obtain the point estimate of the hazard ratio in Table 13.2. For example, the 0.0678 value for epoq2 is exponentiated to get the HR value of 1.07 in Table 13.2 for the 2nd EPO dose quartile in the full model.

Table 13.2 Estimates of Hazard Ratios for Different Models and Different Levels of Weight Truncation

Treatment Model*	Weight Truncation Level	Maximum Weight	Zero Dose	EPO Dose Quartiles			
				1st	2nd	3rd	4th
Simple	2%	32	1.69 (1.06, 2.39)	1	1.09 (0.92, 1.31)	1.27 (1.02, 1.60)	1.51 (1.08, 1.89)
Expanded	2%	28	1.62 (1.16, 2.09)	1	1.09 (0.94, 1.35)	1.24 (1.05, 1.56)	1.49 (1.22, 1.91)
Full	2%	82	1.56 (0.98, 2.02)	1	1.07 (0.91, 1.33)	1.21 (1.00, 1.53)	1.39 (1.08, 1.91)
Simple	1%	133	1.71 (1.00, 2.55)	1	1.01 (0.83, 1.26)	1.07 (0.89, 1.42)	1.15 (0.94, 1.68)
Expanded	1%	117	1.81 (0.87, 2.51)	1	1.02 (0.82, 1.29)	1.11 (0.85, 1.41)	1.21 (0.90, 1.70)
Full	1%	471	1.72 (0.84, 2.59)	1	0.97 (0.79, 1.33)	1.00 (0.81, 1.45)	0.98 (0.76, 1.74)

*Treatment models, as discussed in Section 13.3, include baseline covariates and the following time-dependent covariates:

Simple = Hb level and EPO dose 2, 4, 6, and 8 weeks prior to exposure

Expanded = Covariates in the simple model plus the following covariates: Days in Hospital, Number of Non-Hospital EPO Dose, Albumin, Ferritin, TSAT, Vascular Access Type, Hypertension, and Dialysis Adequacy 2 weeks prior to exposure

Full = Covariates in the expanded model plus the following covariates: Interaction between Hb level and EPO dose 2 weeks prior to exposure

Hazard ratio estimates use the lowest non-zero Epoetin alfa dose quartile as the reference group. The zero dose category consistently showed higher mortality rates than the reference category, as evidenced by hazard ratios ranging from 1.56 to 1.81 across the three treatment models and the two levels of weight truncation. For dose quartiles 2, 3, and 4, the hazard ratios for every Epoetin alfa dose quartile in general decreased toward the null as the treatment model moved from simple to expanded to full and as IPTW truncation was less restrictive. The degree of change in the hazard ratios tended to increase by dose category, suggesting that control of confounding for high-dose subjects would be hindered by an inadequate treatment model or excessive truncation of IPTWs. The full model with 1% truncation would suggest increased risk for those in the zero dose group and near null hazard ratios for the higher dose categories.

An important thing to check together with the structural model results is the fit of the treatment (and censoring) models. The three treatment models, as predicted, worked progressively well, with the full model offering the best treatment prediction due to more closely mimicking clinical practice. The most influential variables in predicting subsequent EPO doses were previous EPO dose, previous Hb, and the interaction between the two. The other variables (for example, vascular access and hospitalization) added a considerable amount of accuracy to the predictions and were important to take into consideration.

Because the confidence intervals (CIs) provided by PROC GENMOD are not adequate for MSM estimates, CIs of the hazard ratio estimates were generated using bootstrapping, sampling with replacement from all available patients. Each bootstrapped CI was based on 200 samples. See Program 13.5.

Program 13.5 Bootstrap Confidence Intervals

```
%macro bootstrap(infile, out);

*** get the number of subjects;
data infile;
   set &infile;
   by pat;
   if first.pat;
run;

data filerecs;
   set infile end=_last_;
   rec=_n_;
   if _last_=1 then output filerecs;
run;

%global filrecs;
data _null_;
   set filerecs;
   call symput("filrecs",put(rec,8.));
run;

*** sample with replacement;
data sample;
   do i=1 to &filrecs;
   rec=int((ranuni(-1)*&filrecs)+1);
   output;
   drop i;
   end;
run;
```

```
proc sort data=sample;
by rec;
run;

proc freq data=sample noprint;
table rec/out=norecs (keep=rec count);
run;

*** unique sample;
data uniquesample;
   set sample;
   by rec;
   if first.rec;
   selected=1;
run;

data infile2;
   set &infile;
   by pat;
   retain rec;
   if _n_=1 then rec=0;
   if first.pat then rec+1;
run;

data mysample;
   merge infile2 (in=one) uniquesample (in=two);
   by rec;
   if one and two;
run;

data mysample;
   set mysample;
   pat2=pat;
run;

*** subjects sampled more than once;
data extrapats;
   merge infile2 (in=one) norecs(in=two where=(count>1));
   by rec;
   if one and two;
run;

proc sort data=extrapats;
   by pat;
run;

*** subjects sampled more than twice;
data extrapats3;
   set extrapats;
           retain irec;
           if _n_=1 then irec=0;
        exrecs=count-1;
        do i=1 to exrecs;
        index=i;
        irec=irec+1;
        selected=1;
        pat2=pat+(0.0001*i);
        output;
        end;
        drop i exrecs;
run;
```

```
proc sort data=extrapats3;
   by pat biweekno;
run;

data &out;
   set mysample extrapats3;
   drop pat;
run;

proc sort data=&out(rename=(pat2=pat));
   by pat biweekno;
run;

%mend bootstrap;

%bootstrap(studyperioddata, newstudydata);
```

Note that in Table 13.2 the hazard ratios have very wide confidence intervals, reflecting considerable uncertainty in estimating the relative mortality risk with increasing EPO dose. Also note that as the quartiles increase, the confidence intervals become wider, pointing to the fact that confounding is especially problematic at higher doses.

The difference between the simple model and the full model was the additional variables available in our granular database. These are not typically available in other databases (for example, hospital days and hospital EPO use). In our analysis, we tried to examine the impact of these additional variables on the MSM analysis by holding all other aspects of the MSM implementation constant. As evidenced in Table 13.2, the impact of these additional data resulted in better prediction of the EPO doses, which, in turn, generated more accurate weights for the MSM. For example, the hazard ratio estimate for the 4th dose quartile was dropped from 1.15 to 0.98 with the introduction of the additional data in the full model compared with the simple model.

Based on the fact that hazard ratios were progressively moving toward the null using the expanded and full models versus the simple model, we hypothesize that data availability or granularity may correlate with the amount of residual confounding due to the resulting model misspecification. That is, the lack of explanatory variables in the simpler models does not help in reducing the confounding problems, but being able to include more variables in expanded models does reduce the confounding, which enables us to generate more realistic estimates of the hazard ratios.

It is worth noting that for this particular application, the hazard ratio estimates were for the most part similar if the maximum weights were similar after truncation, suggesting the importance of controlling for weight outliers due to model misspecification. In other words, controlling the maximum weight through weight truncation seems an efficient way to mitigate the risk of model misspecification.

13.5 Discussion

This chapter presents an example of using MSM to assess safety information, mortality specifically, from a large health care database. Health care databases are often huge in size and rich in data elements, presenting great advantages over small clinical trials. They are also usually collected in a real-world setting, reflecting more actual clinical practice data compared with clinical trials. On the other hand, the lack of randomization and tight control make the databases susceptible to confounding. Sometimes the confounding is time-dependent and severe enough to render the conventional analysis assessing dose relationship useless. More sophisticated methods like marginal structural models, structural nested models, or instrumental variables should be considered when dealing with these databases. However, these methods have only been introduced to the clinical world in the last couple of decades and have been used only in the last few years. Due to their complexity, both in concept and in implementation, they have not been widely used. We hope this chapter serves the purpose of making the methods readily available to general statisticians who practice in the health care database domain. Like any other statistical procedure, assumptions have to be carefully checked before results are accepted. This is especially true for MSM because it's easy to generate unreasonable results unknowingly. It would be even worse to make causal claims based on them.

References

Bárány, P., J. C. Divino Filho, and J. Bergström. 1997. "High C-reactive protein is a strong predictor of resistance to erythropoietin in hemodialysis patients." *American Journal of Kidney Diseases* 29(4): 565–568.

Bradbury, B. D., O. Wang, C. W. Critchlow, et al. 2008. "Exploring relative mortality and epoetin alfa dose among hemodialysis patients." *American Journal of Kidney Diseases* 51(1): 62–70.

Cotter, D. J., K. Stefanik, Y. Zhang, M. Thamer, D. Scharfstein, and J. Kaufman. 2004. "Hematocrit was not validated as a surrogate end point for survival among epoetin-treated hemodialysis patients." *Journal of Clinical Epidemiology* 57(10): 1086–1095.

Feldman, H. I., M. Joffe, B. Robinson, et al. 2004. "Administration of parenteral iron and mortality among hemodialysis patients." *Journal of the American Society of Nephrology* 15(6): 1623–1632.

Hernán, M. A., B. Brumback, and J. M. Robins. 2000. "Marginal structural models to estimate the causal effect of zidovudine on the survival of HIV-positive men." *Epidemiology* 11: 561–570.

Kausz, A. T., C. Solid, B. J. G. Pereira, A. J. Collins, and W. St. Peter. 2005. "Intractable anemia among hemodialysis patients: a sign of suboptimal management or a marker of disease?" *American Journal of Kidney Diseases* 45(1): 136–147.

Regidor, D. L., J. D. Kopple, C. P. Kovesdy, et al. 2006. "Associations between changes in hemoglobin and administered erythropoiesis-stimulating agent and survival in hemodialysis patients." *Journal of the American Society of Nephrology* 17(4): 1181–1191.

Roberts, T. L., G. T. Obrador, W. L. St. Peter, B. J. G. Pereira, and A. J. Collins. 2004. "Relationship among catheter insertions, vascular access infections, and anemia management in hemodialysis patients." *Kidney International* 66(6): 2429–2436.

Robins, J. M., M. A. Hernán, and B. Brumback. 2000. "Marginal structural models and causal inference in epidemiology." *Epidemiology* 11: 550–560.

Rossert, J., C. Gassmann-Mayer, D. Frei, and W. McClellan. 2007. "Prevalence and predictors of epoetin hyporesponsiveness in chronic kidney disease patients." *Nephrology Dialysis Transplantation* 22: 794–800.

Rothman, K. J., and C. E. Wentworth, III. 2003. "Mortality of cystic fibrosis patients treated with tobramycin solution for inhalation." *Epidemiology* 14(1): 55–59.

Teng, M., M. Wolf, M. N. Ofsthun, et al. 2005. "Activated injectable vitamin D and hemodialysis survival: a historical cohort study." *Journal of the American Society of Nephrology* 16(4): 1115–1125.

Teruel, J. L., R. Marcen, J. Ocana, M. Fernandez-Lucas, et al. 2005. "Clinical significance of C-reactive protein in patients on hemodialysis: a longitudinal study." *Nephron* 100: c140–145.

U.S. Renal Data System, USRDS. 2004. "Annual data report: atlas of end-stage renal disease in the United States." National Institutes of Health, National Institute of Diabetes and Digestive and Kidney Diseases, Bethesda, MD.

U.S. Renal Data System, USRDS. 2007. "Annual data report: atlas of end-stage renal disease in the United States." National Institutes of Health, National Institute of Diabetes and Digestive and Kidney Diseases. Bethesda, MD.

Zhang, Y., M. Thamer, K. Stefanik, J. Kaufman, and D. J. Cotter. 2004. "Epoetin requirements predict mortality in hemodialysis patients." *American Journal of Kidney Diseases* 44(5): 866–876.

Part 5

Pharmacoeconomics

Chapter 14

Costs and Cost-Effectiveness Analysis Using Propensity Score Bin Bootstrapping

Douglas E. Faries
Xiaomei Peng
Robert L. Obenchain

Abstract

Analysis of cost and cost-effectiveness data is of increasing importance among health care decision-makers in today's economic climate. Propensity score bin bootstrapping is a new analytical approach that addresses three fundamental challenges of observational cost data analysis:

1. the typical skewness of cost distributions
2. the need to estimate mean rather than median or other robust measures
3. the need to adjust for selection bias

In this chapter, an overview of various methodologies for analyzing cost data is presented along with SAS code to perform a propensity score bin bootstrapping analysis comparing the mean cost and cost-effectiveness of competing interventions.

14.1 Introduction

14.1.1 Overview

As the cost of health care in the United States continues to grow, cost and cost-effectiveness analyses have become key factors in medical decision-making. For instance, health care payers have great interest in analyses such as comparing the total costs of care from two or more competing treatment regimens. However, the appropriate analysis for comparing cost data between groups can be complex because it must address the potential skewness in the data, estimate mean costs, and adjust for important baseline treatment group differences.

Cost data from medical studies are typically skewed because a subset of patients may have very high costs due to resource-intensive treatments (such as hospitalizations), while another subset may perform very well and utilize few or less costly medical resources. Second, medians or trimmed means are commonly used statistical measures of central tendency for describing populations with outliers. Unfortunately, these measures are unrealistic and misleading for payers responsible for all of the costs incurred by a patient population. Mean costs are more relevant here; the population size times the median cost is not representative of the total liability to the payer (Ramsey et al., 2005; Doshi et al., 2006). Third, the most realistic (generalizable) cost data typically come from naturalistic research. Randomized, clinical trials use protocols with regularly scheduled health care provider visits (often more frequent than actual practice), free access to many resources, structured dosing, strict entry criteria, and mandated compliance. All of these issues clearly limit the generalizability of the clinical trial cost estimates (Grimes and Schulz, 2002; Revicki and Frank, 1999; Roy-Byrne et al., 2003). On the other hand, naturalistic studies lacking randomization to treatment are subject to treatment selection bias on baseline patient characteristics that needs to be accounted for in analyses (Rosenbaum and Rubin, 1983).

Several approaches to the analyses of cost data appear in the published literature (Doshi et al., 2006):

- *t*-tests/ANOVA
- rank-based nonparametric tests
- transformation approaches
- generalized linear models
- bootstrapping

In this chapter, we review published guidance on analysis and reporting of economic data, briefly review commonly used methodology, introduce and discuss a new approach—propensity score bin bootstrapping (PSBB)—and demonstrate an analysis of cost data from a schizophrenia trial using SAS software. Given the availability of multiple approaches and the fact that the validity of each is based on different assumptions, it is critical that researchers understand and evaluate the assumptions behind cost analyses, perform appropriate sensitivity analyses, and provide transparency in presenting their work. This will allow consumers to fully assess the robustness of the findings and appropriately utilize the information in decision-making.

Last, medical payer decision-makers are often faced with a tradeoff—that is, a new medication may have some advantage over a competing medication, but that advantage comes at a higher financial cost. Cost-effectiveness analyses, where one estimates the incremental cost necessary to gain some unit of benefit (for example, quality-of-life years) by using the more expensive treatment options, typically involve the assessment of either an incremental cost-effectiveness ratio (ICER) or an incremental net benefit (INB) (Willan and Briggs, 2006). Because the INB approach is demonstrated in the following chapter, we will demonstrate the ICER approach here.

14.1.2 Economic Analysis Guidelines

Over the past years, many guidelines have been published on the study design, data collection, data analysis, and reporting of economic analyses (Bouckaert and Crott, 1997; Ramsey et al.,

2005; Rutten-van Mölken et al., 1994). Recently, the International Society of Pharmacoeconomics and Outcomes Research (ISPOR) commissioned several task forces to provide guidance on topics related to economic analyses. For instance, Drummond and colleagues (2003) provided a review of 15 previous guidelines for reporting economic analyses. The previous guidelines were consistent on topics such as cost/resource measurement, discounting, target audience, and perspective of the analyses. However, Drummond and colleagues cited a need for additional guidance on multiple topics, including transparency of reporting, extensive use of assumptions, and extrapolations. Subsequently, a task force was chartered to create updated guidance based on consensus of good practices for the design, conduct, analysis, and reporting of economic studies alongside clinical trials (Ramsey et al., 2005). Garrison and colleagues (2007) have also recently provided guidance for the use of real-world data for coverage and payment decisions. For checklists and more detailed discussion of these issues, refer to these references.

Regarding specific statistical approaches, detailed information is typically not provided in such guidance documents. However, Rutten-van Mölken and colleagues (1994) stressed the need to perform Duan "smearing" to eliminate downwards bias in mean cost estimates resulting from retransforming log cost estimates. The ISPOR guidelines stress the importance of assessing uncertainty, performing sensitivity analyses, and addressing missing data (Ramsey et al., 2005). In addition, they emphasize the need to assess mean costs—and mention bootstrapping as a robust analytical approach. The general issue of the need to assess uncertainty in estimates is a common basic theme across all guidance documents.

14.1.3 Current Methodology Overview

Despite the existence of such guidelines, a recent survey of analytical methods used for cost analyses in the literature revealed a lack of consistent application of quality methods. Doshi and colleagues (2006) evaluated statistical methods utilized for economic analyses for 115 manuscripts reported in the MEDLINE database in 2003. They concluded that the quality of statistical methods used in economic evaluations was poor in the majority of studies. For instance, over 40% failed to report an estimate of uncertainty in their results, and less than 25% of the studies making statistical comparisons utilized nonparametric estimates of mean costs (for example, nonparametric bootstrapping). The most commonly used statistical approach for comparing costs between groups per Doshi (2006) was the simple *t*-test. The *t*-test does assess the differences in mean costs and, with the use of ANCOVA, can adjust for linear effects of covariates. However, the distribution of costs in the majority of cases is highly skewed and non-normal. Thus, the validity of the test relies on the central limit theorem and the estimates of the means. The test can be adversely affected by outliers. There are no clear guidelines on when the sample size is large enough relative to the observed level of skewness for a *t*-test to be appropriate, though one simulation study has suggested 500 per group is sufficient (Lumley et al., 2002). Thus, while the use of such tests may be appropriate in a given setting, sensitivity analyses are clearly warranted.

Rank tests, such as the Wilcoxon-ranked sum test, are nonparametric and simple to perform using SAS (with PROC NPAR1WAY). However, these approaches assess location differences, which, in general, are not differences in mean costs unless the unrealistic assumption of symmetry is met (in which case the median and mean coincide). Medians and other robust estimators are useful for describing the distribution of costs; however, such approaches are not relevant for statistical cost comparisons.

A common simple approach for comparing group costs is to transform the data to address the skewness and normalize the data using a log, square root, or other transformation. Standard, normal statistical methods such as *t*-tests and ANOVA can then be utilized to compare the groups. Such an approach is easily implemented using SAS functions (for example, the LOG function) and PROC GLM or PROC MIXED. However, a transformation approach can result in misleading results unless key assumptions are satisfied. One obvious assumption is that the transformation produces normality (or at least relies on the central limit theorem). While perhaps less obvious, what is actually more important is that standard test statistics assume that variances of the transformed costs for each treatment group are equal.

To illustrate the basic difficulty, suppose that treatment H with a high acquisition cost is compared, on a cost basis, with treatment L with a low acquisition cost. The low cost (left-hand) tail of the distribution of total accumulated cost over any fixed period of time will then be dominated by patients treated with L. The only way that H could effectively compete on cost with L would be for H to reduce, relative to L, the likelihood of high accumulated costs. In other words, the high cost (right-hand) tail of the distribution of total accumulated cost would then also be dominated by patients treated with L. To be remotely competitive on mean cost, treatment H must (greatly) reduce the variability in accumulated costs. Obviously, if a cost analyst fails to examine these distributions and perhaps unknowingly assumes that variances are equal, treatment H has been unfairly placed at a great disadvantage.

When variances are not equal, comparison of transformed means, which are functions of both the means and the variances on the initial cost scale, can yield badly biased results. This helps explain retransformation problems that have been discussed extensively in the literature (Duan, 1983; Manning, 1998; Mullahy, 1998; Gianfrancesco et al., 2002).

Generalized linear models—which can be fitted using PROC GENMOD—are an additional approach to assessing cost data. Within PROC GENMOD, one can specify a link function and distribution directly, avoiding these retransformation issues. This method obviously requires a distributional assumption, but it allows for easy adjustment of covariates. The *SAS/STAT User's Guide* (1999; Example 29.3) provides example code for an analysis of data assuming a gamma distribution using PROC GENMOD that could be applied to cost data. Refer to Lindsey and Jones (1998) for details about choosing between various generalized linear models.

Nonparametric bootstrapping is a technique where an empirical distribution of the test statistic (for example, the mean cost difference between groups) is constructed through resampling with replacement from the observed data. Though computationally intensive, bootstrapping is an attractive alternative for analysis of cost data because it is a nonparametric approach that can directly address arithmetic means. Inferences can be drawn from the empirical distribution using confidence intervals (CIs) formed by the percentile method, bias corrected method, bias corrected and accelerated method, or the percentile–*t* method (Briggs et al., 1997; DiCiccio and Efron, 1996). While more detailed arguments are possible (Chernick, 1999), a general recommendation is that 5,000 to 10,000 replications be utilized when forming confidence intervals. The validity of the bootstrap approach does rely on asymptotic assumptions—because the observed data must adequately represent the population distribution. While there is no clear guidance on what sample size is sufficient, Chernick provides a general rule of thumb (n>50) and states that sample size considerations should not be altered when using bootstrapping compared with other approaches. While the bootstrap approach allows for estimation of means without making assumptions about the shape of the distribution, by itself it does not allow for adjustment for the confounding variables necessary for addressing group differences. However, this shortcoming can be addressed by incorporating propensity score stratification, as described in the next section.

Combined assessments of both cost and effectiveness typically utilize either an ICER or an INB approach. In this chapter, we consider the use of the ICER approach. The ICER is simply the ratio of the treatment group difference in cost divided by the treatment group difference in effectiveness. Added statistical complexity comes when measures of uncertainty in the ICER point estimate are needed to draw inferences. Several different approaches have been utilized, including a Taylor Series method, Fieller Theorem method, and bootstrapping (Obenchain et al., 1997; Polsky et al., 1997; Willan and Briggs, 2006). For consistency, we focus on the bootstrap approach for determining degrees of dominance using observed incremental cost-effectiveness quadrant confidence levels (Obenchain et al., 2005). When using bootstrapping, one can assess uncertainty in the cost difference, the effectiveness difference, and the cost-effectiveness ratio simultaneously. For each bootstrap sample, one retains both the cost difference and the effectiveness difference from the selected patients—thus retaining any implied correlation structure between cost and effectiveness in the actual data.

14.2 Propensity Score Bin Bootstrapping

The PSBB approach is a potentially useful tool for cost-related analyses because it addresses arithmetic means, adjusts for confounding factors, and does not make distributional assumptions (Obenchain, 2003–2006). The first step in a PSBB analysis is to compute the propensity score for each patient using logistic regression and then group the propensity scores into five strata of equal size determined by estimated propensity score quintiles (Rosenbaum and Rubin, 1984). A thorough assessment should then be made to verify that one's propensity score estimates produce balanced covariate distributions between treatments within each stratum and that there is sufficient overlap of propensity score estimates between the treatment groups. Because the details of assessing the quality of a propensity model are covered in Chapters 2 through 4, they are not repeated here.

Second, within each treatment group, bootstrap resamples of fixed size are drawn within each stratum—with the total number of samples equaling the total number of patients. For instance, if $N = 100$ for treatment 1 and $N = 200$ for treatment 2, then 20 bootstrap samples of treatment 1 patients are taken from each strata, and 40 bootstrap samples of treatment 2 patients are taken from each of the five strata (regardless of the actual number of patients in each strata for each treatment group). For analyses comparing costs, the difference in mean total costs between treatment groups is computed for each replication, and a large number of replications generates the bootstrap distribution of mean cost differences. The percentile method, which identifies the 2.5% and 97.5% points of the distribution of bootstrap order statistics, is one simple way to generate a 95% two-sided confidence interval of the difference in mean costs. Other alternatives include the bias corrected and accelerated (BCa) method (Briggs et al., 1997; DiCiccio and Efron, 1996).

When assessing cost-effectiveness using PSBB, both the cost measure and the effectiveness measure are retained from each patient selected by the resampling, and the ICER is computed for each bootstrap sample. A display of the uncertainty of the ICER is then provided as a bivariate scatter plot of these differences on the cost-effectiveness plane, as described by Obenchain and colleagues (2005).

14.3 Example: Schizophrenia Effectiveness Study

To illustrate PSBB using SAS, we will analyze simulated cost and effectiveness data based on a 1-year, randomized, open-label, naturalistic study of patients with schizophrenia or schizoaffective disorder who were randomly assigned to initial treatment with one of three treatment regimens as reported by Tunis and colleagues (2006). The study was naturalistic in the sense that after randomization patients were treated as in a usual treatment setting and allowed to switch or stop medications and remain in the study. For simplicity, the analysis here focuses on the comparison of total 1-year costs (intent to treat) and cost-effectiveness (with effectiveness defined as estimated days in response [Nyhuis et al., 2003]) between two treatment groups labeled A and B. There were no significant differences in any baseline measure between groups—due to the randomization. However, because most analyses of observational data require adjustment for treatment-selection bias, we illustrate this adjustment using the same covariates examined by Tunis and colleagues (2006). To illustrate distinctions between alternative approaches, we compare the PSBB results to those from the log-transformation and the generalized linear modeling approaches. SAS code for these comparisons is not provided because it is easily accomplished using PROC GLM, PROC MIXED, or PROC GENMOD with PROC PLOT.

Before running the PSBB analysis, we examined the distribution of costs and we present summary statistics for the simulated data (see Program 14.1). The histogram (Output from Program 14.1) shows the high level of skewness and the large variability of the cost data. Summary statistics reveal that treatment A had a slightly lower mean cost and a slightly higher median cost as compared to treatment B.

Program 14.1 Display of Data and Summary Statistics

```
**************************************************;
** key variables from data set                  **;
**   therapy - randomized treatment group       **;
**   totcost - total 1-year costs               **;
**   respdays - estimated responder days(BPRS)  **;
**   inv - investigational site number          **;
**   bs_bprsc - baseline bprs level             **;
**   age - age in years                         **;
**   inpatst - inpatient status at baseline     **;
** subsabdx - substance abuse diagnosis         **;
** psycdur - duration of psychiatric problems   **;
** hospestmo - duration of hosp in past year    **;
** insured - insurance status                   **;
**************************************************;

ods rtf file="D:\Temp\ICER_SumCostEff.rtf"
        style=minimal;

proc tabulate data = icer;
  class therapy;
  var respdays totcost;
  tables therapy,
    (totcost='Total Costs' respdays='Response Days (BPRS)')*
    (N*FORMAT=3. P25 MEDIAN P75 MEAN STD);
  title 'Summary of costs and effectiveness measures by therapy';
  run;

ods rtf close;
```

```
proc sort data = ICER;
  by therapy; run;

proc univariate data =ICER noprint;
  by therapy;
  var totcost;
  histogram / lognormal(fill l=b) cfill=yellow midpoints =
     2500 to 152500 by 5000;
  title h=2.5 lspace=1 "Test histogram: raw costs - lognormal
distribution";
run;

data icer2; set icer;
  group=floor(totcost/10000);
run;

proc sort data=icer2; by therapy group;
run;

filename MYFILE "D:\Temp\ICER_TOTCOST.gif";

goptions reset=all device=gif gsfname=MYFILE gsfmode=replace htext=1
ftext=swiss rotate=landscape;

proc format;
 value charge 0='<1';
 run;

legend1 label=none across=3 value=(height=1.3) cborder=black cblock=gray;

pattern1 v=solid c=black;
pattern3 v=solid  c=LIBRGR ;
pattern2 v=L1  c=black;

footnote1  h=1.5 'Total Costs (10 thou. $)';

title 'Summary of Total Costs by Initial Therapy';
AXIS1 LABEL=none value=(H=1.5 C=BLACK);
AXIS2 LABEL=(H=2 C=BLACK angle=90 "Frequency" J=CENTER) value=(H=1.5
C=BLACK);
AXIS3 label=none value=none;

PROC GCHART data=ICER2;
format group charge.;
VBAR therapy/patternid=subgroup subgroup=therapy group=group space=0
            ref=(10 to 120 by 10) gaxis=axis1 raxis=axis2 maxis=axis3
legend=legend1;
run;
quit;
```

Output from Program 14.1

```
Summary of costs and effectiveness measures by therapy
```

	Total Costs					
	N	P25	Median	P75	Mean	Std
THERAPY						
A	223	4841.09	8467.46	22796.24	20863.59	28995.86
B	210	2899.83	7633.27	25269.44	21227.37	30992.32

	Response Days (BPRS)					
	N	P25	Median	P75	Mean	Std
THERAPY						
A	218	20.48	97.66	229.70	129.23	117.63
B	200	10.38	96.63	212.06	123.74	118.29

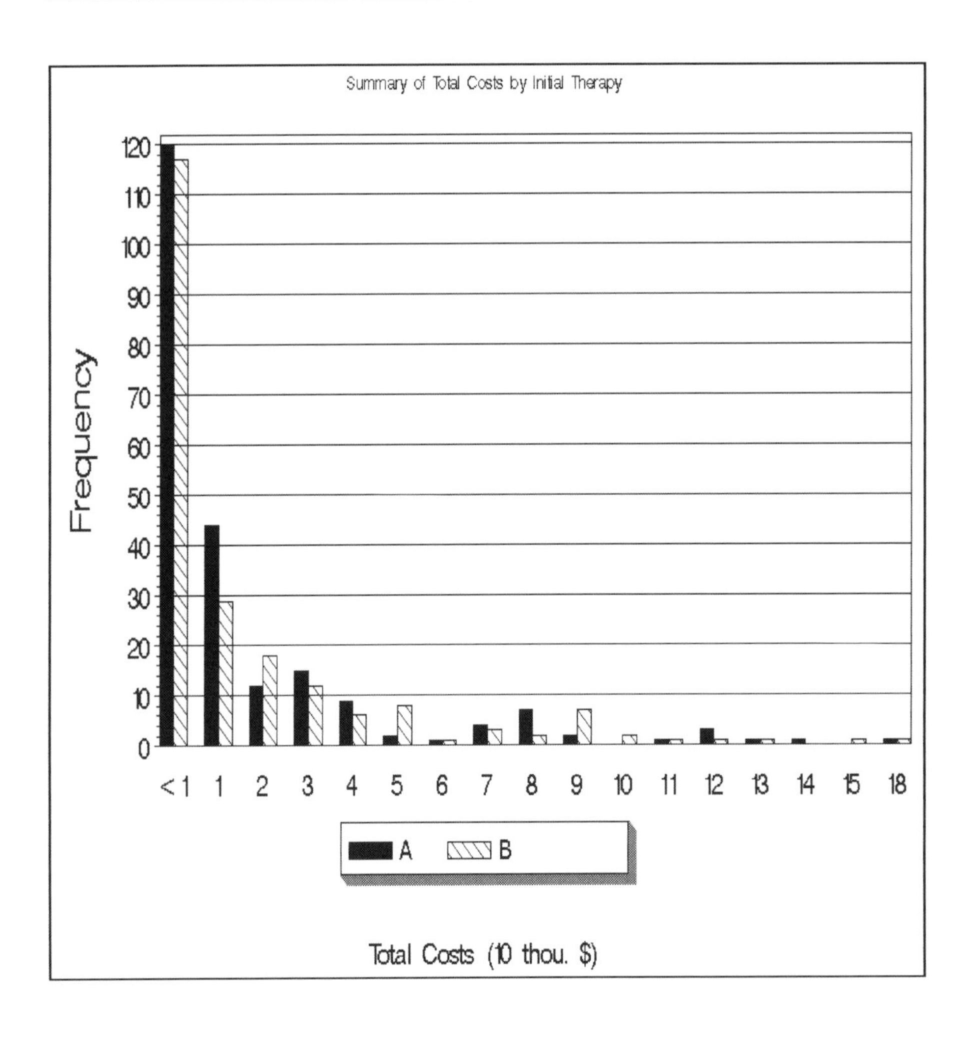

Program 14.2 provides the SAS code for the PSBB analysis. After preliminary calculation of the summary statistics necessary for later computation of confidence intervals, the first main step in the analysis is to compute the propensity score for each patient and form the propensity score strata (using quintiles). This is accomplished using the GENMOD and RANK procedures. Only a brief assessment of the quality of the propensity model is made here—simply utilizing PROC FREQ to confirm adequate numbers of patients per treatment group within each stratum. A lack of patients from either treatment group within a stratum is an indication that there is insufficient overlap (common support) between the two groups to make reliable comparisons (Rosenbaum and Rubin, 1984). Macro PSBB then creates a stratified bootstrap sample of both cost and effectiveness measure values. The inputs to the macro are the number of replications desired, the cost measure, the effectiveness measure, the input data set, and the treatment indicator variable. We used 10,000 bootstrap samples as confidence intervals of interest. The bootstrap distribution for each measure, the confidence intervals for each measure using both the percentile and BCa approaches, the bootstrap distribution of the ICER, and a graphical display of the variability in the ICER are produced.

From the Output from Program 14.2 (scatter plot), the bootstrap distribution for total cost difference is centered near zero and shows the large variability in mean costs. The estimated mean treatment difference was $–173 (treatment A–treatment B) and neither the percentile method, 95% CI of (–5777, 5345), nor the bias corrected and accelerated approach, 95% CI of (–6190, 4908), suggests a significant difference in mean costs. Similarly, non-significant differences were observed in the effectiveness measure (9.1 more days of response on treatment A with a 95% CI of –13.4 to +31.3 days).

Program 14.2 SAS Code for Propensity Score Bin Bootstrapping Analysis

```
TITLE 'PSBB ANALYSIS';

PROC PRINTTO LOG='D:\TEMP\PSBBLog.log' NEW; RUN;

** Assign summary statistics utilized in analysis code below **;
** Values not computed here to focus code on cost analysis steps **;

%let nc1 = 210;   * Sample size for group B with cost data *;
%let nc2 = 223;   * Sample size for group A with cost data *;
%let ne1 = 200;   * Sample size for group B with effectiveness data *;
%let ne2 = 218;   * Sample size for group A with effectiveness data *;
%let mc1 = 21227;   * Mean of cost variable for group B *;
%let mc2 = 20864;   * Mean of cost variable for group A *;
%let me1 = 123.74;   * Mean of effectiveness variable for group B *;
%let me2 = 129.23;   * Mean of effectiveness variable for group A *;

  ** Compute statistic used later in bootstrap CI calculations **;

data icer;
  set icer;
      * Compute score statistic *;
  if therapy = 'A' then do;
    mnc1 = (&nc2*&mc2 - totcost) / (&nc2 - 1);
          * Mean of group without current obs *;
    mne1 = (&ne2*&me2 - respdays) / (&ne2 - 1);
          * Mean of group without current obs *;
    diffc1 = mnc1 - &mc2;
          * Mean diff between groups without current obs *;
    diffe1 = mne1 - &me2;
          * Mean diff between groups without current obs *;
```

```
    uc = (&mc2 - &mc1 - diffc1);
    ue = (&me2 - &me1 - diffe1);
       * Diff between overall and estimate without curren obs *;
  end;

  if therapy = 'B' then do;
    mnc1 = (&nc1*&mc1 - totcost) / (&nc1 - 1);
          * Mean of group without current obs *;
    mne1 = (&ne1*&me1 - respdays) / (&ne1 - 1);
          * Mean of group without current obs *;
    diffc1 = &mc1 - mnc1;
          * Mean diff between groups without current obs *;
    diffe1 = &me1 - mne1;
          * Mean diff between groups without current obs *;
    uc = (&mc2 - &mc1 - diffc1);
    ue = (&me2 - &me1 - diffe1);
       * Diff between overall and estimate without current obs *;
  end;
  if therapy = 'A' then ther = 1;
  if therapy = 'B' then ther = 0;
run;

/** Compute acceleration constant for later BCa CI calculations **/

data accel;
  set icer;
  dm = 1;
  uc_cub + uc**3;
  ue_cub + ue**3;
  uc_sqr + uc**2;
  ue_sqr + ue**2;
  keep patient dm uc ue uc_cub ue_cub uc_sqr ue_sqr;
run;

proc sort data = accel; by dm;
run;

data accel2;
  set accel;
  by dm;
  if last.dm;
  c_aconst = uc_cub / (((uc_sqr**1.5))*6);
  e_aconst = ue_cub / (((ue_sqr**1.5))*6);
run;

**Assign the c_aconst and e_aconst to macro variables for BCa calculation
in macro PSBB **;

data _null_; set accel2;
 call symput('c_aconst', trim(left(c_aconst)));
 call symput('e_aconst', trim(left(e_aconst)));
run;

%put c_aconst=&c_aconst e_aconst=&e_aconst;

/*******************************************************************
** Compute propensity score strata                               **
*******************************************************************/

option spool;
ods listing close;
```

```
proc genmod data = icer;
  class inv inptatst subsabdx bs_bprsc insured;
  model therapy = inv bs_bprsc age inptatst subsabdx psycdur hospestmo
                  insured   / dist = bin link = logit type3 obstats;
  output out=pred6 pred = prdct;
  run;

ods listing;

data premab;
  set pred6;
  predmo = 1-prdct;
  predmc = prdct;
  keep patient predmo predmc therapy ther totcost respdays age
       gender inptatst subsabdx insured hospestmo psycdur bs_bprsc;
run;

proc rank data = premab groups = 5 out = rankmab;
  ranks rnkm_ab;
  var predmo;
run;

data rankmab;
  set rankmab;
  bin_ps = rnkm_ab + 1;
run;

proc sort data = rankmab;
  by therapy;
run;

proc univariate data = rankmab;
  by therapy;
  var predmo;
  title 'Distribution of propensity scores: oc';
run;

proc freq data = rankmab;
  tables bin_ps*therapy;
  title 'Therapy distribution among bins';
run;

proc tabulate data = rankmab;
  class therapy bin_ps;
  var respdays totcost;
  tables bin_ps*therapy,(respdays totcost)*(n*format=3. mean std);
  title 'Summary of costs/responder days by bin and therapy';
run;

/******************************************************************
Macro PSBB is for a propensity score bin bootstrap analysis

Inputs:

REP    = Number of bootstrap samples
AVARC  = Variable for Total Costs
AVARE  = Variable for Effectiveness (response days calculated for BPRS)
INDAT  = Data set to be analyzed
GRPVAR = Variable for therapy group number
FSEED0 = Starting randomization seed for therapy group 0
FSEED1 = Starting randomization seed for therapy group 1
******************************************************************/
```

```
%MACRO
  PSBB(rep=,avarc=,avare=,indat=,grpvar=,fseed0=887583,fseed1=566126);

data temp; set &indat;
run;

proc freq data=temp noprint;
   tables &grpvar / out=freqnums;
   where not(&grpvar=.);
run;

data _null_; set freqnums;
 call symput('val'||compress(put(_n_, 4.)), trim(left(&grpvar)));
 call symput('ssize'||compress(put(_n_, 4.)), trim(left(count)));
run;

%* Create data sets for each treatment *;
data trt0 trt1;
  set temp;
  if (&grpvar=&val1) then output trt0;
  else if (&grpvar=&val2) then output trt1;
  keep &grpvar &avarc &avare bin_ps;
run;

data bssumm;    %* Empty data set to add to later *;
 if _n_ eq 1 then stop;
run;

proc sort data=trt0; by &grpvar bin_ps;
  run;

proc sort data=trt1; by &grpvar bin_ps;
  run;

%do i=1 %to &rep;
   %** Generate random bootstrap sample data set for therapy0**;
      %* Perform bootstrap resampling *;
   %let btnum=%qsysfunc(round(&ssize1/5,1));
   %let rseed=%qsysfunc(round(&i + &fseed0, 1));

  proc surveyselect data=trt0 method=urs outhits rep=1
                   n=&btnum. seed=&rseed. noprint out=trt0out;
    strata &grpvar bin_ps;
   run;

   %** Generate random bootstrap sample data set for therapy1**;
   %let btnum=%qsysfunc(round(&ssize2/5,1));
   %let rseed=%qsysfunc(round(&i + &fseed1, 1));

  proc surveyselect data=trt1 method=urs outhits rep=1
                   n=&btnum. seed=&rseed. noprint out=trt1out;
    strata &grpvar bin_ps;
   run;

  data bothgrps;
   set trt0out trt1out;
  run;

  %** Compute overall statistics for the sample **;
  proc means data=bothgrps noprint;
   class &grpvar;
   var &avarc &avare;
   output out = mn mean = out_avgc out_avge;
```

```
  data mn; set mn end=eof;
   label &avarc._avg1 = "Average for &AVARC, Group=&VAL1"
         &avare._avg1 = "Average for &AVARE, Group=&VAL1"
         &avarc._avg2 = "Average for &AVARC, Group=&VAL2"
         &avare._avg2 = "Average for &AVARE, Group=&VAL2";
   dumm= 1;
   retain &avarc._avg1 &avare._avg1 &avarc._avg2 &avare._avg2;
   if &grpvar=0 then do;
   &avarc._avg1=out_avgc;
   &avare._avg1=out_avge;
   end;
   if &grpvar=1 then do;
   &avarc._avg2=out_avgc;
   &avare._avg2=out_avge;
   end;
   keep dumm &avarc._avg1 &avare._avg1 &avarc._avg2 &avare._avg2;
   if eof then output;
  run;

%** Update data set with statistics from this sample **;
  data bssumm;
   set bssumm mn;
  run;

%**Clean work library**;
  proc datasets library=work memtype=data nolist;
   delete trt0out trt01ut bothgrps mn;
  run;
  quit;

%end;    %* End of %do loop *;

%** Compute differences and test statistics **;
data bssumm;
  set bssumm;
   &avare._diff = &avare._avg2 - &avare._avg1;
   &avarc._diff = &avarc._avg2 - &avarc._avg1;
    if &avarc._diff ne . and &avare._diff ne . then do;
    if &avarc._diff ge 0 and &avare._diff ge 0 then ce_quad = '++';
    if &avarc._diff ge 0 and &avare._diff lt 0 then ce_quad = '+-';
    if &avarc._diff lt 0 and &avare._diff ge 0 then ce_quad = '-+';
    if &avarc._diff lt 0 and &avare._diff lt 0 then ce_quad = '--';
    end;
    if &avarc._diff lt (&mc2 - &mc1) then zzeroctc + 1;
    if &avare._diff lt (&me2 - &me1) then zzerocte + 1;
    label &avare._diff="Average for &AVARE Diff: Grp2-Grp1"
       &avarc._diff="Average for &AVARC Diff: Grp2-Grp1";
run;

*Calculate quadrants percentage and assign macro variable for graph **;

ods output OneWayFreqs=quadrt(keep=ce_quad percent);

proc freq data = bssumm;
  tables ce_quad;
  title2 "Quadrants distribution for cost effectiveness";
  title3 "Variables &avarc and avare";
run;
data _null_; set quadrt;
 if ce_quad='++' then call symput('pospos', compress(percent));
 if ce_quad='+-' then call symput('posneg', compress(percent));
```

```
 if ce_quad='-+' then call symput('negpos', compress(percent));
 if ce_quad='--' then call symput('negneg', compress(percent));
 run;

proc univariate data=bssumm freq noprint;
   var &avarc._diff &avare._diff;
   output out=pctls pctlpts=2.5 97.5 pctlpre = &avarc &avare
            pctlname=_lcl _ucl;
run;

proc print data=pctls;
  title2 "Bootstrap Percentile 95% confidence limits for &avarc and
         &avare";  run;

** Compute BCa confidence intervals **;

data zerodat;
  set bssumm;
  by dumm;
  if last.dumm;
  keep zzeroctc zzerocte;
run;

data bcacalc;
  set zerodat;
  zzeroc = probit( zzeroctc / &rep );
  zzeroe = probit( zzerocte / &rep );
  zzl = probit(.025);
  zzh = probit(.975);
  bcaclo = zzeroc + ((zzeroc + zzl) / (1 - &c_aconst.*(zzeroc + zzl)));
  bcachi = zzeroc + ((zzeroc + zzh) / (1 - &c_aconst.*(zzeroc + zzh)));
  bcaelo = zzeroe + ((zzeroe + zzl) / (1 - &e_aconst.*(zzeroe + zzl)));
  bcaehi = zzeroe + ((zzeroe + zzh) / (1 - &e_aconst.*(zzeroe + zzh)));

  bcacl = probnorm(bcaclo);
  bcach = probnorm(bcachi);
  bcael = probnorm(bcaelo);
  bcaeh = probnorm(bcaehi);
run;

data _null_; set bcacalc;
  call symput('bcacl', trim(left(bcacl*100)));
  call symput('bcach', trim(left(bcach*100)));
  call symput('bcael', trim(left(bcael*100)));
  call symput('bcaeh', trim(left(bcaeh*100)));
  run;

%put bcacl=&bcacl bcach=&bcach bcael=&bcael baceh=&bcaeh;

proc univariate data=bssumm freq noprint;
   var &avarc._diff;
   output out=pctls2 pctlpts=&bcacl. &bcach. pctlpre = &avarc
      pctlname=_lcl _ucl;
run;

proc print data=pctls2;
   title2 "BCa bootstrap 95% confidence limits for &avarc";
run;
```

```
proc univariate data=bssumm freq noprint;
   var &avare._diff;
   output out=pctls3 pctlpts=&bcael. &bcaeh. pctlpre = &avare
      pctlname=_lcl _ucl;
run;

proc print data=pctls3;
   title2 "BCa bootstrap 95% confidence limits for &avare";
run;


%** Create graph of bootstrap ce **;

axis1 label=(h=1.5 c=black a=90 "Effectiveness Difference: A - B"
              J=CENTER) value=(h=1.5 c=black) ;
axis2 label=(h=1.5 c=black "Cost Difference: A - B" J=CENTER)
      value=(h=1.5 c=black) ;

proc gplot data=bssumm;
  plot &avare._diff*&avarc._diff = '*'/nolegend haxis=axis2
                                        vaxis=axis1
                                        href=0
                                        vref=0 ;
%**Add quadrant frequency percentage **;
  note height=1.75 m=(80pct,80pct) "&pospos.%";
  note height=1.75 m=(80pct,30pct) "&posneg.%";
  note height=1.75 m=(20pct,30pct) "&negneg.%";
  note height=1.75 m=(20pct,80pct) "&negpos.%";

  title1 h=2.5 lspace=1 "Quadrant distribution for cost effectiveness";
run;  quit;

%**Clean work library**;
proc datasets library=work memtype=data nolist;
   delete temp freqnums trt0 trt1 pctls pctls2 pctls3 zerodat;
run;  quit;

goptions reset=all;

%MEND PSBB;           /* End of macro psbb */


/* Call the bootstrap macro */

filename myfile1 "D:\Temp\ICER_TOTCOST_RDBPRS_DIFF2.gif";

goptions reset=all device=gif gsfname=MYFILE1 gsfmode=replace htext=1
ftext=swiss rotate=landscape noborder;

%PSBB(rep=10000,avarc=totcost,avare=respdays,indat=rankmab,grpvar=ther);

quit;
goptions reset=all;

***Draw histogram of mean difference in costs***;

data bssumm; set bssumm;
 totcost_diff1=totcost_diff/1000;
     **resize the cost to show in the graph x-axis**;
run;

filename myfile2 "D:\Temp\ICER_TOTCOST_DIFF2.gif";
```

```
goptions reset=all device=gif gsfname=MYFILE2 gsfmode=replace htext=1.25
ftext='arial/bo' rotate=landscape noborder;
title ' ';
footnote ' ';
pattern1 v=solid c=black;
footnote1  h=1.5 "Mean Difference in Costs: A - B (thousand $)";

AXIS1 LABEL=(H=2 C=BLACK angle=90 "Frequency" J=CENTER) value=(H=1.5
   C=BLACK) order=(0 to 1600 by 200);
AXIS2 LABEL=(H=2 C=BLACK  J=CENTER ' ') ;

PROC GCHART data=bssumm;
  VBAR totcost diff1/ref=(0 to 1600 by 200) midpoints=(-12 to 12 by 1)
raxis=axis1 maxis=axis2 space=5 width=2;
run;  quit;
goptions reset=all;

PROC PRINTTO; RUN;
```

Output from Program 14.2

Table of bin_ps by THERAPY

bin_ps Frequency Percent Row Pct Col Pct	THERAPY(THERAPY) A	B	Total
1	54 12.47 62.79 24.22	32 7.39 37.21 15.24	86 19.86
2	48 11.09 55.17 21.52	39 9.01 44.83 18.57	87 20.09
3	41 9.47 47.13 18.39	46 10.62 52.87 21.90	87 20.09
4	43 9.93 49.43 19.28	44 10.16 50.57 20.95	87 20.09
5	37 8.55 43.02 16.59	49 11.32 56.98 23.33	86 19.86
Total	223 51.50	210 48.50	433 100.00

(continued)

Output from Program 14.2 *(continued)*

Summary of costs/responder days by bin and therapy

		Response Days calculated for BPRS			TOTALCOST		
		N	Mean	Std	N	Mean	Std
bin_ps	THERAPY						
1	A	53	110.25	95.95	54	26888.70	40157.77
	B	31	106.45	105.16	32	20484.75	38666.46
2	A	47	113.29	112.52	48	12551.58	14638.41
	B	38	113.49	115.44	39	15421.72	21692.73
3	A	40	125.38	122.55	41	17913.06	22861.74
	B	45	103.18	121.55	46	28424.47	36420.49
4	A	42	163.39	129.75	43	20371.88	25649.21
	B	42	120.86	109.20	44	22364.51	27221.33
5	A	36	142.40	128.56	37	26694.28	31476.58
	B	44	168.55	127.57	49	18555.59	29170.77

PSBB Estimated Mean Treatment Differences for Cost and Effectiveness

Obs	psbb_meandiff_cost	psbb_meandiff_effect
1	-172.904	9.06927

Bootstrap Percentile 95% confidence limits for Cost and Effectiveness Treatment Differences

Obs	totcost_lcl	totcost_ucl	respdays_lcl	respdays_ucl
1	-5777.38	5344.59	-13.4060	31.3172

(continued)

Output from Program 14.2 *(continued)*

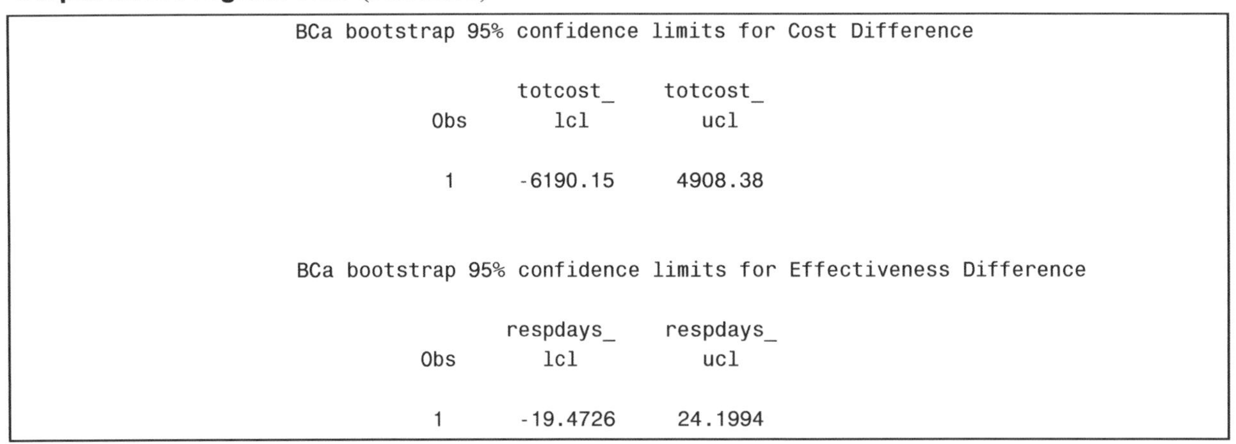

```
BCa bootstrap 95% confidence limits for Cost Difference

             totcost_     totcost_
Obs            lcl          ucl

  1         -6190.15      4908.38


BCa bootstrap 95% confidence limits for Effectiveness Difference

            respdays_     respdays_
Obs            lcl           ucl

  1         -19.4726      24.1994
```

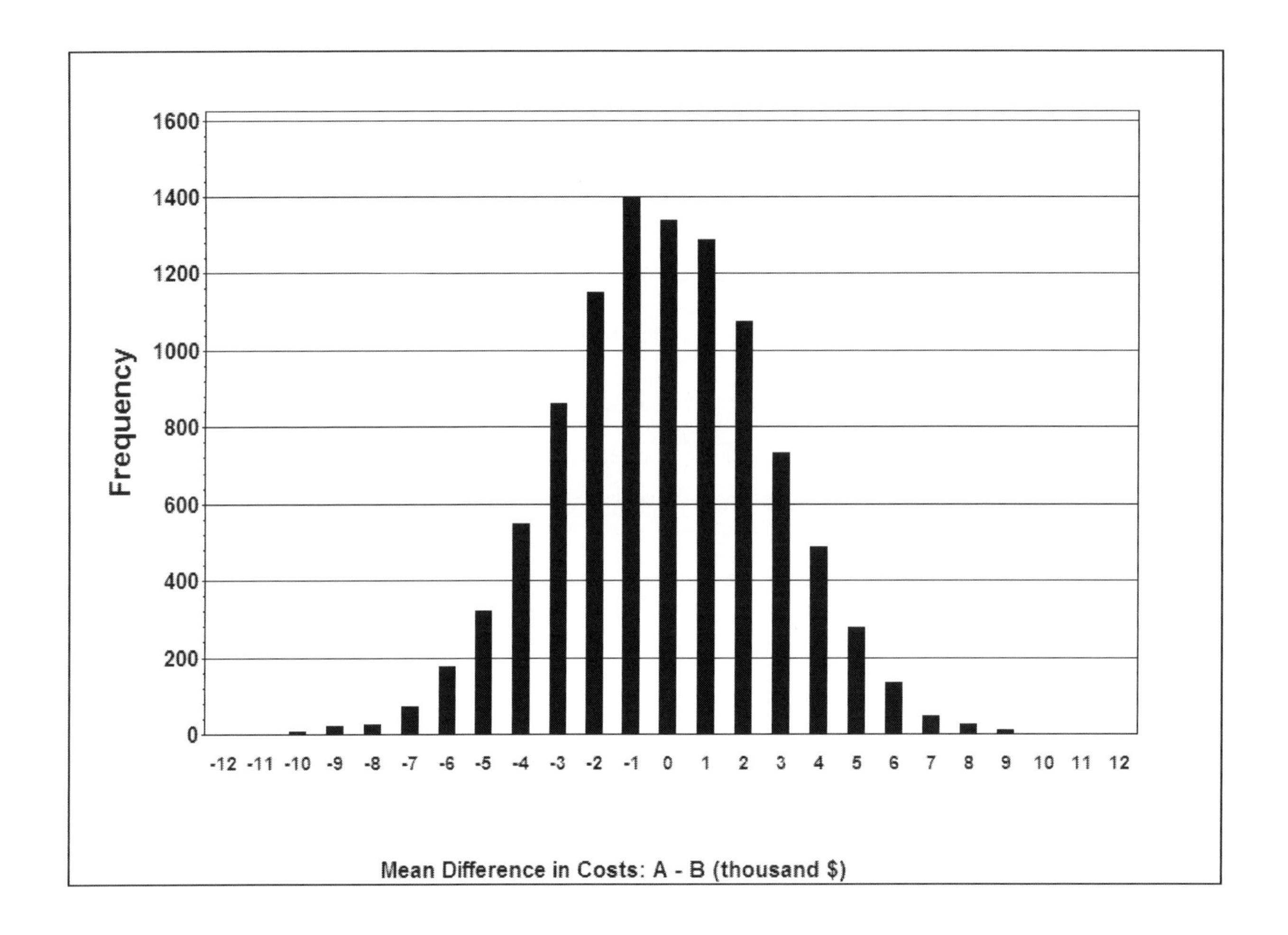

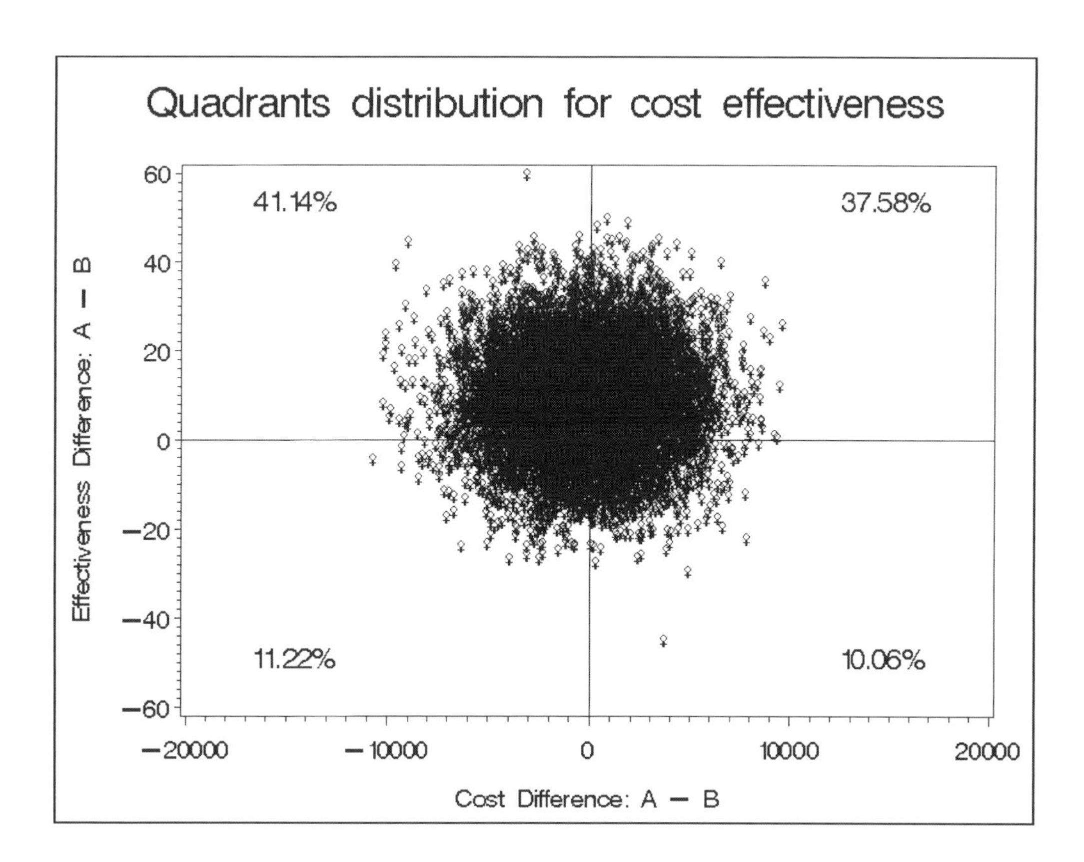

With a small estimated cost savings and a small effectiveness advantage, the point estimate of incremental cost-effectiveness does fall within the dominant region (save $173 with a gain of 9 days of response; not a tradeoff here). Output from Program 14.2 confirms that, relative to its uncertainty, this ICE point estimate is quite near the origin. In fact, the bootstrap distribution of ICE uncertainty spans all four quadrants of the cost-effectiveness plane. Note that one has 41.1% confidence in dominance (indicating better effectiveness and less cost for treatment A), 37.6% in the "A is more costly and more effective" quadrant, and 10%–12% in each of the other two quadrants ("A is less costly and less effective" and "A is more costly and less effective"). Thus, Obenchain and his colleagues' (2005) levels of confidence needed to signal some, much, or strict dominance are not met in this example.

While not presented in detail here, sensitivity analyses utilizing other methods demonstrated some striking results in regard to treatment comparisons of costs. While the simple *t*-test (p=.900) and generalized linear model (gamma distribution) (p=.880) provided similar results to the PSBB analysis, both a log-transformation analysis (p=.007) and a Wilcoxon-ranked sum test (p=.045) resulted in statistically significant lower costs for the treatment B group. This is despite the fact that the observed mean costs were higher for this group. This is a result of the fact that in this situation the log-transformed and ranked tests are not reliable tests for differences in means. The median was lower for treatment B—as picked up by the ranked test—and a simple comparison of the variances of the log-transformed data (as can be obtained through PROC TTEST) demonstrates that the assumptions behind the log-transformed analysis are not valid here. Gianfrancesco and colleagues (2002) have discussed the potential for situations such as this, especially when comparing costs for treatments from different medication classes.

14.4 Discussion

In this chapter, we have discussed the main issues involved in analyzing cost and cost-effectiveness comparisons between groups. SAS code for performing a PSBB analysis was provided along with a simulated example based on a schizophrenia trial. The PSBB approach is an attractive analytical method because it assesses the mean costs, is nonparametric, and adjusts for baseline selection bias through the well-accepted approach of propensity score stratification. PSBB may not be the best method for all situations—as comparative research on methodology to understand under what scenarios various methods perform best is lacking.

We have not fully addressed all issues involved in either the analysis or the presentation of cost data. First, we focused here on the statistical analysis methodology—ignoring issues such as study design, collection of resources or costs, assignment of costs to resource data, and cost discounting—because these have been widely discussed in the referenced guidelines on economic analyses. We also have not discussed the effects of missing or censored cost data. The methods illustrated here assume that unbiased cost estimates or imputed values are available or that the methods for addressing the missing data can be used within the structure of the propensity score bin bootstrap analysis (for example, use a method that adjusts for censoring [such as described in Chapter 16] to estimate cost differences within each propensity stratum—instead of a simple mean difference within each stratum as presented here). For other references on dealing with missing data specific to cost analyses, see Willan and Briggs (2006) or Young (2005). In addition, we did not present a full discussion of issues and options surrounding cost-effectiveness approaches (see Chapter 15).

Our objectives here were to use a specific example to illustrate that propensity score bin bootstrapping is relatively easy for researchers to implement and to demonstrate the importance of understanding the basic assumptions behind statistical methods for analysis of cost data. Given the variety of methods available, the different assumptions necessary for the different methods to be valid, the fact that different results follow from the same data using different methods, and the importance of cost analyses to health care payer decision-makers, what should outcomes researchers do? We contend that quality analyses and presentation of cost data must include at least the following three components:

1. a thorough assessment of the reasonableness of all assumptions made and the implications if the assumptions are not met;
2. documented proof that sensitivity analyses were performed; and
3. transparency in reporting all results.

Studies by Obenchain and Johnstone (1999) and Kereiakes and colleagues (2000) are two good examples of quality cost and cost-effectiveness analyses in this sense.

References

Bouckaert, A., and R. Crott. 1997. "The difference in mean costs as a pharmacoeconomic outcome variable: power considerations." *Controlled Clinical Trials* 18: 58–64.

Briggs, A. H., D. E. Wonderling, and C. Z. Mooney. 1997. "Pulling cost-effectiveness analysis up by its bootstraps; a non-parametric approach to confidence interval estimation." *Health Economics* 6(4): 327–340.

Chernick, M. R. 1999. *Bootstrap Methods—A Practitioner's Guide*. New York: John Wiley & Sons, Inc., p. 264.

D'Agostino, Jr., R. B. 1998. "Propensity score methods for bias reduction in the comparison of a treatment to a non-randomized control group." *Statistics in Medicine* 17: 2265–2281.

Davies, L. M., S. Lewis, P. B. Jones, T. R. E. Barnes, F. Gaughran, K. Hayhurst, A. Markwick, H. Lloyd, and the CUtLASS team. 2007. "Cost-effectiveness of first- v. second-generation antipsychotic drugs: results from a randomised controlled trial in schizophrenia responding poorly to previous therapy." *British Journal of Psychiatry* 191(1): 14–22.

DiCiccio, T. J., and B. Efron. 1996. "Bootstrap confidence intervals." *Statistical Science* 11: 189–228.

Doshi, J. A., H. A. Glick, and D. Polsky. 2006. "Analyses of cost data in economic evaluations conducted alongside randomized controlled trials." *Value in Health* 9(5): 334–340.

Drummond, M., R. Brown, A. M. Fendrick, P. Fullerton, P. Neumann, R. Taylor, and M. Barbieri, Marco; the ISPOR scientific task force. 2003. "Use of pharmacoeconomics information—report of the ISPOR task force on the use of pharmacoeconomic/health economic information in health-care decision making." *Value in Health* 6(4): 407–416.

Duan, N. 1983. "Smearing estimate: a nonparametric retransformation method." *Journal of the American Statistical Association* 78: 605–610.

Duggan, M. 2005. "Do new prescription drugs pay for themselves? The case of second-generation antipsychotics." *Journal of Health Economics* 24(1): 1–31.

Garrison, Jr., L. P., P. J. Neumann, P. Erickson, S. Marshall, and C. D. Mullins. 2007. "Using real-world data for coverage and payment decisions: the ISPOR Real-World Data task force report." *Value in Health* 10(5): 326–335.

Gianfrancesco, F., R. Wang, R. Mahmoud, and R. White. 2002. "Methods for claims-based pharmacoeconomic studies in psychosis." *PharmacoEconomics* 20(8): 499–511.

Grimes, D. A., and K. F. Schulz. 2002. "Bias and causal associations in observational research." The *Lancet* 359: 248–252.

Kereiakes, D. J., R. L. Obenchain, B. L. Barber, A. Smith, M. McDonald, T. M. Broderick, J. P. Runyon, T. M. Shimshak, J. F. Schneider, C. R. Hattemer, E. M. Roth, D. D. Whang, D. Cocks, and C. W. Abbottsmith. 2000. "Abciximab provides cost- effective survival advantage in high-volume interventional practice." *American Heart Journal* 140(4): 603–610.

Lindsey, J. K., and B. Jones. 1998. "Choosing among generalized linear models applied to medical data." *Statistics in Medicine* 17: 59–68.

Liu, G. G., S. X. Sun, D. B. Christensen, and Z. Zhao. 2007. "Cost analysis of schizophrenia treatment with second-generation antipsychotic medications in North Carolina's Medicaid program." *Journal of the American Pharmacists Association* 47(1): 77–81.

Lumley T., P. Diehr, S. Emerson, and L. Chen. 2002. "The importance of the normality assumption in large public health data sets." *Annual Review of Public Health* 23: 151–169.

Manning, W.G. 1998. "The logged dependent variable, heteroscedacsticity, and the retransformation problem." *Journal of Health Economics* 17: 283–295.

Mullahy, J. 1998. "Much ado about two: reconsidering retransformation and the two-part model in health econometrics." *Journal of Health Economics* 17(3): 247–281.

Nyhuis, A. W., M. D. Stensland, and D. E. Faries. 2003. "Calculating responder days for cost-effectiveness studies." *Schizophrenia Research* 60(1) (Supplement 1): 341.

Obenchain, R. L. 2003–2006. "ICEpsbbs: a Windows application for incremental cost-effectiveness inference via propensity score bin boot strapping (two biased samples)." Available at http://members.iquest.net/~softrx/ICErefs.htm

Obenchain, R. L., and B. M. Johnstone. 1999. "Mixed-model imputation of cost data for early discontinuers from a randomized clinical trial." *Drug Information Journal* 33: 191–209.

Obenchain, R. L., C. A. Melfi, T. W. Croghan, and D. P. Buesching. 1997. "Bootstrap analyses of cost effectiveness in antidepressant pharmacotherapy." *PharmacoEconomics* 11(5): 464–472.

Obenchain, R. L., R. L. Robinson, and R. W. Swindle. 2005. "Cost-effectiveness inferences from bootstrap quadrant confidence levels: three degrees of dominance." *Journal of Biopharmaceutical Statistics* 15(3): 419–436.

Oostenbrink, J. B., and M. J. Al. 2005. "The analysis of incomplete cost data due to dropout." *Health Economics* 14(8): 763–776.

Polsky, D., H. A. Glick, R. Willke, and K. Schulman. 1997. "Confidence intervals for cost-effectiveness ratios: a comparison of four methods." *Health Economics* 6(3): 243–252.

Polsky, D., J. A. Doshi, M. S. Bauer, and H. A. Glick. 2006. "Clinical trial based cost-effectiveness analyses of antipsychotic use." The *American Journal of Psychiatry* 163: 2047–2056.

Ramsey, S., R. Willke, A. Briggs, R. Brown, M. Buxton, A. Chawla, J. Cook, H. Glick, B. Liljas, S. Petitti, and S. Reed. 2005. "Good research practices for cost-effectiveness analysis alongside clinical trials: the ISPOR RCT-CEA task force report." *Value in Health* 8(5): 521–533.

Revicki, D. A., and L. Frank. 1999. "Pharmacoeconomic evaluation in the real world: effectiveness versus efficacy studies." *PharmacoEconomics* 15(5): 423–434.

Rosenbaum, P. R., and D. B. Rubin. 1983. "The central role of the propensity score in observational studies for causal effects." *Biometrika* 70: 41–55.

Rosenbaum, P. R., and D. B. Rubin. 1984. "Reducing bias in observational studies using subclassification on a propensity score." *Journal of the American Statistical Association* 79: 516–524.

Rosenheck, R., D. Perlick, S. Bingham, W. Liu-Mares, J. Collins, S. Warren, D. Leslie, E. Allan, E. C. Campbell, S. Caroff, J. Corwin, L. Davis, R. Douyon, L. Dunn, D. Evans, E. Frecska, J. Grabowski, D. Graeber, L. Herz, K. Kwon, W. Lawson, F. Mena, J. Sheikh, D. Smelson, and V. Smith-Gamble; Department of Veterans Affairs Cooperative Study Group on the Cost-Effectiveness of Olanzapine. 2003. "Effectiveness and cost of olanzapine and haloperidol in the treatment of schizophrenia: a randomized controlled trial." *The Journal of the American Medical Association* 290(20): 2693–2702.

Rosenheck, R. A., D. L. Leslie, J. Sindelar, E. A. Miller, H. Lin, T. S. Stroup, J. McEvoy, S. M. Davis, R. S. Keefe, M. Swartz, D. O. Perkins, J. K. Hsiao, and J. Lieberman; CATIE Study Investigators. 2006. "Cost-effectiveness of second-generation antipsychotics and perphenazine in a randomized trial of treatment for chronic schizophrenia." The *American Journal of Psychiatry* 163(12): 2080–2089.

Roy-Byrne, P. P., C. D. Sherbourne, M. G. Craske, M. B. Stein, W. Katon, G. Sullivan, A. Means-Christensen, and A. Bystritsky. 2003. "Moving treatment research from clinical trials to the real world." *Psychiatric Services* 54(3): 327–332.

Rutten-van Mölken, M. P., E. K. van Doorslaer, R. C. van Vliet. 1994. "Statistical analysis of cost outcomes in a randomized controlled clinical trial." *Health Economics* 3(5): 333–345.

Tollefson, G. D., C. M. Beasley, Jr., C.M. Jr., P. V. Tran, J. S. Street, J.S., J. A. Krueger, R. N. Tamura, K. A. Graffeo, and M. E. Thieme. 1997. "Olanzapine versus haloperidol in the treatment of schizophrenia and schizoaffective and schizophreniform disorders: results of an international collaborative trial." The *American Journal of Psychiatry* 154(4): 457–465.

Tunis, S. L., D. E. Faries, A. W. Nyhuis, B. J. Kinon, H. Ascher-Svanum, and R. Aquila. 2006. "Cost-effectiveness of olanzapine as first-line treatment for schizophrenia: results from a randomized, open-label, 1-year trial." *Value in Health* 9(2): 77–89.

Willan, A. R., and A. H. Briggs. 2006. *Statistical Analysis of Cost-Effectiveness Data.* West Sussex, England: John Wiley & Sons Ltd., p. 196.

Young, T. A. 2005. "Estimating mean total costs in the presence of censoring: a comparison assessment of methods." *PharmacoEconomics* 23(12): 1229–1242.

Zhu, B., S. L. Tunis, Z. Zhao, R. W. Baker, M. J. Lage, L. Shi, and M. Tohen. 2005. "Service utilization and costs of olanzapine versus divalproex treatment for acute mania: results from a randomized, 47-week clinical trial." *Current Medical Research and Opinion* 21(4): 555–564.

Chapter 15

Incremental Net Benefit

Andrew R. Willan

Abstract

Since the early 1990s, motivated by the availability of patient-level cost data in clinical studies for comparing patient groups, researchers have made rapid developments in statistical methods for cost-effectiveness data. Initial efforts concentrated on inference about the incremental cost-effectiveness ratio, but due to difficulties associated with ratio statistics, interest has settled more recently on incremental net benefit. Regardless of the approach, five parameters need to be estimated: the between-treatment arm differences in mean effectiveness and mean cost and the corresponding variances and covariance. With these parameter estimates, the analyst can estimate the incremental cost-effectiveness ratio and calculate the corresponding confidence limits. Due to concerns regarding ratio statistics, the analyst may choose to focus on the incremental net benefit. Taking a traditional Frequentist's approach, the incremental net benefit can be estimated, with the uncertainty being characterized by the corresponding confidence limits. Alternatively, taking a Bayesian approach, the cost-effectiveness acceptability curve can be used to display the magnitude of the between-group contrast and to characterize its uncertainty. A review of these methods is given. The particular statistical procedure used for estimating the five parameters depends on:

- whether censoring is present
- whether covariates are adjusted for
- whether random effects, such as country, are adjusted for
- what the assumptions are regarding the distribution for cost

A brief review of the statistical procedures, particular to each combination of these conditions, is given, where they exist. An example of a randomized clinical trial is provided.

15.1 Introduction

Since the early 1990s, it has become more common for resource utilization data to be collected in clinical studies. The resource data, combined with unit price weights, provide a measure of total cost at the patient level, in addition to measures of effectiveness. Having measures of effectiveness and cost at the patient level permits the use of conventional methods of statistical inference for quantifying the uncertainty due to sampling and measurement error. Numerous articles have been published on the statistical analysis of cost-effectiveness data. Initial efforts concentrated on providing confidence intervals for the incremental cost-effectiveness ratio (ICER), which is the between-treatment difference in mean cost divided by the between-treatment difference in mean effectiveness. However, due to concerns regarding ratio statistics, the concept of incremental net benefit (INB) has been adopted as an alternative. The INB is the increase in effectiveness, expressed in monetary terms, minus the increase in cost. The purpose of this chapter is to provide a structured review of commonly proposed methods for a statistical cost-effectiveness analysis (CEA), with emphasis on the INB. The context used throughout the paper is that of a two-arm randomized clinical trial where patients are randomized to treatment (arm *T*) or standard (arm *S*). However, the methods apply to the comparison of any two groups, subject to the concerns one might have regarding bias due to the lack of random group allocation (see Section 15.5 for further discussion).

In a parametric approach, the essential task of a CEA is to jointly model effectiveness and cost to estimate five parameters. Two of the parameters are the between-treatment arm differences in mean effectiveness, denoted by Δ_e, and the between-treatment arm differences in mean cost, denoted by Δ_c. The other three parameters are the variance of the estimator of Δ_e, denoted by $V(\hat{\Delta}_e)$; the variance of the estimator of Δ_c, denoted by $V(\hat{\Delta}_c)$; and the covariance of the estimators of Δ_e and Δ_c, denoted by $C(\hat{\Delta}_e, \hat{\Delta}_c)$, where $\hat{\theta}$ indicates the estimator of θ. Effectiveness and cost must be modeled jointly to enable the estimation of the covariance. The particular statistical procedure used for estimating the five parameters depends on the following:

- whether censoring is present
- whether covariates are adjusted for
- whether random effects such as country are adjusted for
- what the assumptions are regarding the distribution for cost

With the estimators of these five parameters, a CEA, based on either the incremental cost-effectiveness ratio or the incremental net benefit, can be performed. Throughout the rest of this chapter, it is assumed that the estimators of Δ_e and Δ_c are normally distributed. This assumption relies on the central limit theorem, which holds that the sum of a large number of independent random variables will tend to follow a normal distribution.

In Section 15.2, the methods used to display a CEA, based on the five parameter estimates, are illustrated. The statistical procedures used to estimate the parameters, which depend on the issues discussed earlier, are reviewed in Section 15.3. An example using data from a randomized clinical trial is given in Section 15.4. Section 15.5 discusses the issues specific to observational studies. A summary of the chapter follows in Section 15.6.

15.2 Cost-Effectiveness Analysis

A general introduction to the cost-effectiveness analysis associated with the comparison of two groups is given in this section. Typically, though not necessarily, the measure of effectiveness in a CEA is associated with a clinical event experienced by the patient, such as death, relapse, or reaching a pre-specified level of symptom relief. The three measures of effectiveness associated with an event, death for example, are

1. whether the patient survived for the duration of interest
2. the survival time over the duration of interest
3. the quality-adjusted survival time over the duration of interest

Correspondingly, Δ_e is

1. the between-treatment difference in the probability of surviving
2. the between-treatment difference in the mean survival time
3. the between-treatment difference in the mean quality-adjusted survival time

All means are restricted to the duration of interest and the difference is taken as $T-S$, so that positive differences favor *T*. The ICER is defined by Δ_c/Δ_e, where the difference for Δ_c is taken as $T-S$. Therefore the ICER is, respectively,

1. the additional cost of saving a life from using *T* rather than *S*
2. the additional cost of an extra year of life gained from using *T* rather than *S*
3. the additional cost of a quality-adjusted life-year (QALY) from using *T* rather than *S*

The ICER can be illustrated on the cost-effectiveness plane, as shown in Figure 15.1, as the slope of the line between the origin and the point (Δ_e, Δ_c).

In Figures 15.1 through 15.5, we have assumed that the measure of effectiveness is quality-adjusted survival time and the unit of effectiveness is quality-adjusted life-years (QALYs). Also shown in Figure 15.1 is a line, referred to as the threshold, through the origin with the slope equal to the threshold willingness-to-pay (WTP) for a unit of effectiveness, denoted as λ. The threshold divides the cost-effectiveness plane into two regions. For points on the plane below and to the right of the threshold (shaded), *T* is considered cost-effective, but for those above and to the left, it is not. Because λ is positive, points in the SE quadrant, where *T* is more effective and less costly, are always below the threshold and therefore correspond to comparisons for which *T* is cost-effective. On the other hand, points in the NW quadrant, where *T* is less effective and more costly, are always above the threshold and correspond to comparisons for which *T* is not cost-effective. It is in the NE and SW quadrants that the concept of threshold WTP allows for a tradeoff between effectiveness and cost. In the NE quadrant, the slope of any point below the line is less than λ (that is, for any point below the threshold $\frac{\Delta_c}{\Delta_e} < \lambda$), which implies that $\Delta_c < \Delta_e \lambda$.

Therefore, the increase in value ($\Delta_e\lambda$) is greater than the increase in cost, making *T* cost-effective. In the SW quadrant, the slope of any point below the line is greater than λ, and because Δ_e and Δ_c are both negative (that is, treatment is less effective and less costly), we have $\frac{\Delta_c}{\Delta_e} = \frac{|\Delta_c|}{|\Delta_e|} > \lambda$, which implies that $|\Delta_c| > |\Delta_e\lambda|$. Therefore, the value lost ($|\Delta_e\lambda|$) is less than the amount saved ($|\Delta_c|$), making *T* cost-effective. In summary, *T* is cost-effective if, and only if,

$$A:\ \frac{\Delta_c}{\Delta_e} < \lambda \ \text{ if } \Delta_e > 0; \ \text{ or } \ \frac{\Delta_c}{\Delta_e} > \lambda \ \text{ if } \Delta_e < 0. \quad (1)$$

Equation 1 (Hypothesis *A*) defines the region below the threshold and can be thought of as the alternative hypothesis for the null hypothesis *H*, given by:

$$H:\ \frac{\Delta_c}{\Delta_e} \geq \lambda \ \text{ if } \Delta_e > 0; \ \text{ or } \ \frac{\Delta_c}{\Delta_e} \leq \lambda \ \text{ if } \Delta_e < 0. \quad (2)$$

Rejecting *H* in favor of *A* would provide evidence to adopt *T*. These equations are somewhat awkward and can be simplified considerably by the introduction of INB.

Figure 15.1 The Cost-Effectiveness Plane

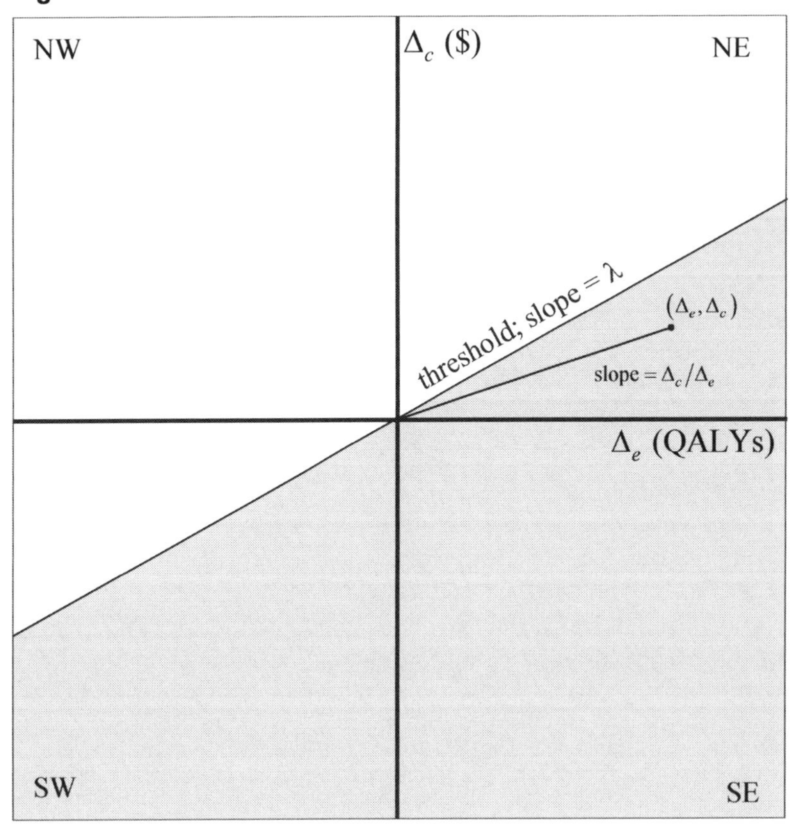

The INB is a function of λ and is defined as $b_\lambda \equiv \Delta_e\lambda - \Delta_c$. b_λ is the incremental net benefit because it is the difference between the incremental value ($\Delta_e\lambda$) and the incremental cost (Δ_c). *T* is cost-effective if, and only if, $b_\lambda > 0$, regardless of the sign of Δ_e. To see this, both inequalities involving the ICER in Equation 1 can be rearranged to the inequality $\Delta_e\lambda - \Delta_c > 0$. Similarly, both inequalities involving the ICER in Equation 2 can be rearranged to the inequality $\Delta_e\lambda - \Delta_c \leq 0$. Therefore, in terms of INB the null and alternative hypotheses become simplified as:

$$H : b_\lambda \leq 0 \quad versus \quad A : b_\lambda > 0. \tag{3}$$

The formulations of hypotheses *H* and *A* given in Equations 1, 2, and 3 illustrate the close relationship between the ICER and the INB. On the cost-effectiveness plane, b_λ is the vertical distance from the point (Δ_e, Δ_c) to the threshold, being positive if the point is below the line and negative otherwise. Because it has a slope of λ, the point on the threshold with abscissa equal to Δ_e is (Δ_e, $\Delta_e\lambda$) and so the vertical distance between it and (Δ_e, Δ_c) is $\Delta_e\lambda$ - Δ_c (see Figure 15.2).

Figure 15.2 INB (b_λ) on the Cost-Effectiveness Plane

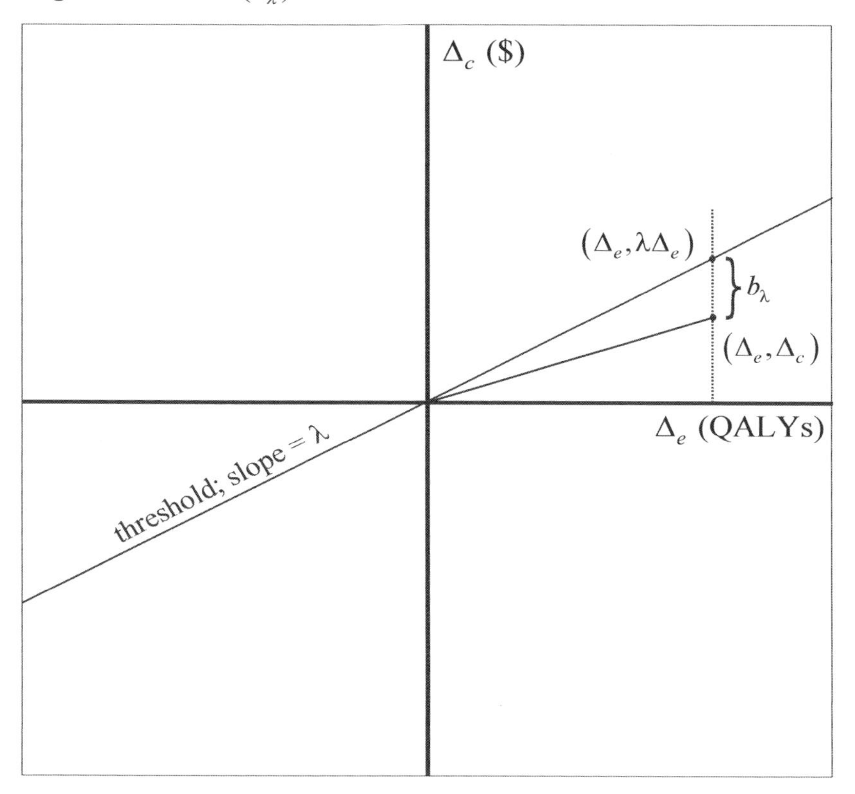

The ICER can be estimated by $\hat{\Delta}_c/\hat{\Delta}_e$, where $\hat{\Delta}_c$ and $\hat{\Delta}_e$ are the estimators of Δ_c and Δ_e, respectively. The estimator $\hat{\Delta}_c/\hat{\Delta}_e$ is biased, but it is consistent if $\hat{\Delta}_c$ and $\hat{\Delta}_e$ are unbiased, meaning that the bias diminishes as the sample size increases (Chaudary and Stearns, 1996; Cochran, 1997). Statistical inference for the ICER has been restricted to calculating its confidence interval. Applying Fieller's theorem [1, 3], the $(1-2\alpha)100\%$ confidence limits are given by

$$R\left\{\left(1 - z_{1-\alpha}^2 c \pm z_{1-\alpha}\sqrt{a + b - 2c - z_{1-\alpha}^2(ab - c^2)}\right)\Big/\left(1 - z_{1-\alpha}^2 a\right)\right\}, \qquad (4)$$

Where $R = \hat{\Delta}_c/\hat{\Delta}_e$, $a = \hat{V}\left(\hat{\Delta}_e\right)/\hat{\Delta}_e^2$, $b = \hat{V}\left(\hat{\Delta}_c\right)/\hat{\Delta}_c^2$, $c = \hat{C}\left(\hat{\Delta}_e, \hat{\Delta}_c\right)/\left(\hat{\Delta}_e\hat{\Delta}_c\right)$, and $z_{1-\alpha}$ is the $100(1-\alpha)$th percentile of the standard normal random variable. The set of points on the cost-effectiveness plane, whose slopes are between the limits defined in Equation 4, define a "bow tie" region on the cost-effectiveness plane (see Figure 15.3), but inference is usually restricted to the region of the bow tie that includes the point $(\hat{\Delta}_e, \hat{\Delta}_c)$. If $a + b - 2c - z_{1-\alpha}^2(ab - c^2) < 0$, then Equation 4 has no solution and neither limit is defined, meaning that the data are too close in probability to the origin for an analysis to provide, with high confidence, inference regarding the value of the ICER. The ICER has other weaknesses. It cannot be interpreted without specifying the sign of either Δ_e or Δ_c. Also, the estimator of the ICER has an undefined mean and variance.

Figure 15.3 Bow Tie ICER Confidence Region

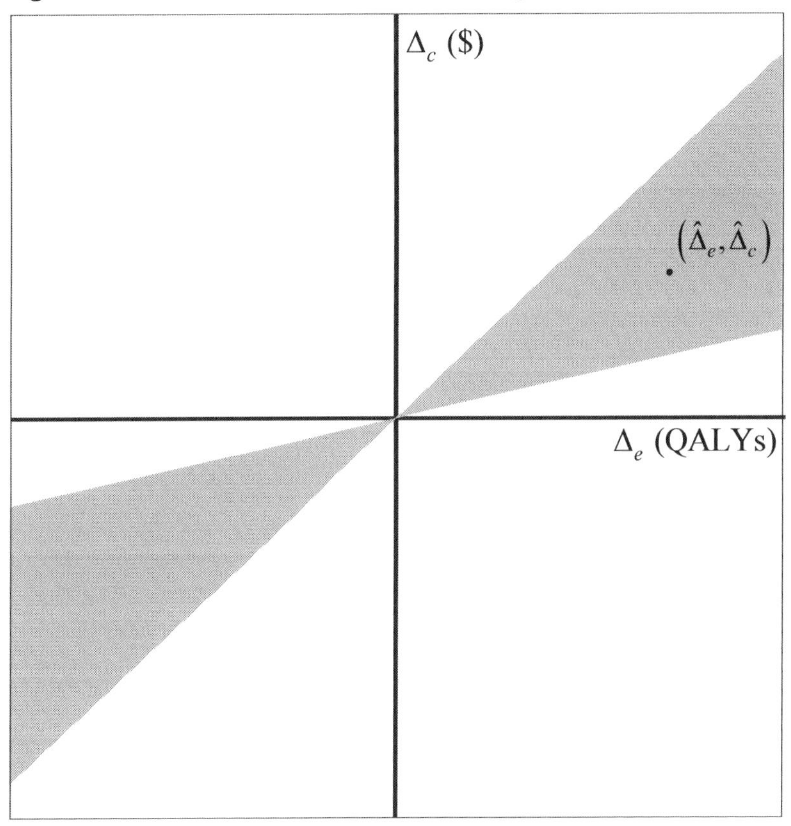

These difficulties, plus the fact that the ICER is not properly ordered on the non-tradeoff (SE and NW) quadrants of the cost-effectiveness plane, have led analysts to make inferences regarding cost-effectiveness with respect to INB as an alternative. As stated previously, T is cost-effective if, and only if, $b_\lambda > 0$, and taking a Bayesian approach, the cost-effectiveness acceptability curve (CEAC) is a plot of the probability that $b_\lambda > 0$ as a function of λ. Assuming no prior information, the CEAC can be given by $\text{CEAC}(\lambda) = \Phi\left(\hat{b}_\lambda / \text{SE}(\hat{b}_\lambda)\right)$, where $\Phi(\cdot)$ is the cumulative distribution function for the standard normal random variable and $\hat{b}_\lambda = \hat{\Delta}_e \lambda - \hat{\Delta}_c$ is the estimator of b_λ with standard error $\text{SE}(\hat{b}_\lambda)$, given by $\sqrt{\lambda^2 \hat{V}(\hat{\Delta}_e) + \hat{V}(\hat{\Delta}_c) - 2\lambda \hat{C}(\hat{\Delta}_e, \hat{\Delta}_c)}$. Estimating the CEAC by $\Phi\left(\hat{b}_\lambda / \text{SE}(\hat{b}_\lambda)\right)$ assumes that $\hat{\Delta}_e$ and $\hat{\Delta}_c$ are normally distributed. This assumption relies on the central limit theorem. For a more complete discussion of the Bayesian framework in cost-effectiveness, see O'Hagan and Stevens (2001).

The CEAC has the advantage of capturing both the magnitude and uncertainty of the observed cost-effectiveness. It also allows readers to apply the threshold WTP that is most appropriate for them. As illustrated in Figure 15.4, the CEAC passes through 0.5 at λ equal to the ICER and through α and 1 - α at λ equal to the ICER Fieller limits defined here. Therefore, the CEAC, although based on the INB, provides inference regarding the ICER. For more on CEACs, see Fenwick, O'Brien, and Briggs (2004). More direct inference based on INB is provided by plotting its estimate and confidence limits as a function of λ (see Figure 15.5). Confidence limits for the INB are given by $\hat{b}_\lambda \pm z_{1-\alpha} \text{SE}(\hat{b}_\lambda)$. The close relationship between b_λ and the ICER is illustrated in Figure 15.5. The plot of $\hat{b}_\lambda$ crosses the horizontal axis at the ICER. If $\hat{\Delta}_e$ is positive, the lower limit for b_λ crosses the horizontal axis at the upper Fieller limit for the ICER and the upper limit for b_λ at the lower Fieller limit for the ICER. On the other hand, if $\hat{\Delta}_e$ is negative, the lower limit for b_λ crosses the horizontal axis at the lower Fieller limit for the ICER and the upper limit for b_λ at the upper Fieller limit for the ICER.

Figure 15.4 The Cost-Effectiveness Acceptability Curve

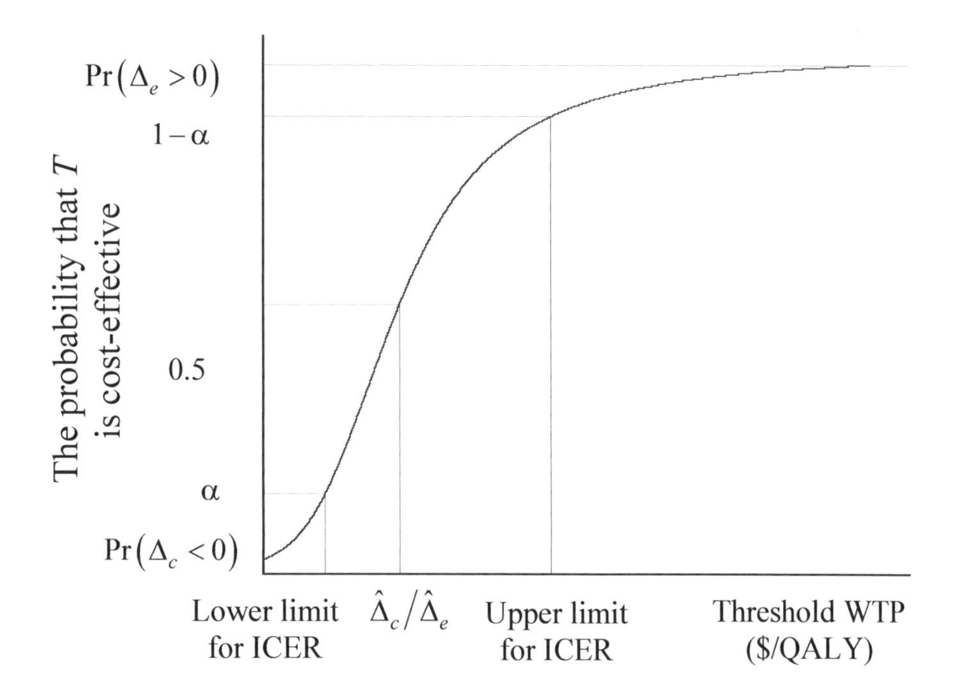

Figure 15.5 Incremental Net Benefit as a Function of WTP (λ)

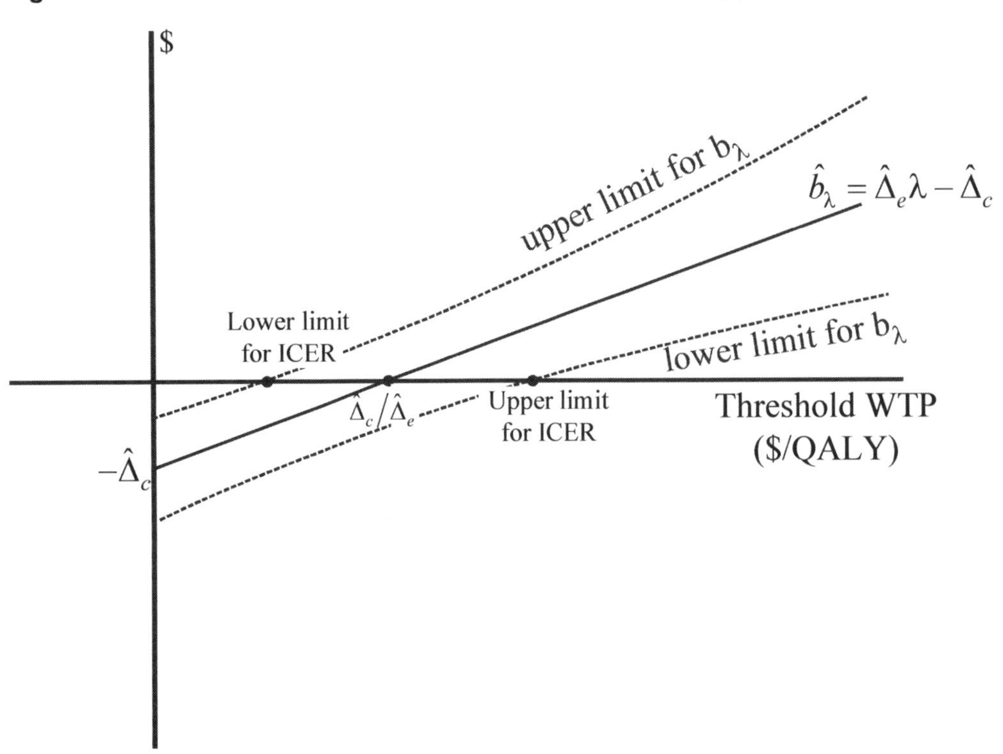

The CEAC and the plot of b_λ and its confidence limits provide a comprehensive summary of the cost-effectiveness analysis of comparison of two groups. Both graphs can be determined using only the estimators of Δ_e, Δ_c, $V(\hat{\Delta}_e)$, $V(\hat{\Delta}_c)$ and $C(\hat{\Delta}_e, \hat{\Delta}_c)$. As discussed previously, how these estimators are determined depends on the nature and sampling of the data. The estimation procedures are reviewed in Section 15.3. The validity of the CEAC and the plots based on INB depend on the assumption that the threshold is a straight line through the origin (that is, λ is invariant to Δ_e). For a discussion of the relaxation of this assumption, see O'Brien and colleagues (2002) and Willan, O'Brien, and Leyva (2001).

15.3 Parameter Estimation

Methods used to estimate the parameters required in a CEA are given in this section. A general introduction is given in Section 15.3.1, with more details provided in Section 15.3.2.

15.3.1 Introduction to Parameter Estimation

The methods for parameter estimation depend on

- whether censoring is present
- whether covariates are adjusted for
- whether random effects such as center or country are accounted for
- what the assumptions are regarding the distribution for cost

Only simple sample statistics are required for non-censored data with no covariates or random effects and assuming symmetric cost distributions. However, the methods get more complex as fewer of these conditions apply (Willan and Briggs, 2006). The following subsections provide a review of some of the approaches taken. Bootstrap methods, which are often used in a CEA, are not discussed here because their use is intended for situations where no acceptable closed form solution exists [9]. For more on bootstrap methods in cost-effectiveness analysis, see Briggs, Wonderling, and Mooney (1997) and Chapter 4 of Willan and Briggs (2006).

15.3.1.1 Right-Skewing of Cost Data

Because of right-skewing, which is usually in cost data, use of least squares methods such as sample means and variances is often criticized (O'Hagan and Stevens, 2003; Briggs and Gray, 1998; Thompson and Barber, 2000; Nixon and Thompson, 2004; and Briggs et al., 2005). Transformations, such as the logarithm and square root, are sometimes proposed as an alternative. However, such transformations provide estimates on a scale not relevant to decision-makers (Manning and Mullahy, 2001, and Thompson and Barber, 2000). Additionally, a number of investigations into the issue of skewed data, using mostly simulated data, have drawn the conclusion that least squares methods provide valid estimates of mean cost and the between-treatment difference in mean cost. Lumley and colleagues (2002) provide a review of such investigations. Nonetheless, the blind application of sample means and variances to cost data with extreme outliers could lead to misleading conclusions. Faith in the robustness of least squares methodology is no substitute for careful examination of the data using box-plots and histograms. Furthermore, although least squares methods may provide consistent estimators of mean cost, the estimators may be inefficient in the presence of right-skewing.

15.3.1.2 Covariate Adjustment

In randomized clinical trials (RCTs), because covariates tend to be balanced across treatment arms, covariate adjustment may not be necessary, although regression models may be used for improving precision or examining for subgroup effects with the use of interaction terms. However, for observational studies, covariate adjustment is generally considered essential.

15.3.1.3 Censoring

In many clinical trials, some patients are not followed for the entire duration of interest. Some may be lost to follow up, either because they refuse to attend follow-up clinic visits or because they move out of the jurisdiction covered by trial management resources. Also, because of staggered entry and long follow-up times, analysis may be performed before all patients are followed for the entire duration of interest. When censoring is uninformative (that is, the time to death is independent of the time to censoring), life-table methods can be used to provide unbiased estimates of the probability of surviving the duration of interest and the mean survival time. However, for cost and quality-adjusted survival time, the censoring is informative, even if the time to censoring and the time to death are independent, and the use of life-table methods will yield biased estimates (Willan et al., 2002). Consequently, more complex methods must be used to estimate mean quality-adjusted survival time and mean cost. Throughout this chapter, the terms *mean survival time*, *mean quality-adjusted survival time*, and *mean cost* refer to the mean, restricted to the duration of interest. In a cardiology trial, the duration of interest may be 30 days or 12 months; however, in a cancer trial, it could be as long as 5 or 10 years.

15.3.1.4 Random Effects

Many studies are often conducted in more than one country. The advantages are an increase in statistical power, resulting from an increase in sample size, and the perception of greater generalizability. However, the analyses of multinational studies often ignore the possibility of a treatment by country interaction, in which the treatment effects vary between countries. In the presence of an interaction, estimates of treatment effects (that is, between-treatment differences in mean cost and effectiveness) that ignore country effects will have inappropriately small variances and lead to inflated type I errors. Models that treat country as a fixed effect (Wilke et al., 1998; Cook et al., 2003) to account for the interaction have no parameter for the overall treatment effect and provide estimates of the country-specific treatment effects that are based solely on the individual country's data. A number of recent publications (see Grieve et al., 2005; Willan et al., 2005; Manca et al., 2005; Pinto et al., 2005; and Nixon and Thompson, 2005) address this issue by proposing hierarchal models that treat country as a random effect. These models have the advantage of providing an overall estimate of treatment effect and country-specific estimates that use the data from all countries.

15.3.2 Details of Parameter Estimation

Let E_{ji} and C_{ji} be the observed measure of effectiveness and cost, respectively, for patient i on treatment arm j, where $i = 1, 2, \ldots n_j, j = T, S$. E_{ji} is scaled so that larger values correspond to better health outcomes. For a binary outcome, E_{ji} is 1 for a success and 0 for a failure. As discussed in Section 15.1.4, it is generally recognized that cost data are skewed to the right. In Sections 15.3.2.1 to 15.3.2.4, methods that ignore the issue of skewed cost data are reviewed, and in Section 15.3.2.5, a review is given for methods that accommodate skewed cost data.

15.3.2.1 No Censoring, No Random Effects, No Covariates

If there is no censoring, no random effects, and no covariates, the parameter estimators are simple functions of sample statistics, such as mean, variances, and proportions. The estimated difference in mean effectiveness and cost are given by

$$\hat{\Delta}_e = \bar{E}_T - \bar{E}_S = \frac{\sum_{i=1}^{n_T} E_{Ti}}{n_T} - \frac{\sum_{i=1}^{n_S} E_{Si}}{n_S} \text{ and } \hat{\Delta}_c = \bar{C}_T - \bar{C}_S = \frac{\sum_{i=1}^{n_T} C_{Ti}}{n_T} - \frac{\sum_{i=1}^{n_S} C_{Si}}{n_S}.$$

The estimated variance of $\hat{\Delta}_c$ is given by

$$\hat{V}(\hat{\Delta}_c) = \frac{\sum_{i=1}^{n_T} (C_{Ti} - \bar{C}_T)^2}{n_T(n_T - 1)} + \frac{\sum_{i=1}^{n_S} (C_{Si} - \bar{C}_S)^2}{n_S(n_S - 1)} \quad \text{or}$$

$$\hat{V}(\hat{\Delta}_c) = \left(\frac{n_T + n_S}{n_T n_S}\right) \frac{\sum_{i=1}^{n_T} (C_{Ti} - \bar{C}_T)^2 + \sum_{i=1}^{n_S} (C_{Si} - \bar{C}_S)^2}{(n_T + n_S - 2)}$$

for homogeneous variance.

If the measure of effectiveness is continuous, then the estimated variance of $\hat{\Delta}_e$ is given by

$$\hat{V}\left(\hat{\Delta}_e\right)=\frac{\sum_{i=1}^{n_T}\left(E_{Ti}-\bar{E}_T\right)^2}{n_T(n_T-1)}+\frac{\sum_{i=1}^{n_S}\left(E_{Si}-\bar{E}_S\right)^2}{n_S(n_S-1)} \text{ or}$$

$$\hat{V}\left(\hat{\Delta}_c\right)=\left(\frac{n_T+n_S}{n_T n_S}\right)\frac{\sum_{i=1}^{n_T}\left(E_{Ti}-\bar{E}_T\right)^2+\sum_{i=1}^{n_S}\left(E_{Si}-\bar{E}_S\right)^2}{(n_T+n_S-2)}$$

for homogeneous variance.

The estimated covariance between $\hat{\Delta}_e$ and $\hat{\Delta}_c$ is given by

$$\hat{C}\left(\hat{\Delta}_e,\hat{\Delta}_c\right)=\frac{\sum_{i=1}^{n_T}\left(E_{Ti}-\bar{E}_T\right)\left(C_{Ti}-\bar{C}_T\right)}{n_T(n_T-1)}+\frac{\sum_{i=1}^{n_S}\left(E_{Si}-\bar{E}_S\right)\left(C_{Si}-\bar{C}_S\right)}{n_S(n_S-1)} \text{ or}$$

$$\hat{C}\left(\hat{\Delta}_e,\hat{\Delta}_c\right)=\left(\frac{n_T+n_S}{n_T n_S}\right)\frac{\sum_{i=1}^{n_T}\left(E_{Ti}-\bar{E}_T\right)\left(C_{Ti}-\bar{C}_T\right)+\sum_{i=1}^{n_S}\left(E_{Si}-\bar{E}_S\right)\left(C_{Si}-\bar{C}_S\right)}{(n_T+n_S-2)}$$

for homogeneous covariance.

If the measure of effectiveness is binary, then the estimated variance of $\hat{\Delta}_e$ is given by

$$\hat{V}\left(\hat{\Delta}_e\right)=\frac{\bar{E}_T\left(1-\bar{E}_T\right)}{n_T}+\frac{\bar{E}_S\left(1-\bar{E}_S\right)}{n_S},$$

and the estimated covariance between $\hat{\Delta}_e$ and $\hat{\Delta}_c$ is given by

$$\hat{C}\left(\hat{\Delta}_e,\hat{\Delta}_c\right)=\frac{\left(\sum_{i=1}^{n_T}E_{Ti}C_{Ti}\Big/n_T\right)-\bar{E}_T\bar{C}_T}{n_T}+\frac{\left(\sum_{i=1}^{n_S}E_{Si}C_{Si}\Big/n_S\right)-\bar{E}_S\bar{C}_S}{n_S}.$$

15.3.2.2 No Censoring, No Random Effects, with Covariates

To adjust for covariates when there is no censoring or random effects, Willan, Briggs, and Hoch (2004) propose using seemingly unrelated regression equations. Let there be p_e covariates for effectiveness and p_c covariates for costs. The regression model is given by

$$E(y) = X\beta,$$

where $y = \begin{pmatrix} e \\ c \end{pmatrix}$ and e and c are the vectors of length $n_T + n_S$ of the observed effectiveness and costs, respectively. The matrix $X = \begin{pmatrix} Z & \underset{\sim}{0} \\ \underset{\sim}{0} & W \end{pmatrix}$, where Z is of dimension $n_T + n_S$ by $p_e + 2$ and contains the covariate values for effectiveness. The first column of Z is a dummy indicator for treatment group (1 for T and 0 for S) and the second column contains all ones to provide an intercept. Similarly, W is of dimension $n_T + n_S$ by $p_c + 2$ and contains the covariate values for costs. The symbol $\underset{\sim}{0}$ represents a matrix of zeroes with the appropriate dimensions. The vector $\beta = \begin{pmatrix} \omega \\ \theta \end{pmatrix}$ is the vector of parameters, where the first components of ω and θ are Δ_e and Δ_c, respectively. If the covariates for effectiveness and cost are the same, then the ordinary least squares solution provides the best linear unbiased estimators. If one set of covariates is a subset of the other, then the ordinary least squares solution provides the best linear unbiased estimators for the smaller set. In all other situations, efficiency gains are possible from the generalized least squares solution. For estimation details, see Willan, Briggs, and Hoch (2004) and Chapter 6 of Willan and Briggs (2006).

The regression methods given here are most appropriate for continuous measures of effectiveness. One approach for covariate adjustment, when the measure of effectiveness is binary, is to combine the methods proposed by Thompson, Warn, and Turner (2004) for binary regression, which allow for the estimation of risk differences (rather than odds ratios) with those of Nixon and Thompson (2005) for jointly modeling effectiveness and cost. The approach requires the use of Markov chain Monte Carlo simulation. A more accessible, albeit slightly ad hoc, method for binary measures of effectiveness is to use the SAS GENMOD procedure (see Section 15.4).

15.3.2.3 No Censoring, Random Effects, and Covariates

To account for random country effects in a multinational RCT, two general approaches are proposed. The first approach, proposed by Pinto, Willan, and O'Brien (2005) and Willan and colleagues (2005), has two stages. In the first stage, each country is treated as a separate trial and the appropriate methods are used to estimate the five parameters of interest. The appropriate methods may include those that account for censoring or covariates. The country-specific estimates are then combined for overall trial estimates using empirical Bayes procedures in what is, essentially, a bivariate (effectiveness and cost) meta-analysis. The second approach (Grieve et al., 2005; Manca et al., 2005; and Nixon and Thompson, 2005) models effectiveness and cost at the patient level, using a hierarchal model to account for the two sources of error (patient and country).

15.3.2.4 Censoring

If the parameter of interest for effectiveness is the probability of survival or mean survival, then life-table methods using the Kaplan-Meier survival curves can be used to estimate Δ_e (Willan et al., 2003, 2002). For quality-adjusted survival and costs, the censoring is informative even if the time to censoring and the time to death are independent, and the use of life-table methods will yield biased estimates. There are primarily two methods for handling this issue. The first, known as the Lin or direct method, is given in Lin and colleagues (1997) and Willan and Lin (2001). The other, based on inverse probability weighting, is given in Bang and Tsiatis (2000), Lin (2000), Zhao and Tian (2001), and Willan and colleagues (2002). Details for both methods are given in Willan and Briggs (2006), Chapter 3.

For parameter estimation in the presence of covariates, see Lin (2000) and Willan, Lin, and Manca (2005). To account for random country effects in a multinational trial with censored data, the analysis could be stratified by country, yielding estimates of Δ_e and Δ_c and the corresponding variances and covariances for each country. These estimates can then be combined for overall trial estimates using empirical Bayes procedures (Willan et al., 2005; Pinto et al., 2005) as discussed in Section 15.3.2.3.

15.3.3 Accounting for Skewness in Cost Data

Jointly modeling cost and effectiveness with asymmetrical distributions for cost can be facilitated using Markov chain Monte Carlo methods, a complete discussion of which is given in Nixon and Thompson (2005). Often a gamma distribution is used to model cost. The gamma distribution appears to be sufficiently flexible for fitting cost data in most situations. The models can handle adjustment for covariates, interaction terms for subgroup analysis, and random effects for country. Again, a more accessible method is facilitated by using PROC GENMOD, as illustrated in Section 15.4.

15.4 Example

A detailed example is given in this section. The measure of effectiveness is binary and the cost data are somewhat skewed. Further, there is a binary covariate, which, for cost, has a statistically significant interaction with treatment group.

15.4.1 The CD Trial

At the request of the principal investigators, the data for this example have been disguised to eliminate any conflict with previous publications. This RCT is referred to as the *CD Trial*. In the CD Trial, 1,356 patients were recruited and randomly allocated between two treatment groups, denoted by T and S. There was a single binary baseline covariate, denoted as X, with levels labeled 0 and 1. The primary measure of effectiveness was 30-day survival. Health care utilization data were collected on all patients and combined with price weights to provide patient-level cost data. The proportion of patients surviving 30 days and the average cost, broken down by treatment group and the covariate, are given in Table 15.1. The overall observed increase in 30-day survival for those patients receiving T is around 0.05 and is consistent between the levels of the covariate. The overall cost saving for those receiving T is around \$800. The observed difference in mean cost depends on the covariate, being approximately \$1,200 for $X = 0$ and \$300 for $X = 1$. A histogram of cost, broken down by treatment group, is given in Figure 15.6. The width of each pair of rectangles is \$2,000, with the last pair representing costs in excess of \$44,000. A high degree of skewing is evident from this figure.

Table 15.1 Proportion Surviving and Average Cost by Treatment Group and *X* for the CD Trial

	Proportion Surviving 30 Days		Average Cost (CAD)	
	T	*S*	*T*	*S*
X = 0	0.9345	0.8847	8976.36	10203.31
X = 1	0.9271	0.8746	8859.37	9137.26
All Patients	0.9309	0.8802	8919.76	9725.48

Figure 15.6 Histogram of Cost from the CD Trial

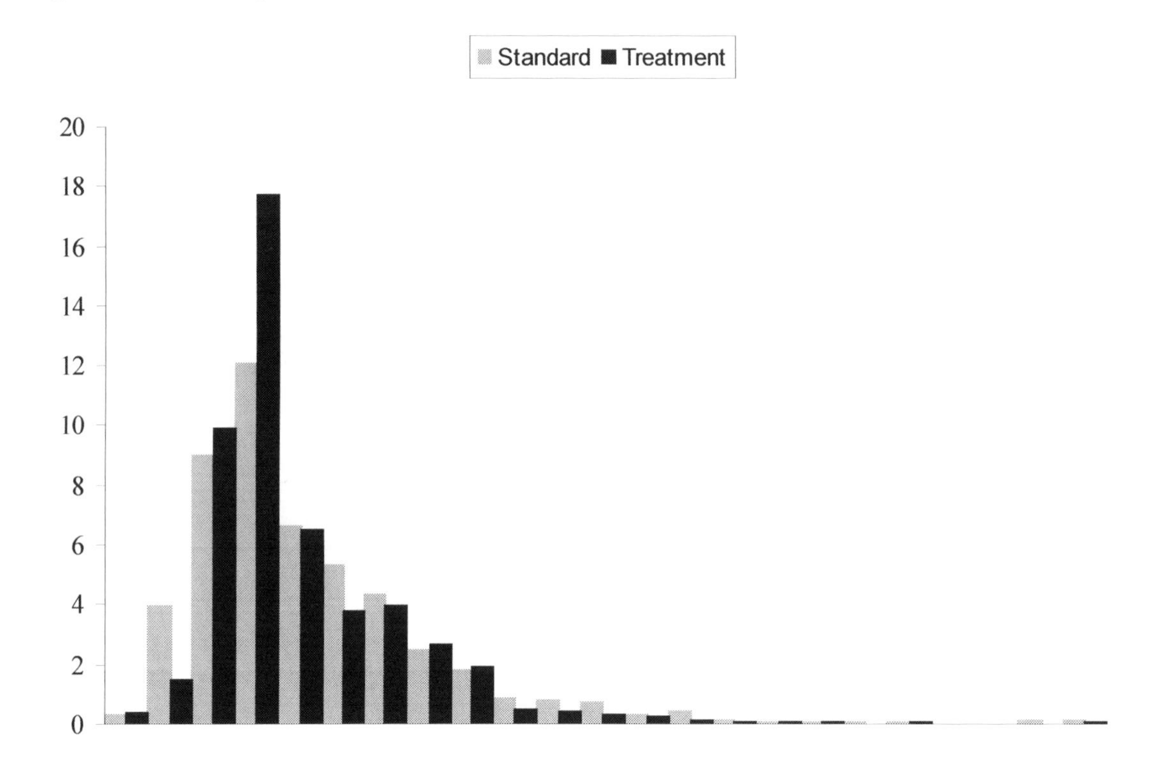

Estimates of the five parameters, ignoring any influence of the covariate, are given in Table 15.2. The estimates in the first column are derived from the formulae given in Section 15.3.2.1 using the pooled formulae for the variance and covariance. The estimates in the second column are derived from specifically modeling cost using a normal distribution. See Program 15.1 for details. As expected, the estimates in this column are almost identical to the estimates in the first. The estimates in the third column are derived from modeling cost using a gamma distribution. See Program 15.2 for details. Although the estimates of the Δ_e and Δ_c are very similar to those in the first two columns, the estimate of variance of $V\left(\hat{\Delta}_c\right)$ is more than 25% smaller, indicating that the gamma distribution provides a much better fit of the data. The impact of this increase in efficiency is demonstrated in Figures 15.7 and 15.8. Plots of the estimates and confidence limits of b_λ, as a function of λ, are given in Figure 15.7 for both the normal and gamma model assumptions. The CEACs are given in Figure 15.8. Although the gamma model provides a significant decrease in the variance of the estimated difference in mean cost, the confidence limits for the INB for the normal and gamma models are essentially equivalent, especially for values of λ that are appropriate for preventing a death. Some separation can be seen in the plot of the CEACs for low values of λ, but the curves are indistinguishable for larger, more appropriate values.

The following SAS code provides the estimates of the five required parameters, where *arm* is the treatment group indicator (1 for *T* and 0 for *S*), *effectiveness* equals 1 if the patient survived 30 days and 0 otherwise, and *cost* is the total cost for each patient.

Program 15.1 Modeling Cost Using a Normal Distribution

```
proc genmod data=yourDataset;
   model cost = arm / dist=normal link=identity;
   output out=c predicted=pred_c;
run;

proc genmod data= yourDataset desc;
   model effectiveness= arm / dist=bin link=identity;
   output out=e predicted=pred_e;
run;

data temp; merge e c;
   resid_e = effectiveness - pred_e;
   resid_c = cost - pred_c;
   keep resid_e resid_c;
run;

proc corr data=temp; var resid_e resid_c; run;
```

Output from Program 15.1

Parameter	DF	Estimate	Standard Error	Wald 95% Confidence Limits		Chi-Square	Pr > ChiSq
Intercept	1	9725.479	210.9007	9312.121	10138.84	2126.50	<.0001
arm	1	-805.724	297.8197	-1389.44	-222.008	7.32	0.0068

$\hat{\Delta}_c = -805.724$; $\hat{V}(\hat{\Delta}_c) = (297.8197)^2$.

Parameter	DF	Estimate	Standard Error	Wald 95% Confidence Limits		Chi-Square	Pr > ChiSq
Intercept	1	0.8802	0.0125	0.8557	0.9047	4965.68	<.0001
arm	1	0.0507	0.0158	0.0197	0.0817	10.26	0.0014

$\hat{\Delta}_e = 0.0507$; $\hat{V}(\hat{\Delta}_e) = (0.0158)^2$.

Pearson Correlation Coefficients, N = 1356

	resid_e	resid_c
resid_e	1.00000	-0.31306
resid_c	-0.31306	1.00000

$\hat{C}(\hat{\Delta}_e, \hat{\Delta}_c) = (-0.31306) * (297.8197) * (0.0158)$.

The following SAS code provides the estimates of the five required parameters. The output (not shown) has the same structure as the Output from Program 15.1.

Program 15.2 Modeling Cost Using a Gamma Distribution

```
proc genmod data=yourDataset;
   model cost = arm / dist=gamma link=identity;
   output out=c predicted=pred_c;
run;

proc genmod data= yourDataset desc;
   model effectiveness= arm / dist=bin link=identity;
   output out=e predicted=pred_e;
run;

data temp; merge e c;
   resid_e = effectiveness - pred_e;
   resid_c = cost - pred_c;
   keep resid_e resid_c;
run;

proc corr data=temp; var resid_e resid_c; run;
```

Table 15.2 Parameter Estimates for the CD Trial

Parameter	Pooled	Normal*	Gamma*
$\hat{\Delta}_e$	0.0507	0.0507	0.0507
$\hat{\Delta}_c$	-805.72	-805.72	-805.72
$\hat{V}(\hat{\Delta}_e)$	0.0002506	0.0002496	0.0002496
$\hat{V}(\hat{\Delta}_c)$	88,828	88,697	65,839
$\hat{C}(\hat{\Delta}_e, \hat{\Delta}_c)$	-1.482	-1.473	-1.268

* distribution used for cost

Figure 15.7 Incremental Net Benefit and Confidence Limits Using the Normal and Gamma Distributions for the CD Trial

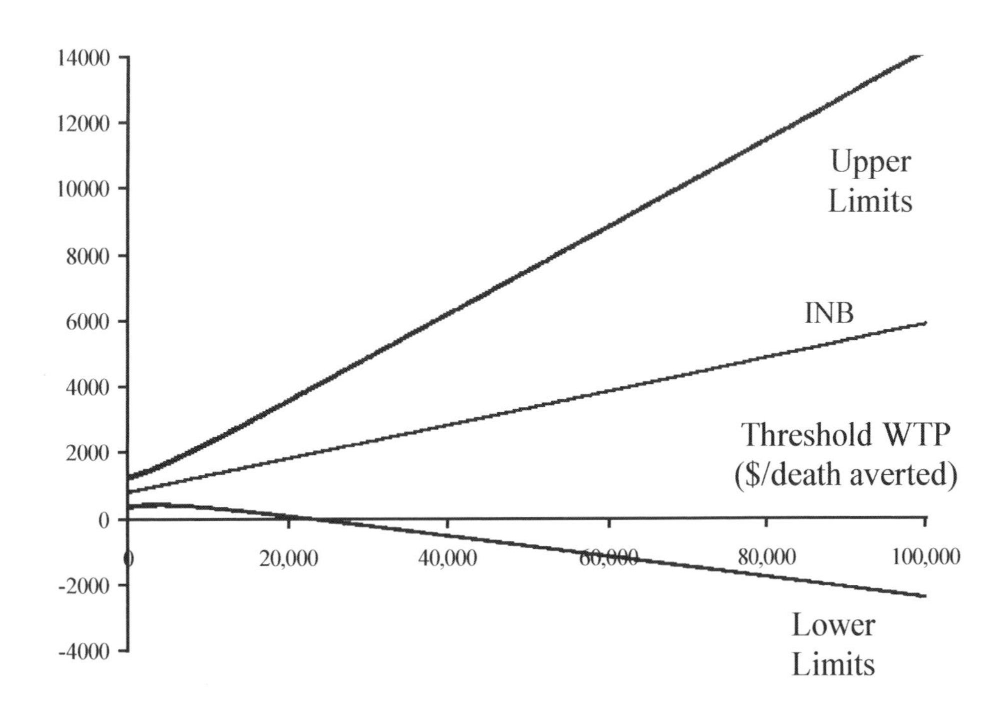

Figure 15.8 Cost-Effectiveness Acceptability Curves Using the Normal and Gamma Distributions for the CD Trial

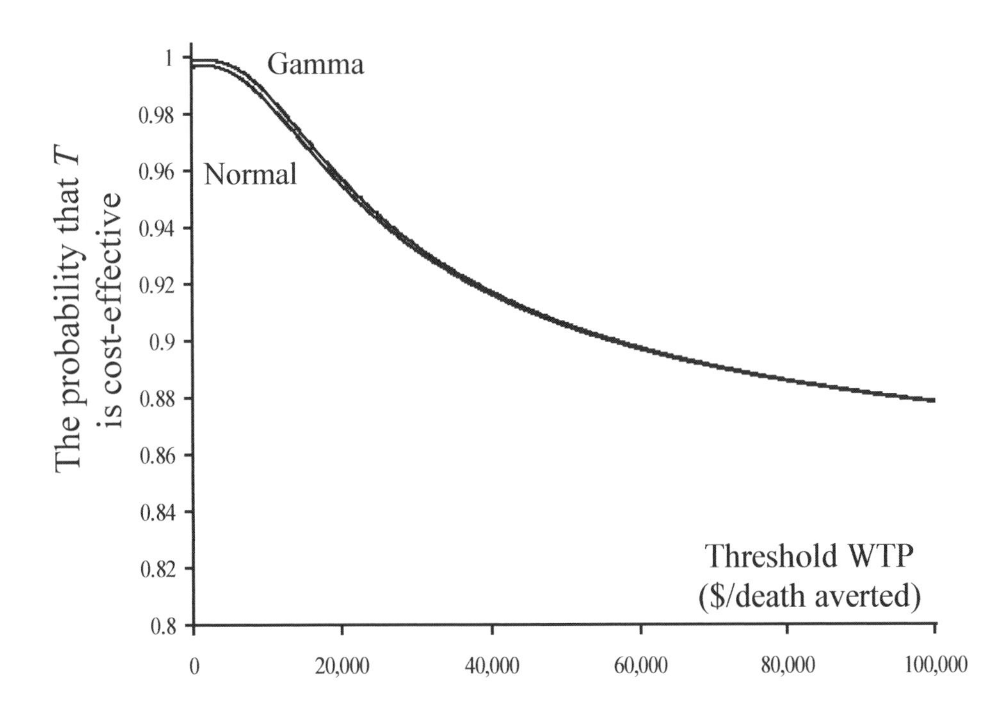

Using a gamma distribution for cost, we examined the effect of the covariate on cost and 30-day survival. There was no significant effect ($p = 0.5843$) of the covariate on 30-day survival, but there was a significant overall affect (0.0315) and a marginally significant interaction (0.0630) with treatment group for cost. Final models, which include treatment group, *X*, and the interaction for cost and treatment group only for 30-day survival, were used to provide parameter estimates. See Program 15.3 for details. The parameter estimates are given in Table 15.3. Because of the interaction term between treatment group and *X* for the cost model, estimates of Δ_c and the associated variance and covariance depend on the level of *X*. The cost saving is much higher for $X = 0$, and consequently treatment will be more cost-effective in that subgroup of patients. The plot of incremental net benefit and the CEAC are given in Figures 15.9 and 15.10. The CEAC exceeds 0.9 for $X = 0$ for all values of λ, and it exceeds 0.85 for $X = 1$ for values of λ greater than \$10,000 per life saved. This provides strong evidence in support for the cost-effectiveness of *T*.

A Microsoft EXCEL file for generating the plots of the CEAC and the INB (with confidence intervals) is available at http://www.andywillan.com/downloads. The only inputs required are the five parameter estimates, the minimum and maximum values for λ and the confidence level.

The following code shows the final models. The model for effectiveness included arm as the only covariate and the model for cost included arm, *X*, and their interaction.

Program 15.3 Covariate Adjustment

```
proc genmod data=yourData;
   model cost = arm X arm*X/ dist=gamma link=identity;
   output out=c predicted=pred_c;
run;

proc genmod data=yourData desc;
   model effectiveness = arm / dist=bin link=identity;
   output out=e predicted=pred_e;
run;

data temp; merge e c;
   resid_e = effectiveness - pred_e;
   resid_c = cost - pred_c;
   keep resid_e resid_c;
run;

proc corr data=temp; var resid_e resid_c; run;
```

Output from Program 15.3

Parameter	DF	Estimate	Standard Error	Wald 95% Confidence Limits		Chi-Square	Pr > ChiSq
Intercept	1	10203.31	266.7096	9680.571	10726.05	1463.54	<.0001
arm	1	-1226.95	360.0549	-1932.65	-521.259	11.61	0.0007
X	1	-1066.06	375.9776	-1802.96	-329.153	8.04	0.0046
arm*X	1	949.0657	510.5547	-51.6032	1949.735	3.46	0.0630

For $X = 0$: $\hat{\Delta}_c = -1226.95$; $\hat{V}\left(\hat{\Delta}_c\right) = (360.0549)^2$.

For $X = 0$: $\hat{C}\left(\hat{\Delta}_e, \hat{\Delta}_c\right) = (-0.31470)*(360.0549)*(0.0158)$.

```
                              Standard        Wald 95%            Chi-
Parameter  DF  Estimate        Error    Confidence Limits      Square  Pr > ChiSq

Intercept   1    0.8802       0.0125     0.8557     0.9047  4965.68      <.0001
arm         1    0.0507       0.0158     0.0197     0.0817    10.26      0.0014
```

$\hat{\Delta}_e = 0.0507$; $\hat{V}\left(\hat{\Delta}_e\right) = (0.0158)^2$.

```
Pearson Correlation Coefficients, N = 1356

              resid_e       resid_c

resid_e       1.00000      -0.31470

resid_c      -0.31470       1.00000
```

For parameter estimates for $X = 1$, the values of X can be reversed and the program rerun, yielding the following output:

```
                                  Standard        Wald 95%            Chi-
Parameter       DF  Estimate        Error    Confidence Limits      Square   Pr > ChiSq

Intercept        1  9137.256    265.0003   8617.865   9656.647   1188.88       <.0001
arm              1  -277.888    361.9759   -987.348   431.5715      0.59       0.4427
X                1  1066.056    375.9776   329.1531   1802.958      8.04       0.0046
arm*X            1  -949.066    510.5547   -1949.73    51.6032      3.46       0.0630
```

For $X = 1$: $\hat{\Delta}_c = -227.89$; $\hat{V}\left(\hat{\Delta}_c\right) = (361.9759)^2$.

For $X = 1$: $\hat{C}\left(\hat{\Delta}_e, \hat{\Delta}_c\right) = (-0.31470)*(361.9759)*(0.0158)$.

Table 15.3 Parameter Estimates by Levels of the Covariate for the CD Trial

Parameter	$X = 0$	$X = 1$
$\hat{\Delta}_e$	0.0507	0.0507
$\hat{\Delta}_c$	-1226.95	-277.89
$\hat{V}\left(\hat{\Delta}_e\right)$	0.002496	0.0002496
$\hat{V}\left(\hat{\Delta}_c\right)$	129,640	131,027
$\hat{C}\left(\hat{\Delta}_e, \hat{\Delta}_c\right)$	-1.790	-1.800

Figure 15.9 Incremental Net Benefit by Levels of the Covariate for the CD Trial

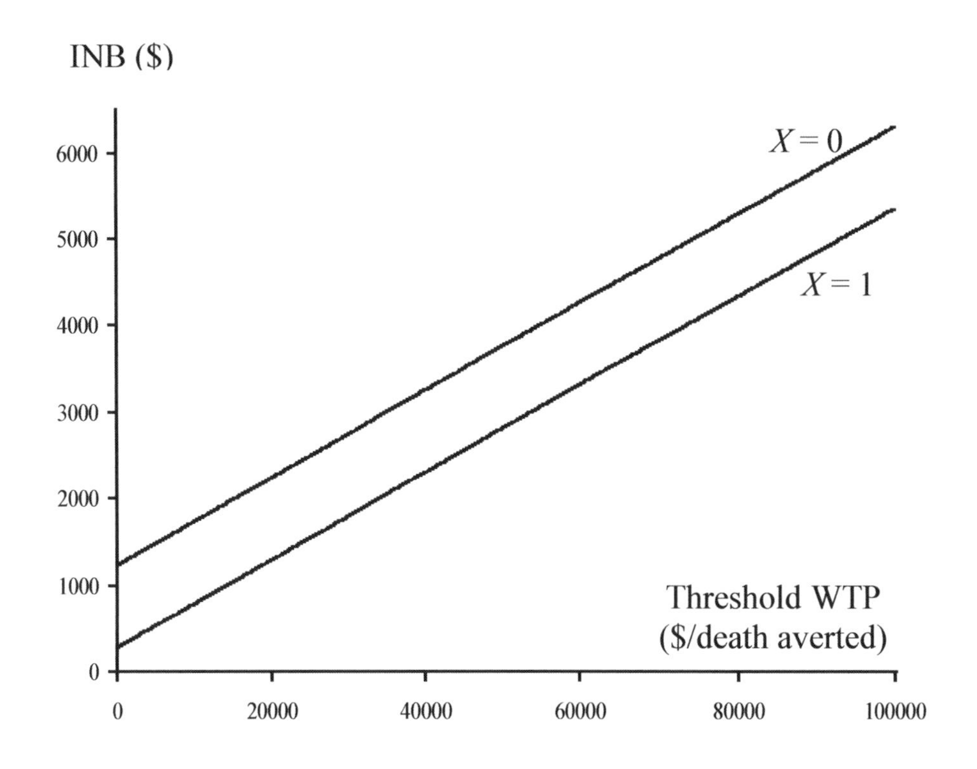

Figure 15.10 Cost-Effectiveness Acceptability Curves by Levels of the Covariate for the CD Trial

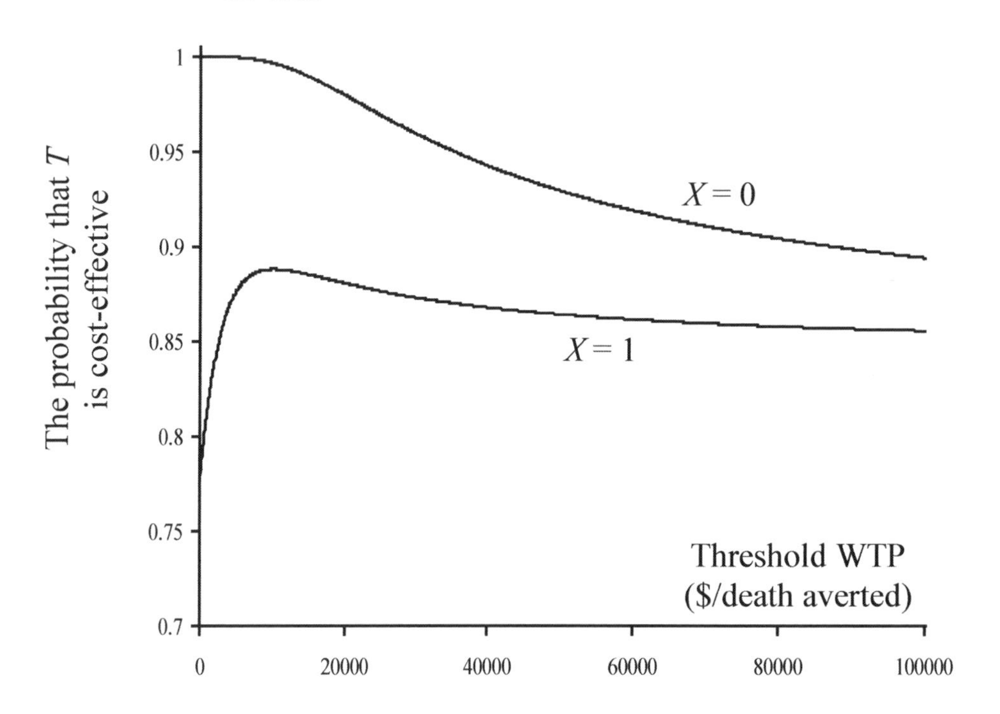

15.5 Observational Studies

Although many cost-effectiveness analyses are performed on data from randomized clinical trials, the methods are also appropriate for the comparison of two groups from observational studies, subject to the concerns one might have regarding bias due to the lack of random group allocation. Typically, an analysis for comparing two groups based on data from an observational study requires adjustment for selection bias. Two general approaches are available: propensity scoring and regression analysis. If the data set is sufficiently large, then propensity matching is a possible option (see Chapter 3). In this case, the propensity match data could be analyzed as if they came from an RCT. Propensity stratification is also an option (see Chapter 2). For propensity stratified data, a regression analysis is required, where effectiveness and cost must be regressed on the treatment indicator variable plus the dummy indicator variables for the propensity stratification (one less than the number of strata). For non-censored data, the analyst can use PROC GENMOD to perform the regression, as demonstrated in the example in Section 15.4. The stratification variable can be included in the CLASS statement, negating the need to create the dummy indicators. For censored data, the regression methods given in Willan, Lin, and Manca (2005) are appropriate. For regression analysis without propensity stratification, refer to Willan, Briggs, and Hoch (2004) for non-censored data and to Willan, Lin, and Manca (2005) for censored data.

15.6 Discussion

Outlined in this chapter is the use of the incremental net benefit for comparing the cost-effectiveness of two groups. An analyst can, as a function of the threshold WTP, estimate the INB and determine its corresponding confidence limits in a Frequentist's approach or, alternatively, in a Bayesian approach plot the cost-effectiveness acceptability curve. The CEAC has the advantage that it both displays the magnitude of the estimated between-group contrast and characterizes its uncertainty. The INB is preferred to the ICER, which suffers from all the problems associated with ratio statistics. Further, the INB ties in directly with Bayesian decision analysis and is used in value of information methods (see, for example, Willan and Pinto, 2006, and other sources under "References"). As with other cost-effectiveness analyses, inference focused on INB requires the estimation of the between-group differences in mean effectiveness and mean cost. In addition, the variances and covariance of these estimators are required. The methods used for parameter estimation depend on

- whether censoring is present
- whether covariates are adjusted for
- whether random effects such as center or country are accounted for
- what the assumptions are regarding the distribution for cost

For situations where there is no censoring, covariates, or random effects and the skewing of cost data is ignored, only simple statistics are required. SAS PROC GENMOD can be used to accommodate covariates and random effects and specify skewed distributions for modeling costs. The presence of censoring adds an additional layer of complexity and is covered elsewhere (for example, Willan and Briggs, 2006; Willan et al., 2002; Willan et al., 2003; and so forth).

Acknowledgments

The author is funded through the Discovery Grant Program of the Natural Sciences and Engineering Research Council of Canada (grant number 44868-03).

References

Bang, H., and A. A. Tsiatis. 2000. "Estimating medical costs with censored data." *Biometrika* 87(2): 329–343.

Briggs, A. H., and A. M. Gray. 1998. "The distribution of health care costs and their statistical analysis for economic evaluation." *Journal of Health Services Research & Policy* 3(4): 233–345.

Briggs A. H., D. E. Wonderling, and C. Z. Mooney. 1997. "Pulling cost-effectiveness analysis up by its bootstraps; a non-parametric approach to confidence interval estimation." *Health Economics* 6(4): 327–340.

Briggs, A., R. Nixon, S. Dixon, and S. Thompson. 2005. "Health economics letter: parametric modeling of cost data: some simulation evidence." *Health Economics* 14: 421–428.

Chaudhary, M. A., and S. C. Stearns. 1996. "Estimating confidence intervals for cost-effectiveness ratios: an example from a randomized trial." *Statistics in Medicine* 15: 1447–58.

Cochran, W. G. 1997. *Sampling Techniques*. New York: John Wiley & Sons, Inc.

Cook, J. R., M. Drummond, H. Glick, and J. F. Heyse. 2003. "Assessing the appropriateness of combining economic data from multinational clinical trials." *Statistics in Medicine* 22: 1955–76.

Eckermann, S., and A. R. Willan. 2007. "Expected value of information and decision making in HTA." *Health Economics* 16: 195–209.

Eckermann, S., and A. R. Willan. 2008. "The option value of delay in health technology assessment." *Medical Decision Making* 28(3): 300–305.

Eckermann, S., and A. R. Willan. 2008. "Time and expected value of sample information wait for no patient." *Value in Health* 11(3): 522–526.

Eckermann, S., and A. R. Willan. 2009. "Globally optimal trial design for local decision making." *Health Economics* 18:203–216.

Efron, R. B., and B. R. J. Tibshirani. 1993. *An Introduction to the Bootstrap*. New York: Chapman & Hall.

Fenwick, E., B. J. O'Brien, and A. H. Briggs. 2004. "Cost-effectiveness acceptability curves—facts, fallacies and frequently asked questions." *Health Economics* 13: 405–415.

Grieve, R., R. Nixon, S. G. Thompson, and C. Normand. 2005. "Using multilevel models for assessing the variability of multinational resource use and cost data." *Health Economics* 14: 185–196.

Lin, D.Y. 2000. "Linear regression analysis of censored medical costs." *Biostatistics* 1:35–47.

Lin, D. Y., E. J. Feuer, R. Etzioni, and Y Wax. 1997. "Estimating medical costs from incomplete follow-up data." *Biometrics* 53: 419–34.

Lumley, T., P. Diehr, S. Emerson, and L. Chen. 2002. "The importance of the normality assumption in large public health data sets." *Annual Review of Public Health* 23: 151–169.

Manca, A., N. Rice, M. J. Sculpher, and A. H. Briggs. 2005. "Assessing generalisability by location in trial-based cost-effectiveness analysis: the use of multilevel models." *Health Economics* 14: 471–475.

Manning, W. G., and J. Mullahy. 2001. "Estimating log models: to transform or not to transform?" *Journal of Health Economics* 20: 461–94.

Nixon, R. M., and S. G. Thompson. 2004. "Parametric modeling of cost data in medical studies." *Statistics in Medicine* 23: 1311–1331.

Nixon, R. M., and S. G. Thompson. 2005. "Methods for incorporating covariate adjustment, subgroup analysis and between-centre differences into cost-effectiveness evaluations." *Health Economics* 14: 1217–1229.

O'Brien, B. J., K. Gertsen, A. R. Willan, and A. Faulkner. 2002. "Is there a kink in consumers' threshold value for cost-effectiveness in health care?" *Health Economics* 11(2): 175–180.

O'Hagan, A., and J. W. Stevens. 2001. "A framework for cost-effectiveness analysis from clinical trial data." *Health Economics* 10(4): 303–315.

O'Hagan, A., and J. W. Stevens. 2003. "Assessing and comparing costs: how robust are the bootstrap and methods based on asymptotic normality?" *Health Economics* 12(1): 33–49.

Pinto, E. M., A. R. Willan, and B. J. O'Brien. 2005. "Cost-effectiveness analysis for multinational clinical trials." *Statistics in Medicine* 24: 1965–1982.

Thompson, S. G., D. E. Warn, and R. M. Turner. 2004. "Bayesian methods for analysis of binary outcome data in cluster randomized trials on the absolute risk scale." *Statistics in Medicine* 23: 389–410.

Thompson, S. G., and J. A. Barber. 2000. "How should cost data in pragmatic randomised trials be analysed?" *British Medical Journal* 320(7243): 1197–1200.

Wilke, R. J., H. A. Glick, D. Polsky, and K. Schulman. 1998. "Estimating country-specific cost-effectiveness from multinational clinical trials. *Health Economics* 7(6): 481–493.

Willan, A. R. 2007. "Clinical decision making and the expected value of information." *Clinical Trials* 4: 279–285.

Willan, A. R., A. H. Briggs, and J. S. Hoch. 2004. "Regression methods for covariate adjustment and subgroup analysis for non-censored cost-effectiveness data." *Health Economics* 13: 461–475.

Willan, A. R., and D. Y. Lin. 2001. "Incremental net benefit in randomized clinical trials." *Statistics in Medicine* 20: 1563–1574.

Willan, A. R., B. J. O'Brien, and R. A. Leyva. 2001. "Cost-effectiveness analysis when the WTA is greater than the WTP." *Statistics in Medicine* 20: 3251–3259.

Willan, A. R., and A. H. Briggs. 2006. *Statistical Analysis of Cost-effectiveness Data.* West Sussex, England: John Wiley & Sons, Ltd.

Willan, A. R., and B. J. O'Brien. 1996. "Confidence intervals for cost-effectiveness ratios: an application of Fieller's theorem." *Health Economics* 5(4): 297–305.

Willan, A.R., D. Y. Lin, and A. Manca. 2005. "Regression methods for cost-effectiveness analysis with censored data." *Statistics in Medicine* 24: 131–145.

Willan, A. R., D. Y. Lin, R. J. Cook, and E. B. Chen. 2002. "Using inverse-weighing in cost-effectiveness analysis with censored data." *Statistical Methods in Medical Research* 11: 539–51.

Willan, A. R., E. B. Chen, R. J. Cook, and D. Y. Lin. 2003. "Incremental net benefit in randomized clinical trials with qualify-adjusted survival." *Statistics in Medicine* 22: 353–62.

Willan, A. R., and E. M. Pinto. 2005. "The expected value of information and optimal clinical trial design." *Statistics in Medicine* 24: 1791–1806.

Willan, A. R., E. M. Pinto, B. J. O'Brien, P. Kaul, R. Goeree, L. Lynd, et al. 2005. "Country-specific cost comparisons from multinational clinical trials using empirical Bayesian shrinkage estimation: the Canadian ASSENT-3 economic analysis." *Health Economics* 14: 327–338.

Willan, A. R., and M. E. Kowgier. 2008. "Determining optimal sample sizes for multi-stage randomized clinical trials using value of information methods." *Clinical Trials* 5: 289–300.

Willan, A. R. 2008. "Optimal sample size determinations from an industry perspective based on the expected value of information." *Clinical Trials* 5: 587–594.

Zhao, H., and L. Tian. 2001. "On estimating medical cost and incremental cost-effectiveness ratios with censored data." *Biometrics* 57: 1002–1008.

Chapter 16

Cost and Cost-Effectiveness Analysis with Censored Data

Hongwei Zhao
Hongkun Wang

Abstract

Cost assessment and cost-effectiveness analysis serve as an essential part in the economic evaluation of medical interventions. In clinical trials and many observational studies, cost data as well as survival data are often incomplete due to patients' loss to follow up or administrative termination of the study. There are numerous well-established statistical methodologies and software available for analyzing censored survival data. However, standard techniques for survival-type data are invalid in analyzing censored cost data, due to the induced informative censoring (dependence between censored costs and potential uncensored costs). In this chapter, we present some statistical methods that have been proposed for estimating medical cost and cost-effectiveness analysis with censored data. An example from a clinical trial comparing the effectiveness of implantable cardiac defibrillators with conventional therapy for individuals at high risk for ventricular arrhythmia is used to illustrate the method. SAS code for performing the analysis is provided. The model assumptions are examined and further development is discussed.

16.1 Introduction

With the advance of medicine, medical costs have escalated. However, due to limited resources, it is of great interest for health care organizations and health policy makers to evaluate medical costs associated with different treatment options. In general, the mean cost per patient is of most concern to us because the total cost of an intervention can be derived from the mean, not from the mode, median, or other quartiles of the cost distribution (Ramsey et al., 2005).

Cost estimation in observational studies is challenging for many reasons. First of all, cost data are highly skewed. However, if a log transformation is used on cost data, the inference on the mean of the log transformed cost is transferred back to the geometric mean, not the arithmetic mean of cost as desired. The smearing method (Duan, 1983) has been proposed to handle this type of problem. Another challenge is that there can be a lot of missing data for medical costs, due to either missing visits or missing information on some types of medical costs (Briggs et al., 2003). Naive methods such as omitting missing data, carrying forward the last observation, or replacing the missing values with mean measures from observed data are often not satisfactory. Instead, multiple imputation (Rubin, 1987) and Bayesian simulation methods (Schafer, 1997; Van Buuren, 1999) have been advocated for computing missing data. In general, missing data can be classified into three categories according to Little and Rubin (1987):

- missing completely at random (MCAR), where missing mechanisms are independent of the variables of our interest
- missing at random (MAR), where missing is dependent only on observed variables
- not missing at random (NMAR), where missing depends on unobserved variables

It is usually easier to handle MCAR and MAR cases; when NMAR is true, inference will rely on the assumptions about the missing mechanisms, which cannot be verified from available data.

One type of missing data is caused by censoring, either due to dropout from the study or to administrative censoring from the design of the study. This chapter mainly concentrates on this problem. Similar to other missing mechanisms, censoring can be classified into three categories as well, according to whether

- censoring is independent of the survival and cost history process (censoring completely at random)
- censoring depends only on observed variables (censoring at random)
- censoring depends on some unobserved variables

We will show that it is challenging to estimate the mean costs, even for the first scenario of censoring, completely at random. Due to the censoring of costs, we cannot estimate the mean cost by simply averaging the medical cost of all the subjects. This would underestimate the true cost by equating the costs after censoring time to be zero. An average of the cost from only complete observations results in an estimator that is biased toward the costs of the patients with shorter survival time. Methods based on standard survival techniques, such as the Kaplan-Meier estimator (Kaplan and Meier, 1958), also result in biased estimators, even when the assumption that censoring is independent of the survival time is valid. This is due to so-called *induced informative censoring*, first noted by Lin and colleagues (1997). As an example, an individual with a higher cost accumulation rate tends to incur more medical cost at both censoring time and potential uncensored survival time, even when the censoring time is completely independent of the failure time.

Different statistical methods have been proposed for estimating mean cost with censored data (Young, 2005). We will focus on estimating the mean costs without using covariate information. Further development on incorporating covariate information in cost estimation is discussed in the last section of this chapter. Realizing that it is impossible to estimate nonparametrically the lifetime cost due to censoring, Huang and Louis (1998) proposed a method to jointly estimate survival time and lifetime costs. An alternative approach for handling the censoring issue is to limit the medical cost estimation to a certain time, which is determined by the availability of the data. Because the focus of an economical study involving cost is often on the marginal distribution of the cost, not the cost distribution conditional on a certain survival time, we concentrate on the second approach in the remainder of this chapter.

All methods for using censored data to estimate mean cost within a time limit can be classified into two types:

1. approaches that use only the information on the final cost observed in each individual that is complete
2. approaches that use additional information from a patient's cost history for both complete and censored individuals

In general, the former approaches are simple but inefficient (that is, the estimator has a larger variance), while the latter are more complicated but produce asymptotically more efficient estimators.

Lin and colleagues (1997) proposed three different estimators for estimating mean costs using either patients' total cost or cost history. Their methods provide consistent estimates only when the censoring times are discrete. Bang and Tsiatis (2000) employed the inverse probability weighting scheme and proposed several estimators that belong to a general class of consistent and asymptotically normal estimators for estimating mean cost with censored data. Their so-called *partitioned estimator* makes use of the cost accumulation data. Thus, it improves the efficiency of the simple weighted estimator, but it requires dividing the health history into subintervals. Later, a more convenient and efficient estimator was suggested by Zhao and Tian (2001), which also belongs to the general class of estimators of Bang and Tsiatis (2000). In a recent article, Zhao and colleagues (2007) established equivalency among the estimators that were introduced by Lin and colleagues (1997), Bang and Tsiatis (2000), and Zhao and Tian (2001). For each type of estimator (with or without utilizing cost history), the estimators are identical under the condition that partition boundaries are chosen at the censoring points.

Cost estimation is frequently used in cost-effectiveness analysis to compare different treatments and evaluate the economic impact of new treatment options. Willan and Lin (2001) and Willan and colleagues (2003) illustrate the use of incremental net benefit (INB), which depends upon a decision maker's willingness to pay (WTP) for an additional unit of effectiveness, denoted as λ. Namely, INB=cost - $\lambda\times$ effect. A major advantage of this measure is that it is more mathematically convenient to deal with simple differences, whereas a major disadvantage is that it depends on λ, which is usually unknown or not well defined. An alternative measure of cost-effectiveness is the incremental cost-effectiveness ratio (ICER), which is defined as the extra costs incurred for saving an additional year of (quality-adjusted) life. The ICER is very useful for comparing two treatments when one is more costly but more effective than the other. The ICER has long been considered a standard tool among decision makers (Gold et al., 1996). The ICER and INB approaches are also discussed in Chapters 14 and 15.

For the purpose of illustration, our data analysis uses an example from a clinical trial, the Multicenter Automatic Defibrillator Implantation Trial (MADIT), which compared the effectiveness of implantable cardiac defibrillators vs. conventional therapy in preventing death among people who had prior myocardial infarctions (Mushlin et al., 1998). Methods that utilize either only the total costs or additional cost history are employed to obtain the cost estimator and calculate the incremental cost-effectiveness ratio and its confidence. SAS code is provided together with analysis results.

The outline of this chapter is as follows. Section 16.2 introduces the methodology for estimating the mean cost as well as estimating the ICER and its confidence intervals. It is followed by the MADIT data analysis using SAS in Section 16.3. In Section 16.4, we examine the model assumptions and discuss other approaches available for estimating medical cost and for obtaining confidence intervals for cost-effectiveness ratios.

16.2 Statistical Methods

16.2.1 Notation and Assumptions

We first confine our attention to patients in one arm of the study. For the ith person in the study, let T_i denote his overall survival time and C_i the censoring time. Censoring is assumed to be random and independent of survival time. This assumption is usually satisfied when censoring is mainly caused by administrative reasons, such as the limited duration of a clinical trial or survey data. In the discussion section, we will comment on the case when this assumption is not valid. Due to censoring, T_i and C_i are observed only through the follow-up time $X_i = \min(T_i, C_i)$. Let the censoring indicator be $\Delta_i = I(T_i \leq C_i)$. Then $\Delta_i = 1$ means the ith person's death is observed and $\Delta_i = 0$ means his survival time is censored. Denote $U_i(t)$ as the cost accumulated from time 0 (the point when the patient entered the study) to time t. Because of the presence of censoring, it is impossible to estimate the cost over the entire health history without making some distributional assumptions. Therefore, we consider only cost accumulated up to a prespecified time horizon L, where one has a reasonable amount of data available on the time period [0, L]. Hence, we will consider $T_i^L = \min(T_i, L)$. But for ease of notation, we will suppress the superscript L and continue to use T_i.

Our goal is to estimate the mean of the medical cost $\mu = E\{U_i(T_i)\}$ up to a maximum time of L, from a set of observed data $[X_i, \Delta_i, \{U_i(t), t \leq X_i\}, i = 1, \cdots, n]$. If the cost history is not recorded, we see only the final cost $U_i(X_i)$ for each individual, and those who experience the event of interest before being censored have $U_i = U_i(T_i) = U_i(X_i)$.

16.2.2 Estimating Mean Cost

If every patient is followed up to time L or until his death, then we would have complete costs for each patient and the standard statistical method such as the sample mean could be used for estimating mean costs. However, in most cases, the cost and the survival time are not completely observed for all patients due to censoring. A simple weighted estimator for the mean cost was proposed by Bang and Tsiatis (2000), which has the following form:

$$\hat{\mu}_{WT} = \frac{1}{n} \sum_{i=1}^{n} \frac{\Delta_i U_i}{\hat{K}(T_i)}, \tag{1}$$

where $\hat{K}(T_i)$ is the Kaplan-Meier estimator for $K(t) = \Pr(C > t)$, the survival distribution of the censoring variable C evaluated at time T_i. In this simple weighted estimator, censoring is taken into account by weighting each uncensored individual with their probability of being observed. This inverse probability weighting idea originated with Horvitz and Thompson (1952) in sampling survey methods. This estimator is shown by Bang and Tsiatis (2000) to be consistent and asymptotically normal. Its variance can be consistently estimated by

$$\hat{V}(\hat{\mu}_{WT}) = \frac{1}{n}\left[\frac{1}{n}\sum_{i=1}^{n}\frac{\Delta_i(U_i - \hat{\mu}_{WT})^2}{\hat{K}(T_i)} + \frac{1}{n}\sum_{j=1}^{n}\frac{(1-\Delta_j)}{\hat{K}(C_j)^2}\{G_j(U^2) - G_j^2(U)\}\right] \tag{2}$$

where

$$G_j(U) = \frac{1}{n\hat{S}(X_j)}\sum_{i=1}^{n}\frac{\Delta_i U_i(X_i) I(X_i \geq X_j)}{\hat{K}(X_i)}$$

This estimator has been shown by Zhao and colleagues (2007) to be equivalent to the estimator *T* of Lin and colleagues (1997), if the boundaries of the intervals were chosen to be at those censoring times.

The simple weighted estimator utilizes only data with complete observations. Thus it cannot be efficient, especially when censoring is heavy. One way to improve it is by capturing information from censored observations or from available cost history for both censored and uncensored observations. To improve the efficiency of the simple weighted estimator, Bang and Tsiatis (2000) proposed the partitioned estimator. It partitions the interval [0, L] into smaller intervals, computes the simple weighted estimator for cost incurred in each interval, and then sums over all intervals. Later, a more convenient and efficient estimator was suggested by Zhao and Tian (2001), which belongs to the general class of estimators of Bang and Tsiatis (2000) for mean cost but which does not require partitioning the health history. Pfeifer and Bang (2005) suggested a user-friendly formula for this improved estimator, which can be written as:

$$\hat{\mu}_{IMP} = \frac{1}{n}\sum_{i=1}^{n}\frac{\Delta_i U_i}{\hat{K}(T_i)} + \frac{1}{n}\sum_{j=1}^{n}\frac{(1-\Delta_j)}{\hat{K}(C_j)}\{U_j - \bar{U}(C_j)\} \tag{3}$$

where $\bar{U}(C_j) = \frac{\sum_{i=1}^{n} U_i(C_j) I(X_i \geq C_j)}{\sum_{i=1}^{n} I(X_i \geq C_j)}$ is the average cost at C_j of individuals who are still under observation at time C_j This estimator has been shown by Zhao and colleagues (2007) to be equivalent to the partitioned estimator of Bang and Tsiatis (2000) and the Lin and colleagues (1997) estimators A and B, when the partition boundaries are chosen to be at those censoring times.

The variance estimator for the improved estimator of mean cost is given by

$$\hat{V}(\hat{\mu}_{IMP}) = \hat{V}(\hat{\mu}_{WT})$$

$$-\frac{2}{n^2}\sum_{j=1}^{n}\frac{1-\Delta_j}{Y(C_j)\hat{K}(C_j)}\sum_{i=1}^{n}\frac{\Delta_i I(X_i \geq X_j)}{\hat{K}(T_i)}\{U_i - G_j(U)\}\{U_i(X_j) - \bar{U}(X_j)\} \tag{4}$$

$$+\frac{1}{n^2}\sum_{j=1}^{n}\frac{1-\Delta_j}{Y(C_j)\hat{K}(C_j)}\sum_{i=1}^{n}\frac{\Delta_i I(X_i \geq X_j)}{\hat{K}(T_i)}\{U_i(X_j) - \bar{U}(X_j)\}^2$$

This improved estimator is not guaranteed to always be more efficient than the simple weighted estimator, but under most realistic situations, it will perform better than the simple weighted estimator.

For both estimators, we assume that we can compute a subject's total cost or accumulated cost at a certain time before his censoring or death occurs. When missing cost data are present, an appropriate method for handling them must be employed first (Briggs et al., 2003). Wang and Zhao (2006) discussed the special situation when censoring for cost happens earlier than censoring for survival time for some subjects.

16.2.3 Estimating the Incremental Cost-Effectiveness Ratio and Its Confidence Interval

We now consider a two-arm trial and estimate the incremental cost-effectiveness ratio. For arm $k(k = 0,1)$, denote μ_k^U as the mean cost and μ_k^T as the mean survival time, each limited to a window of time [0, L]. The ICER is estimated by

$$\frac{\hat{\mu}_1^U - \hat{\mu}_0^U}{\hat{\mu}_1^T - \hat{\mu}_0^T}, \qquad (5)$$

where $\hat{\mu}_k^U$ and $\hat{\mu}_k^T$ are the estimators for the mean cost and mean survival time for arm $k(k = 0,1)$, respectively. The mean survival time can be estimated using the area under the Kaplan-Meier curve of the survival function over [0, L], which can be shown to be equivalent to $\hat{\mu}^T = \frac{1}{n}\sum_{i=1}^{n} \frac{\Delta_i T_i}{\hat{K}(T_i)}$. T is truncated at time L.

There are different approaches available to obtain confidence intervals for the ICER. Chapter 14 provides an example with the bootstrap method. Here we use Fieller's Theorem (Fieller, 1954) because asymptotically the numerator $x = \hat{\mu}_1^U - \hat{\mu}_0^U$ and the denominator $y = \hat{\mu}_1^T - \hat{\mu}_0^T$ in (5) are bivariately normally distributed, which satisfies the requirement for this theorem. Hence, the 100(1-α) percent confidence limits for the ICER are

$$\frac{xy - z_{\alpha/2}^2 S_{xy} \pm \{f(x, y, S_{xx}, S_{xy}, S_{yy})\}^{1/2}}{y^2 - z_{\alpha/2}^2 S_{yy}}, \qquad (6)$$

where $f(x, y, S_{xx}, S_{xy}, S_{yy}) = (xy - z_{\alpha/2}^2 S_{xy})^2 - (x^2 - z_{\alpha/2}^2 S_{xx})(y^2 - z_{\alpha/2}^2 S_{yy})$, S_{xx}, S_{yy}, S_{xy} are, respectively, the variances of x and y and the covariance of x and y, and $z_{\alpha/2}$ is the cutoff point with tail area $\alpha/2$ for the standard normal distribution. Because we assume that the two samples are independent, we can obtain the variance of x and y using previous results. Formulae that can be used to consistently estimate the covariance between costs and survival times are given in Zhao and Tian (2001), so they are not presented here.

16.3 Example

16.3.1 Study Description

To illustrate the methods discussed here, we use data collected from the Multicenter Automatic Defibrillator Implantation Trial (MADIT). MADIT was a randomized, fully sequential clinical trial that examined the effectiveness of an implantable cardiac defibrillator (ICD) in prevention of sudden death for patients who were at high risk for ventricular arrhythmia (Moss et al., 1996). Altogether, 181 patients were enrolled from 36 centers, with 89 patients assigned to the treatment group to receive ICDs and 92 assigned to the control group to receive conventional drug therapy. The first enrolled patient was followed for 61 months and the last for less than 1 month, with an average follow up of 27 months. After completion of the study, Moss and colleagues (1996) showed that use of an ICD as prophylactic therapy leads to improved survival compared with conventional medical therapy. Because of the high initial cost associated with the ICDs, cost data were collected for patients from the United States as part of the study. All medical costs incurred during the study were recorded, as described by Mushlin and colleagues (1998).

The original cost analysis was restricted to a 4-year period and performed using a method similar to the one proposed by Lin and colleagues (1997). We reanalyze the data using both the simple weight estimator and the improved estimator discussed earlier. Restricted to a 4-year period, the data were heavily censored, with a 70% censoring rate in the ICD arm and a 48% censoring rate in the conventional therapy arm. The improved estimator allowed us to capture the information from censored observations. For the cost-effectiveness analysis, the ICER was also calculated using the improved method in estimating the mean cost. As customarily done in cost-effectiveness analysis, both costs and survival time were discounted at 3% annual rate (Gold et al., 1996).

Although this example comes from a clinical trial, not an observational study, the same calculation can be used for a censored observational study as long as the assumption of independent censoring is still valid. In the discussion section, we talk about how to handle the case when censoring depends on observed variables and how to adjust for baseline imbalance for observational studies.

16.3.2 Data Analysis

The data for each treatment arm came from two separate files, one containing the survival information and the other containing the cost information. The survival data included three variables: subject ID, survival time (in days), and survival status (1=death; 0=censored). Because many costs, such as hospitalization costs, were accumulated over a certain period of time, they were recorded by start time, stop time, and total costs within the period (in dollars). These costs were already discounted at a 3% annual rate. The SAS code and output examining the first 10 observations of the two files from the ICD arm follow.

Program 16.1 SAS Code for Examining the Survival File

```
libname local "C:\Documents and Settings\My Documents\Example";

proc print data=local.surv1 (obs=10);
run;
```

Output from Program 16.1

Obs	id	delta	surv
1	1	0	167
2	2	0	1582
3	3	0	1792
4	4	0	1303
5	5	0	1204
6	6	0	763
7	7	0	453
8	8	0	1644
9	9	0	1818
10	10	0	804

Program 16.2 SAS Code for Examining the Cost File

```
proc print data=local.cost1 (obs=10);
run;
```

Output from Program 16.2

Obs	cid	start	stop	cost
1	1	1	29	133.12
2	1	1	29	16.44
3	1	1	158	421.75
4	1	1	158	28.94
5	1	1	158	25.28
6	1	1	158	29.80
7	1	1	158	2.79
8	1	5	7	32764.22
9	1	29	158	79.48
10	1	30	120	150.99

SAS/IML software was used in the analysis. Because our formula involves the Kaplan-Meier estimator, we need to call the SAS LIFETEST procedure within SAS/IML. SAS Stat Studio (now SAS/IML Studio) enables us to perform this task. The following program was run in this environment. For each set of survival and cost data, a user-defined value of time limit L, and a discount rate r, the program calculates and prints the cost estimator (simple weighted and improved), the mean (discounted) the survival time, and their estimated variances and covariance.

Program 16.3 SAS Code for Performing Cost Analysis

```
libname local "C:\Documents and Settings\hongwei\My
Documents\Home\SASbook\Example";

/* Read survival data */
use local.surv1;
read  all var {id delta surv};
/*Subject ID, death indicator, and survival time;*/
close local.surv1;

/* Read cost data */
use local.cost1;
read  all var {cid start stop cost};
/* Subject ID, cost starting date, stop date, cost incurred */
show names;
close local.cost1;
```

```
/* Define global variables */
n=nrow(id); /* number of subjects */
nobs=nrow(cid); /* total number of observations for cost data*/
L=1461; /* time limit */
r=0.03; /* annual discount rate */

/* Truncate survival time to L, name new variables tsurv and tdelta */
run TrunSurv(delta, surv, tdelta, tsurv);

/* Make the largest observation a failure */
do i= 1 to n;
  if (tsurv[i] = L)  then tdelta[i]=1;
end;

/* Calculate the percentage of data that is censored */
percens=CalCensor(tdelta);
print , "Percent of censoring =" percens;

/* Calculate the Kaplan Meier estimator for K(t)=Pr(C>t), name it kc */
run KmCal(tsurv,tdelta,kc);

/* Calculate the Kaplan Meier estimator for S(t)=Pr(C>t), name it s */
censor=j(n,1,0);
do i= 1 to n;
   censor[i]=1-tdelta[i];
end;
run KmCal(tsurv,censor,s);

/* Calculate the total cost for each subject, which is needed for the
simple weighted estimator */
run CalTCost(cid, start,stop, cost, id, tsurv, tcost);

/* Calculate the mean cost using the simple weighted estimator */
mean_sw=CalOurMean(tdelta, kc, tcost);
print , "Simple weighted estimator for mean cost =" mean_sw;

/* Calculate the standard error of the simple weighted estimator */
var_sw=CalOurVar(tsurv, tdelta, s, kc, tcost, mean_sw);
se_sw=sqrt(var_sw);
print , "Standard error estimate for the simple weighted estimator ="
se_sw;

/* Calculate the mean discounted survival time and its standard error*/
dsurv=j(n,1,0);
do i= 1 to n;
  dsurv[i] = 365.25/r * (1.0-exp(-r*(double)tsurv[i]/365.25));
end;
mean_T = CalOurMean(tdelta, kc, dsurv);
var_T = CalOurVar(tsurv, tdelta, s, kc, dsurv, mean_T);
se_T = sqrt(var_T);
print , "Mean survival time =" mean_T;
print , "Standard error for the mean survival time =" se_T;

/* Calculate cumulative cost at each censored time, which is needed for the
improved estimator */
run CalCulCost(cid, start, stop, cost, id, tsurv, tdelta, culcost);
```

```
/* Calculate improved estimator for mean cost and its standard error*/
run CalMeanAdd(tsurv, tdelta, kc, s, tcost, culcost, meanadd, varsub);
mean_imp = mean_sw+meanadd;
se_imp = sqrt(var_sw-varsub);
print , "Imporved estimator for mean cost =" mean_imp;

print , "Standard error of the improved estimator =" se_imp;
/* Calculate the covariance between mean survival time and simple weighted
cost estimator */
cov_sw = CalOurCov(tdelta, tsurv, s, kc, tcost, mean_sw, dsurv, mean_T);
print , "Covariance between mean survival time and the simple weighted cost
estimator =" cov_sw;

/* Calculate the covariance between mean survival time and improved cost
estimator */
covsub=CalCovSub(tdelta, tsurv, s, kc, culcost, dsurv);
cov_imp=cov_sw-covsub;
print , "Covariance between mean survival time and the improved cost
estimator =" cov_imp;

/* Subroutine to truncate the survival time to L */
start TrunSurv(delta, surv, tdelta, tsurv) global (L,n);
  tsurv=surv;
  tdelta=delta;
  do i= 1 to n;
    if surv[i]>L then do;
      tsurv[i]=L;
      tdelta[i]=1;
    end;
  end;
finish TrunSurv;

/* Subroutine to calculate the percentage of data that is censored */
start CalCensor(tdelta) global (L,n);
  cens=1-tdelta;
  percens = sum(cens)/n;
  return(percens);
finish CalCensor;

/* Subroutine to calculate the Kaplan Meier estimator for K(t)=Pr(C>t) */
start KmCal(surv, delta,kc);
  create InputDataSet var {surv delta};
  append;
  close InputDataSet;

  submit;
    proc lifetest data=InputDataSet noprint outsurv=OutputData;
    time surv*delta(1);
    run;

    data Out;
    set OutputData;
   tpdelta=1-CENSOR_;
   tpsurv=surv;
    run;
  endsubmit;
```

```
    use Out;
    read all var {tpsurv tpdelta survival};
    run ChangeKmSurv(tpsurv, tpdelta, survival, surv, delta, kc);
    close Out;
  finish KmCal;

  /* Subroutine to carry forward the survival function estimate at the last
  failure time */
  start ChangeKmSurv(tpsurv, tpdelta, survival, surv, delta, kc) global
  (L,n);
    minkc=1000;
    nn=nrow(tpsurv);
    kc=j(n,1,0);

    do j= 1 to nn;
           if (survival[j]>=0 & survival[j]<minkc) then do;
        minkc=survival[j];
        maxtime=tpsurv[j];
           end;
    end;

    do i= 1 to n;
     if (surv[i]>maxtime) then kc[i]=minkc;
      else do;
        do j = 1 to nn;
           if (surv[i]=tpsurv[j]) then kc[i]=survival[j];
        end;
      end;
    end;
  finish ChangeKmSurv;

  /* Subroutine to calculate the total cost */
  /* This subroutine takes less time to run compared to the routine
  calculating cumulative cost */
  start CalTCost(cid, start, stop, cost, id, tsurv, tcost) global (n, nobs);
    tcost=j(n,1,0);
    do i= 1 to n;
      do k=1 to nobs;
        if (cid [k] = id[i] & start [k] <= tsurv[i]) then do;
           if (stop[k] > tsurv[i]) then
              tcost[i]=tcost[i]+cost[k]*(tsurv[i]-start[k]+1.0)/(stop[k]-
  start[k]+1.0);
           else tcost[i] = tcost[i] + cost[k];
        end;
      end;
    end;
  finish CalTCost;

  /* Subroutine to calculate the simple weighted estimator for the mean cost
  */
  start CalOurMean(tdelta, kc, tcost) global (n);
    mymean=0.;
    do i= 1 to n;
      if (tdelta[i]=1) then mymean = mymean + tcost[i]/kc[i];
    end;
    mymean = mymean/n;
    return(mymean);
  finish CalOurMean;
```

```
/* Subroutine to calculate the variance of the simple weighted estimator */
start CalOurVar(tsurv, tdelta, s, kc, tcost, mymean)global (n);
  temp1 = 0.; /* part 1 of equation (2) */
  temp2 = 0.; /* part 2 of equation (2) */
  do i= 1 to n;
    if (tdelta[i]=1) then temp1 =temp1 + (tcost[i]-mymean)**2/kc[i];
  end;
  temp1 =temp1/n;

  do j= 1 to n;
    e=0.;
    f=0.;
    if (tdelta[j]=0) then do;
      do i= 1 to n;
        if(tdelta[i]=1 & tsurv[i]>=tsurv[j]) then do;
          e =e + tcost[i]/kc[i];
          f = f + (tcost[i])**2/kc[i];
        end;
      end;
      e = e / (s[j]*n);
      f = f /(s[j]*n);
      temp2 = temp2 + (f-e*e)/(kc[j]*kc[j]);
    end;
  end;
  temp2=temp2/n;

  myvar = temp1+temp2;
  myvar = myvar/n;
  return(myvar);
finish CalOurVar;

/* Subroutine to calculate the cumulative cost */
/* This routine is needed for calculating the improved estimator */
start CalCulCost(cid, start, stop, cost, id, tsurv, tdelta, culcost) global
(n, nobs);
  culcost=j(n,n,0);
  do i= 1 to n;
    do j= 1 to n;
      if (tsurv[i]>=tsurv[j] & tdelta[j]=0) then do;
        do k = 1 to nobs;
          if (cid [k] = id[i] & start [k] <= tsurv[j]) then do;
            if (stop[k] > tsurv[j]) then
              culcost[i,j]=culcost[i,j]+cost[k]*(tsurv[j]-
start[k]+1.0)/(stop[k]-start[k]+1.0);
            else culcost[i,j] = culcost[i,j] + cost[k];
          end;
        end;
      end;
    end;
  end;
finish CalCulCost;

/* Subroutine to calculate the additional terms for the improved estimator
and its variance */
start CalMeanAdd(tsurv, tdelta, kc, s, tcost, culcost, meanadd, varsub)
global (n);
```

```
/* First calculate Ubar[j] and risk set y[j] at censoring places */
  Ubar=j(n,1,0);
  y=j(n,1,0);
  do j= 1 to n;
    if (tdelta[j]=0) then do;
      do i= 1 to n;
        if (tsurv[i]>=tsurv[j]) then do;
          Ubar[j]= Ubar[j]+ culcost[i,j];
          y[j] = y[j]+1;
        end;
      end;
      Ubar[j]= Ubar[j]/y[j];
    end;
  end;

  /* Next calculate the additional terms for the improved estimator and its
variance */
  part1=0.; /* Additional term for the improved estimator */
  part2=0.; /* Second term in the variance formula for the improved
estimator, equation (4) */
  part3=0.; /* Third term in the variance formula for the improved
estimator, equation (4) */
  do j= 1 to n;
    if (tdelta[j]=0) then do;
      part1 = part1+ (tcost[j]-Ubar[j])/kc[j];

      gu=0.;
      par2temp=0.;
      par3temp=0.;
      do i= 1 to n;
        if(tdelta[i]=1 & tsurv[i]>=tsurv[j]) then
        gu = gu + tcost[i]/kc[i];
      end;
      gu = gu/( s[j]*n);

      do i= 1 to n;
        if(tdelta[i]=1 & tsurv[i]>=tsurv[j]) then
          par2temp = par2temp+ (tcost[i]-gu)*(culcost[i,j]-Ubar[j])/kc[i];
      end;
      part2 = part2 + par2temp/(y[j]*kc[j]);

      do i= 1 to n;
        if(tsurv[i]>=tsurv[j])then
          par3temp = par3temp +(culcost[i,j]-Ubar[j])**2;
      end;
      part3 = part3+ par3temp/(y[j]*kc[j]*kc[j]);
    end;
  end;
  part1 = part1/n;
  meanadd=part1;
  varsub=(2.0*part2-part3)/(n*n);
finish CalMeanAdd;

/* Subroutine to calculate the covariance between mean survival time and
simple weighted cost estimator */
start CalOurCov(tdelta, tsurv, s, kc, tcost, mymean, dsurv, tmean) global
(n);
  temp1 = 0.;
  temp2 = 0.;
```

```
    do i= 1 to n;
      if (tdelta[i]=1) then temp1 = temp1 + tcost[i]*dsurv[i]/kc[i];
    end;

    temp1 = temp1/n;
    temp1 = temp1 - mymean * tmean;

    do j= 1 to n;
      gtc=0.;
      gt=0.;
      gc=0.;
      if (tdelta[j]=0) then do;
        do i= 1 to n;
          if(tdelta[i]=1 & tsurv[i]>=tsurv[j]) then do;
            gtc = gtc + tcost[i]*dsurv[i]/kc[i];
            gt = gt + dsurv[i]/kc[i];
           gc = gc + tcost[i]/kc[i];
          end;
        end;
        gtc = gtc / (s[j]*n);
        gt = gt/(s[j]*n);
        gc = gc/(s[j]*n);
        temp2 = temp2 +(gtc-gt*gc)/(kc[j]*kc[j]);
      end;
    end;
    temp2 =temp2/n;
    mycov = temp1+temp2;
    mycov = mycov/n;
    return(mycov);
  finish CalOurCov;

  /* Subroutine to calculate the additional term for covariance between mean
  survival time and improved cost estimator */
  start CalCovSub(tdelta, tsurv, s, kc, culcost, dsurv) global (n);

    /* First calculate Ubar[j] and risk set y[j] at censoring places */
    Ubar=j(n,1,0);
    y=j(n,1,0);
    do j= 1 to n;
      if (tdelta[j]=0) then do;
        do i= 1 to n;
          if (tsurv[i]>=tsurv[j]) then do;
            Ubar[j] = Ubar[j] + culcost[i,j];
            y[j] = y[j] + 1;
          end;
        end;
        Ubar[j] =Ubar[j]/y[j];
      end;
    end;

    /* Next calculate the additional term for the covariance using improved
  cost estimator */
    part2=0.;
    do j= 1 to n;
      if (tdelta[j]=0) then do;
        par2temp=0.;
        gt = 0.;
        do i= 1 to n;
          if(tdelta[i]=1 & tsurv[i]>=tsurv[j]) then
            gt = gt +  dsurv[i]/kc[i];
        end;
```

```
        gt = gt/(s[j]*n);

        do i= 1 to n;
          if(tdelta[i]=1 & tsurv[i]>=tsurv[j]) then
            par2temp = par2temp+(culcost[i,j]-Ubar[j])*(dsurv[i]-gt)/kc[i];
        end;
        part2 = part2 + par2temp/(y[j]*kc[j]);
      end;
    end;
    covsub=part2/(n*n);
    return(covsub);
  finish CalCovSub;
```

Output from Program 16.3 for the ICD Group

```
                              PERCENS

Percent of censoring = 0.6966292


                                                  MEAN_SW

Simple weighted estimator for mean cost = 110108.86

                                                                    SE_SW

Standard error estimate for the simple weighted estimator = 6929.7977

                          MEAN_T

Mean survival time = 1261.4032

                                                     SE_T

Standard error for the mean survival time = 35.996617

                                            MEAN_IMP

Improved estimator for mean cost = 99311.725

                                                   SE_IMP

Standard error of the improved estimator =  5481.115


COV_SW

Covariance between mean survival time and the simple weighted cost estimator =
24943.547

                                                                            COV_IMP

Covariance between mean survival time and the improved cost estimator = 30485.773
```

Output from Program 16.3 for the Conventional Treatment Group

```
                                 PERCENS

Percent of censoring = 0.4782609


                                                  MEAN_SW

Simple weighted estimator for mean cost = 70034.696

                                                                   SE_SW

Standard error estimate for the simple weighted estimator = 9267.5059

                                MEAN_T

Mean survival time = 968.77197

                                                     SE_T

Standard error for the mean survival time = 58.370098

                                           MEAN_IMP

Improved estimator for mean cost = 72544.906

                                                  SE_IMP

Standard error of the improved estimator = 8529.8308


COV_SW

Covariance between mean survival time and the simple weighted cost estimator =
24852.951

                                                                              COV_IMP

Covariance between mean survival time and the improved cost estimator = 29764.298
```

Program 16.4 calculates the ICER (in $1,000/year saved) and its confidence interval, using the improved estimators for the costs.

Program 16.4 SAS Code for Obtaining Estimate of ICER and Its 95% Confidence Interval

```
cost1=72544.91/1000;
 secost1=8529.83/1000;
 survt1=968.77/365.25;
 sesurvt1=58.37/365.25;
 covcs1=29764.30/1000/365.25;

 cost2=99311.73/1000;
 secost2=5481.11/1000;
 survt2=1261.40/365.25;
 sesurvt2=36.00/365.25;
 covcs2=30485.77/1000/365.25;

 icer=(cost2-cost1)/(survt2-survt1);
 run CalCIiCER(cost1,secost1,survt1,sesurvt1,covcs1,
cost2,secost2,survt2,sesurvt2,covcs2, lowbd,upperbd);
```

```
  start CalCIiCER(cost1,secost1,survt1,sesurvt1,covcs1,
cost2,secost2,survt2,sesurvt2,covcs2,lowbd,upperbd);
    t=1.96;
    x=cost1-cost2;
    y=survt1-survt2;
    sxx=secost1**2+secost2**2;
    syy=sesurvt1**2+sesurvt2**2;
    sxy=covcs1+covcs2;

    f=(x*y-t**2*sxy)**2-(x**2-t**2*sxx)*(y**2-t**2*syy);
    lowbd=(x*y-t**2*sxy-sqrt(f))/(y**2-t**2*syy);
    upperbd=(x*y-t**2*sxy+sqrt(f))/(y**2-t**2*syy);
  finish CalCIiCER;
print , "Incremental cost-effectiveness ratio =" icer;
print , "Lower 95% confidence limit for icer =" lowbd;
print , "Upper 95% confidence limit for icer =" upperbd;
```

Output from Program 16.4

```
ICER

Incremental cost-effectiveness ratio =  33.40936

                                          LOWBD

Lower 95% confidence limit for icer = 8.6318453

                                        UPPERBD

Upper 95% confidence limit for icer = 73.552101
```

When restricted to a 4-year period, the average cost was $99,312 (standard error [s.e.] $5,481) for the ICD arm and $72,545 (s.e. $8,530) for the conventional therapy arm. The average survival time during the 4-year period was 1,261 (s.e. 36) days for the ICD arm and 969 (s.e. 58) days for the conventional therapy arm. The ICER comparing the ICD arm with the conventional arm was $33,400 per year of life saved, with a 95% confidence interval of (8.6, 73.6). The estimated ICER was less than $50,000 per year of life saved, an often-mentioned threshold under which treatment can be considered cost-effective compared to controls (Gold et al., 1996).

Using the simple weighted estimator, the result for the mean cost for the ICD arm was $110,109 (s.e. $6,930) and the mean cost for the conventional arm was $70,035 (s.e. $9,268). We can clearly see that the simple weighted estimator has a larger standard error, and thus it is less efficient than the improved estimator. Using a method that is similar to Lin and colleagues (1997) and a bootstrap method for the standard error, Mushlin and colleagues (1998) reported a mean cost of $99,310 for the ICD arm and $72,540 for the conventional arm. The estimated ICER is $27,000 per year of life saved, with a 95% confidence interval of (0.2, 68.2). These numbers are very close to the improved estimator.

16.4 Discussion

Throughout this chapter, it is assumed that censoring is random and independent of the survival time and cost-accumulating process. This assumption is usually met in well-conducted clinical trials where censoring is mainly caused by administrative termination of the study. In observational studies, this assumption might not be reasonable. However, if the censoring process can be modeled through some known variables, it is still possible to use the inverse-probability weighted method. In that case, the survival probability for the censoring variable will not be obtained by the non-parametric Kaplan-Meier estimator, but instead it can be estimated by some regression method such as the Cox Proportional Hazards model (Cox, 1972), if the proportional hazard assumption is met. Another alternative is an adjusted Kaplan-Meier estimator where one uses inverse probability of treatment weighting to adjust for the confounding factors for the survival distribution of the censoring (Xie and Liu, 2005).

The weight obtained from the inverse of the survival probability for the censoring variable can turn out to be a very large number when there is considerable censoring near the end of the time limit, L. Consequently, it is possible that a few very small probabilities can inflate this estimator. Under this sort of situation, one may want to reduce the limit, L; it is difficult to estimate costs when there are many censored values near the tail area.

Cost data are usually right-skewed, with some patients accumulating huge costs, while the majority of subjects incur only very little costs. The methods discussed here are fully nonparametric, which means that there is no distributional assumption for either cost history or survival time. However, we do need to use a reasonably large sample because the nonparametric method relies on the large sample theory.

We have discussed how to use Fieller's method to obtain the confidence interval of the incremental cost-effectiveness ratio. Fieller's method always provides us with a confidence set that has a correct coverage probability, as long as the numerator and the denominator in the ICER have a bivariate normal distribution, which was satisfied asymptotically for our method. An alternative way is to implement bootstrapping methods (Efron and Tibshirani, 1986, 1993). See Chapter 14.

The methods demonstrated in this chapter are applicable to observational data when one is interested in estimating costs for a population of patients or in comparing costs or cost-effectiveness between groups and one is not interested in causal inferences. That is, use these methods when you are simply estimating naturalistic treatment differences without needing to adjust for selection bias between groups. Researchers interested in cost comparisons from observational data often need to incorporate covariate information due to baseline imbalance between treatment groups. The methods described in this section may also be helpful in these situations. For instance, if propensity score stratification was used as the method to adjust for selection bias, the methods demonstrated here could be applied within each of the propensity score strata and then a pooled estimator could be obtained by averaging across strata. If one has a propensity score matched population, then the groups are balanced with respect to baseline covariates and the methods demonstrated may be applicable.

Other methodology using regression models with direct covariate adjustment has been proposed by researchers that is applicable to comparative observational research. Among them, Lin (2000a) considered a proportional mean regression model; Jain and Strawderman (2002) proposed a model based on a flexible hazard function of the medical costs; and Lin (2000b) and Willan and colleagues (2005) proposed methods that directly model the mean, using the simple weighted estimator from inverse probability weighting.

Acknowledgments

The authors are very grateful to Dr. Alvin I. Mushlin and Dr. Arthur J. Moss for making the cost data of MADIT available to us.

References

Bang, H., and A. A. Tsiatis. 2000. "Estimating medical costs with censored data." *Biometrika* 87: 329–343.

Briggs, A., T. Clark, J. Wolstenholme, and P. Clarke. 2003. "Missing…presumed at random: cost-analysis of incomplete data." *Health Economics* 12(5): 377–392.

Cox, D. R. 1972. "Regression models and life-tables (with discussion)." *Journal of the Royal Statistical Society* B 34: 187–220.

Duan, N. 1983. "Smearing estimate: a nonparametric retransformation method." *Journal of the American Statistical Association* 78: 605–610.

Efron, B., and R. Tibshirani. 1986. "Bootstrap methods for standard errors, confidence intervals, and other measures of statistical accuracy." *Statistical Science* 1: 54–75.

Efron, B., and R. Tibshirani. 1993. *An Introduction to the Bootstrap.* New York: Chapman & Hall/CRC.

Fieller, E. C. 1954. "Some problems in interval estimation." *Journal of the Royal Statistical Society, Series B* (Statistical Methodology) 16(2): 175–185.

Gold, M. R., J. E. Siegel, L. B. Russell, and M. C. Weinstein, eds. 1996. *Cost-Effectiveness in Health and Medicine.* New York: Oxford University Press.

Horvitz, D. G., and D. J. Thompson. 1952. "A generalization of sampling without replacement from a finite universe." *Journal of the American Statistical Association* 47(260): 663–685.

Huang, Y., and T. A. Louis. 1998. "Nonparametric estimation of the joint distribution of survival time and mark variables. " *Biometrika* 85: 785–798.

Jain, A. K., and R. L. Strawderman. 2002. "Flexible hazard regression modeling for medical cost data." *Biostatistics* 3:101–118.

Kaplan, E. L., and P. Meier. 1958. "Nonparametric estimation from incomplete observations." *Journal of the American Statistical Association* 53: 457–481.

Lin, D. Y. 2000a. "Proportional means regression for censored medical costs." *Biometrics* 56: 775–778.

Lin, D. Y. 2000b. "Linear regression analysis of censored medical costs." *Biostatistics* 1: 35–47.

Lin, D. Y., E. J. Feuer, R. Etzioni, and Y. Wax. 1997. "Estimating medical costs from incomplete follow-up data. *Biometrics* 53: 419–434.

Little, R. J. A., and D. B. Rubin. 1987. *Statistical Analysis with Missing Data.* New York: John Wiley & Sons, Inc.

Moss, A. J., W. J. Hall, D. S. Cannom, J. P. Daubert, S. L. Higgins, H. Klein, J. H.Levine, S. Saksena, A. L. Waldo, D. Wilber, M. W. Brown, and M. Heo. 1996. "Improved survival with an implanted defibrillator in patients with coronary disease at high risk for ventricular arrhythmia." The *New England Journal of Medicine* 335(26): 1933–1940.

Mushlin, A. I., W. J. Hall, J. Zwanziger, E. Gajary, M. Andrews, R. Marron, K. H. Zou, and A. J. Moss for the MADIT Investigators. 1998. "The cost-effectiveness of automatic implantable cardiac defibrillators: results from MADIT." *Circulation* 97(21): 2129–2135.

Pfeifer, P. E., and H. Bang. 2005. "Non-parametric estimation of mean customer lifetime value." *Journal of Interactive Marketing* 19(4): 48–66.

Ramsey , S., R. Willke, A. Briggs, R. Brown, M. Buxton, A. Chawla, J. Cook, H. Glick, B. Liljas, D. Petitti, and S. Reed. 2005. "Good research practices for cost-effectiveness analysis alongside clinical trials: the ISPOR RCT-CEA task force report." *Value in Health* 8(5): 521–533.

Rubin, D. B. 1987. *Multiple Imputation for Nonresponse in Surveys.* New York: John Wiley & Sons, Inc.

Schafer, J. L. 1997. *Analysis of Incomplete Multivariate Data.* London: Chapman & Hall/CRC.

van Buuren, S., H. C. Boshuizen, and D. L. Knook. 1999. "Multiple imputation of missing blood pressure covariates in survival analysis." *Statistics in Medicine* 18(6): 681–694.

Wang, H., and H. Zhao. 2006. "Estimating incremental cost-effectiveness ratios and their confidence intervals with differentially censored data." *Biometrics* 62: 570–575.

Willan, A. R., and D. Y. Lin. 2001. "Incremental net benefit in randomized clinical trials." *Statistics in Medicine* 20: 1563–1574.

Willan, A. R., D. Y. Lin, and A. Manca. 2005. "Regression methods for cost-effectiveness analysis with censored data." *Statistics in Medicine* 24: 131–145.

Willan, A. R., E. B. Chen, R. J. Cook, and D. Y. Lin. 2003. "Incremental net benefit in randomized clinical trials with quality-adjusted survival." *Statistics in Medicine* 22: 353–362.

Xie, J., and C. Liu. 2005. "Adjusted Kaplan-Meier estimator and log-rank test with inverse probability of treatment weighting for survival data." *Statistics in Medicine* 24: 3089–3110.

Young, T. A. 2005. "Estimating mean total costs in the presence of censoring: a comparative assessment of methods." *PharmacoEconomics* 23(12): 1229–1242.

Zhao, H., and L. Tian. 2001. "On estimating medical cost and incremental cost-effectiveness ratios with censored data." *Biometrics* 57: 1002–1008.

Zhao H., H. Bang, H. Wang, and P. E. Pfeifer. 2007. "On the equivalence of some medical cost estimators with censored data." *Statistics in Medicine* 26: 4520–4530.

Part 6

Designing Observational Studies

Chapter 17

Addressing Measurement and Sponsor Biases in Observational Research

Josep Maria Haro

Abstract

Researchers who design, implement, and analyze observational studies must address the potential for multiple types of bias. In this chapter, we focus on methods to minimize measurement and sponsor bias. *Measurement bias* occurs when there are differences in the evaluation of patient outcomes between the groups being compared. *Sponsor bias* is a vague concept that includes many systematic errors that may arise from the interest of the investigator or the sponsor to support a given treatment. The use of easy-to-administer, well-validated assessment scales; the inclusion of objective outcome variables; and the combination of information coming from diverse sources (investigators, patients, databases) may reduce the likelihood of measurement and sponsor bias.

17.1 Introduction

Careful design and implementation of observational studies is needed to provide valid results. Observational studies by nature are subject to the potential for measurement (observer/informational), sponsor (investigator), and selection bias. Selection bias occurs when the intervention groups being compared differ in measured or unmeasured baseline characteristics, which affects prognosis. It usually originates in the way in which participants are selected for the study or assigned to their study groups (Altman et al., 2001). Accounting for selection bias in the analysis of observational study data is discussed in detail in Chapters 2 through 7. In this chapter, we look at addressing bias in observational research—both at the design stage and the analysis stage—with a focus on measurement and sponsor biases. Measurement, or information bias, occurs when the ascertainment of outcomes or other patient characteristics is different in the groups being compared. Sponsor (investigator) bias is a vague term that includes a number of aspects the promoter of a study decides during the design, implementation, or analysis that may influence the results or conclusion of the study.

In randomized clinical trials (RCTs), measurement bias is minimized by blinding the observer/investigator to the treatment the patient is receiving and by the regularly scheduled and structured data collection—which should be the same for all the groups being compared. However, such design features are not always feasible for observational studies. Several other strategies, discussed in Section 17.3, can be used to minimize measurement and sponsor bias when blind assessment is not possible.

Before focusing on strategies to minimize sponsor and observer bias, we provide a brief overview of key issues in the design of observational studies (see Section 17.2). These discussions are not meant to be exhaustive but to raise important issues and provide you with references to more detailed discussions.

17.2 General Design Issues

In observational studies, we often want to describe the relationship between a factor and some outcomes. For simplicity, we will assume for the rest of the chapter that the factor we want to analyze is a treatment provided to patients with a given disease. In order to achieve treatment evaluation, investigators collect information on the individual or patient characteristics, the exposure to the treatment they are analyzing, and the outcomes they are interested in. There are a number of critical aspects that need to be taken into account when designing and conducting observational studies in order to obtain valid results. This includes considerations regarding how to minimize selection bias, measurement bias, sponsor bias, appropriate choice of control groups, and temporal relationships. Each of these issues is discussed briefly here. A discussion of common observational study— designs such as cohort, case-control, and cross-sectional—is not provided. Refer to Szklo and Nieto (2007) and Rosenbaum (2002) for more information.

First, the temporal relationship between the treatment and the outcome needs to be clear (Suissa, 2008). Longitudinal designs are needed in order to analyze treatment effects. *Longitudinal studies* are defined here as those studies in which individuals are assessed when they are exposed to a treatment or risk factor, and later their response to the treatment or the condition being studied is evaluated. Longitudinal studies can be retrospective if available databases can provide information on patient exposure to treatment time before outcome evaluation. In studies with prospective longitudinal designs, we evaluate patient status at the initiation of the treatment, and we analyze the outcomes of that treatment after the patient has been receiving it for some time. Thus, changes in patient status can be related to treatment effects. Cross-sectional studies are not useful in assessing the effects of treatments on outcomes for two reasons. First, in cross-sectional studies, we cannot separate the effects of treatment and the baseline severity of the disease the patient is suffering from. Second, cross-sectional studies do not provide information on the individuals who have been exposed to the factor or treatment in the past but have discontinued the treatment prior to cross-sectional observation. Temporal relationships are one of the Austin Bradford-Hill criteria (Hill, 1965) to evaluate causal associations, along with factors such as consistency, strength, specificity, dose-response relationship, biological plausibility, and coherence.

Second, changes the patients experience due to the treatment need to be distinguished from the natural course of the disorder. For example, if we analyze the effects of the treatment of a self-limiting disease, we need to separate the natural course to cure from the treatment effects. This can be done only if the course of patients receiving the treatment of interest is compared with a proper control group. In observational studies, the selection of the comparison or control group will obviously be determined by the usual practice with patients with the disease we are analyzing. This control group should be formed with patients receiving the most frequently prescribed alternative treatment or with patients receiving no treatment, in settings where patients in routine clinical care usually receive no treatment. In this chapter, we refer only to studies that compare the course of patients receiving a given treatment (treatment group) with patients receiving an alternative treatment or no treatment (control group).

Third, patients receiving different treatments may have different characteristics. Clinicians tend to prescribe treatments believed to be more effective to more severe patients and less invasive or better tolerated treatments to patients who have less severe forms of the disorder. Thus, not taking into account these differences among patients may provide false results. Treatments prescribed to more severe patients who will probably have worse outcomes may appear less effective, although they can actually be more effective than treatments that clinicians may usually prescribe to patients with less severe forms of the disease.

This problem, usually referred to as *selection bias*, is a frequent limitation of observational studies. However, it can be addressed in the design and implementation of the study by carefully collecting information on all those prognostic factors that may influence the outcome and by taking into account in the analysis of the results the possible differences between treatment groups. The collection of these patient characteristics, which will allow the evaluation and control of selection bias, is one advantage of prospective research as compared to retrospective research, such as from health-care claims databases. Causal relationships can only be claimed if all of these factors are recorded and there are no unmeasured confounders that may be modifying the results. In addition, Rubin (2007) argued that observational studies should be designed to mimic randomized trials as much as possible. For instance, where possible, one should finalize any primary bias adjustment model (such as a propensity score model) using background information before accessing the outcome data. This avoids the potential for choosing an adjustment model that provides a desired result and raises the credibility of the study with consumers of the information. Several of the chapters in this book present methods on how to control for this selection bias in the analysis phase.

Finally, the information obtained on the patient needs to faithfully assess patient status. If the evaluation of the patient is not properly conducted and it is influenced by external factors, patient changes during treatment may not reflect real changes. This problem is called *measurement*, *information*, or *observer bias* and occurs when the assessments of the outcomes are not valid (Porta, 2008). Two types of observer bias may be defined: non-differential and differential (Page and Henderson, 2008). In the first case, measurement error occurs similarly and randomly in the treatment and comparison groups. For example, this can occur when patient evaluation is conducted using suboptimal methods. The most frequent consequence of non-differential measurement bias is an increase in measurement error and, thus, a decrease in the ability to detect differences between treatment groups when they exist.

Differential measurement bias occurs when the evaluation of the treatment and control groups is not consistent. In this case, differences in the evaluation process between control and treatment groups may create artificial differences among them. This may occur in non-blinded assessments when prejudices of the investigator may cause a more favorable evaluation of one of the treatment groups. Because this can occur when the investigator or promoter of the study has an interest in demonstrating the benefits of one treatment over the other, this bias is usually called *investigator* or *sponsor bias*. However, there are also a number of other systematic errors that can be included under the definition of sponsor bias. The rest of the chapter presents the origins and effects of this bias and possible ways of assessing, controlling, and eliminating them.

17.3 Addressing Measurement and Sponsor Bias

Treatments are developed and tested by investigators who, obviously, may be interested in showing that the treatment they have created is effective. This may also happen when a pharmaceutical company that is developing or producing a medication tests its efficacy or effectiveness. This desire may also cause investigator or sponsor bias (Harrington and Ohman, 2007), which can include a number of circumstances when designing or implementing a study that may cause the new treatment to appear to have better outcomes than it has. The most typical case occurs when the physicians evaluating patients in the treatment group tend to evaluate them more favorably than patients in the control group (observer bias).

In RCTs, observer bias is minimized by blinding the investigators to the treatment the patient is receiving. If the investigators who evaluate the patients are blind to the treatment the patient is receiving, they cannot rate one differently than the other. Blind assessment is also the first option to avoid observer bias in observational studies. Blind assessment can be implemented by having an investigator who is not the treating physician and who does not know the treatment the patient is receiving evaluate the patient. Although blinding is possible (Pinto-Meza et al., 2008), it has a number of practical difficulties that frequently prevent its use in observational studies.

The most common case in prospective observational studies is that the treating physician or another member of the medical team evaluates the patients using standardized methods. In this case, proper assessment requires several strategies. First, easy-to-administer, well-validated assessment scales are preferred. The investigator brochure or data collection form should include a proper description of the scales. Longer questionnaires may be employed. However, in this case, the total duration of assessment needs to be considered in order to avoid altering the course of treatment. Questionnaires that require in-person training should be avoided because it is usually not feasible to conduct training in observational studies that include a large number of sites. It is especially important to use care when rating the patient with questionnaires that assess the intensity of the symptoms. These questionnaires are based on the subjective appraisal of the clinical status of the patient and thus are more subject to being influenced.

Second, instruments based on the objective patient status (laboratory tests, death) are preferred to instruments based on the subjective appraisal of the symptoms. However, symptom rating is the most relevant assessment of patient severity in several areas of medicine (for example, psychiatry). If that is the case, the evaluation of the patients should include not only the symptom evaluation but also other, more objective measures of patient status (for example, patient functioning in several areas of life). In any case, the answer categories should be clearly defined to minimize interpretation by the evaluator.

A third strategy to decrease the likelihood of observer bias is to complement the patient assessment by the clinician with assessments by other sources. These other sources can be patient or administrative data. Self-rating by the patient has a number of advantages. Because investigator or sponsor bias originates with an interest in showing that one of the treatments is better, this may not be the case for patients. They may be able to provide a more unbiased assessment. Self-rating by the patient may be conducted by generic or disorder-specific health-related quality-of-life instruments or other instruments that self-rate symptoms. However, patient self-evaluation does not measure the same constructs as clinician evaluations. Some differences may arise due not to biases but to the different constructs or outcome measures being evaluated and to the fact that patients acclimate to their symptom severity.

First, analysis can be repeated using patient self-rating instead of clinician rating. If the results are consistent, the conclusions of the study are reinforced. Second, self-rating by the patient may be compared with the investigator assessment. This may inform us of the possible presence of investigator bias (Haro et al., 2006). Specifically, differences between the treatment and control groups as assessed by the patient may be compared to treatment differences as assessed by the investigator. For example, we may compare the percentage of improvement of the treatment versus the control group as assessed by the patient in the patients that experience greater improvement (or a given percentage of improvement) in the treatment group versus the control group. If there is no observer bias, we would expect that the differences between the treatment and control groups in the patient assessment are of similar magnitude in the patient who the investigator rated as improving similarly. If the differences assessed by the investigator show a better outcome than the control group, this could indicate observer bias. In this case, we would also assess whether treatment differences are caused by a reduced number of investigators or distributed homogeneously among them. Haro and colleagues (2006) present a practical example in which changes from baseline to endpoint in Euro-QOL 5D (EQ-5D), a generic quality-of-life scale that was rated by patients, were described in patients who showed the same improvement with the two treatments being compared. (In this case, the patients who were compared experienced a one-point decrease from baseline to endpoint in the Clinical Global Impression scale, a clinician-administered scale that evaluated overall severity from 1 to 7.) Because the differences in EQ-5D between the groups being compared were similar, the authors point out that there was no evidence of observer bias. Finally, in the case that there is some evidence of observer bias because patient self-evaluation differs from investigator evaluation, we may determine whether these mean differences are attributed to a few investigators, who could be driving the observer bias, or are homogeneously distributed among all of them.

Fourth, as in any type of study, treatment and control groups should be evaluated with the same instruments and at similar time intervals. This may be problematic in observational studies because the treatment provided to different patients may be different and they can be cited at different intervals. The study description must clearly specify the intervals at which the patients are to be evaluated, in case regular visits are conducted during the interval, and the way the evaluation must be conducted.

As mentioned previously, investigator or sponsor bias can be present at any stage of study development. During the design of the study, patient outcomes should be widely considered in order to include as many of the areas in which treatment differences may be present as possible. Outcomes should include the clinical and functioning status and also the presence of adverse events. Focusing on outcomes that measure the areas where the new treatment is expected to be superior to existing alternatives may highlight only part of the treatment differences that favor the new treatment.

17.4 Summary

Observational studies, by nature, are subject to a number of systematic errors or biases when used to assess treatment effects. Careful design and implementation, including the inclusion of a control or comparison group, the consideration of the temporal relationship between treatment and outcomes, the control of selection bias, and the avoidance of information bias, are necessary to produce valid results. Observation bias may be reduced by using objective outcomes, by employing simple and valid assessments, and by combining several sources of information.

References

Altman, D. G., K. F. Schulz, D. Moher, M. Egger, F. Davidoff, D. Elbourne, and P. C. Gøtzsche; T. Lang for the CONSORT Group. 2001. "The revised CONSORT statement for reporting randomized trials: explanation and elaboration." *Annals of Internal Medicine* 134(8): 663–694.

Grimes, D. A., and K. F. Schulz. 2002. "Bias and causal associations in observational research." The *Lancet* 359: 248–252.

Harrington, R. A., and E. M. Ohman. 2007. "The enigma of drug-eluting stents: hope, hype, humility, and advancing patient care." *The Journal of the American Medical Association* 297: 2028–2030.

Haro, J. M., S. Kontodimas, M. A. Negrin, M. Ratcliffe, D. Suarez, and F. Windmeijer. 2006. "Methodological aspects in the assessment of treatment effects in observational health outcomes studies." *Applied Health Economics and Health Policy* 5(1): 11–25.

Hill, A. B. 1965. "The environment and disease: association or causation?" *Proceedings of the Royal Society of Medicine* 58: 295–300.

Page, L. A., and M. Henderson. 2008. "Appraising the evidence: what is measurement bias?" *Evidence-Based Mental Health* 11(2): 36–37.

Pinto-Meza, A., A. Fernandez, A. Serrano-Blanco, and J. M. Haro. 2008. "Adequacy of antidepressant treatment in Spanish primary care: a naturalistic six-month follow-up study." *Psychiatric Services* 59: 78–83.

Porta, M. S. 2008. *Dictionary of Epidemiology*. 5th ed. New York: Oxford University Press, Inc.

Rosenbaum, P. R. 2002. *Observational Studies*. 2d ed. New York: Springer-Verlag.

Rubin, D. B. 2007. "The design versus the analysis of observational studies for causal effects: parallels with the design of randomized trials." *Statistics in Medicine* 26: 20–36.

Suissa, S. 2008. "Immeasurable time bias in observational studies of drug effects on mortality." *American Journal of Epidemiology* 168: 329–335.

Szklo, M., and F. J. Nieto. 2006. *Epidemiology: Beyond the Basics*. 2d ed. MA: Jones and Bartlett Publishers.

Chapter 18

Sample Size Calculation for Observational Studies

Sin-Ho Jung
Taiyeong Lee
Elizabeth DeLong

Abstract

For a number of reasons, observational studies are currently being used to provide evidence to support medical decisions. Because these studies do not carry the same level of credibility conferred to randomized trials, appropriate attention to statistical issues is paramount. In particular, considerations of event rate, sample size, and power frequently occur. This chapter provides mechanisms for dealing with these considerations under a variety of scenarios. Additionally, the methods presented here are applicable more generally to clinical trials as well.

18.1 Introduction

The increasing availability of computerized clinical patient data has stimulated greater interest in research on observational data. Individual medical practices and hospitals are now attempting to draw inferences on the basis of data gathered on their own patients. Additionally, the proliferation of large registry databases that harvest clinical data from hundreds of sites has created opportunities to study questions regarding rare diseases and rare events. However, even studies using these large databases, when reduced to the appropriate study populations and endpoints, encounter issues of sample size and power.

Observational studies can be designed to address a variety of objectives. If the primary analysis of the study is simply to estimate some parameter, then one can use standard sample size calculations for requiring a confidence interval of at most a certain width. If the objective involves the comparison of cohorts, then in many cases the statistical analysis will involve some form of selection bias adjustment due to the non-randomized nature of observational research.

Chapters 1 through 11 cover the issues of selection bias adjustment and standard analytical methods for comparing cohorts in these settings, including propensity score regression, stratification, matching, doubly robust adjustment, instrumental variables, local control, and various longitudinal analyses. Regarding the computation of sample sizes in study planning in these scenarios, such complex designs and analyses may require custom sample size and power estimate calculations through simulations. In some cases, the primary hypothesis may be simplified for the purpose of estimating power and sample size, and generalized SAS macros can perform the needed calculations.

In this chapter, we present a series of SAS macros for computing sample sizes for studies with various types of outcomes and comparisons (all for comparisons between two groups):

- *t*-test (Section 18.2.1)
- Wilcoxon Rank Sum test (Section 18.2.2)
- Two-Sample Tests on Binary outcomes (Section 18.3.1)
- Weighted Mantel-Haenszel test (Section 18.3.2)
- Log-Rank test for survival data (Section 18.4)
- Longitudinal Data—Continuous outcomes (Section 18.5.3.3)
- Longitudinal Data—Binary outcomes (Section 18.5.3.3)

The sample size macro for the Weighted Mantel-Haenszel test (provided in Section 18.3.1) is directly applicable for observational studies for which the analysis is based on the commonly utilized propensity score stratification approach. This propensity score stratification analysis methodology is described in detail in Chapter 2. In brief, propensity score stratification involves estimating a propensity score for each study participant, stratifying by this score, estimating the difference in outcomes between the two cohorts within each of the strata, and then combining the estimated cohort differences over strata.

Other sections in this chapter present sample size macros based on analysis methods without specific selection bias adjustments. However, these can be very useful for observational study planning when simple cohort comparisons are planned (for example, such as when causal inference is not the objective) or as a very easy-to-use initial calculation when other methods are being utilized such as propensity score matching. In this example, one would supplement the sample sizes computed in these macros with an estimate of the number of patients excluded from the analysis due to a lack of propensity score matched patients in the other cohort. In addition, most of the sample size calculation methods in this chapter can be used for randomized clinical trials as well.

18.2 Continuous Variables

In this section, we consider two two-sample tests for continuous variables: *t* -test and Wilcoxon rank test.

18.2.1 Two-Sample t-test

Suppose that, for group $k(=1,2)$, $X_{k1},\dots,X_{k,n_k}$ are independent and identically distributed (IID) normal random variables with mean μ_k and variance σ^2. We want to test $H_0:\mu_1=\mu_2$ vs. $H_a:\mu_1\neq\mu_2$. Let $\bar{X}_k=n_k^{-1}\sum_{i=1}^{n_k}X_{ki}$ denote the sample mean for group k, and

$$s_p^2=\frac{\sum_{i=1}^{n_1}(X_{1i}-\bar{X}_1)^2+\sum_{i=1}^{n_2}(X_{2i}-\bar{X}_2)^2}{n_1+n_2-2}$$

denote the pooled sample variance. Then, under H_0,

$$T=\frac{\bar{X}_1-\bar{X}_2}{s_p\sqrt{n_1^{-1}+n_2^{-1}}}$$

follows the t-distribution with n_1+n_2-2 degrees of freedom. Hence, given type I error probability α, we reject H_0 if $|T|>t_{n_1+n_2-2,1-\alpha/2}$, where $t_{v,\gamma}$ is the 100γ-th percentile of the t-distribution with v degrees of freedom.

If n_1 and n_2 are large, then we do not require the normal distribution assumption, and the critical value from the t-test, $t_{n_1+n_2-2,1-\alpha/2}$, can be approximated by the 100γ-th percentile of the standard normal distribution, $z_{1-\alpha/2}$. How large the sample sizes should be for the large approximation depends on how close the distribution of the observations for each group is to a normal distribution. To improve the normality, we often apply a transform to the raw data, such as a log-transformation for positive variables (Carroll and Ruppert, 1988). We derive the sample size formula based on the large sample approximation.

We consider a specific alternative hypothesis $H_a:|\mu_1-\mu_2|=\Delta\sigma$. Note that $\Delta=\sigma^{-1}(\mu_1-\mu_2)$ denotes a standardized effect size under the alternative hypothesis. Without loss of generality, we assume that $\mu_1>\mu_2$ under H_a. Then, under H_a,

$$T\approx\frac{\bar{X}_1-\bar{X}_2-\sigma\Delta}{\sigma\sqrt{n_1^{-1}+n_2^{-1}}}+\frac{\Delta}{\sqrt{n_1^{-1}+n_2^{-1}}}$$

$$=Z+\Delta\sqrt{nr_1r_2},$$

where $Z:N(0,1)$, $r_k=n_k/n$, and $n=n_1+n_2$. For a given n, the power is calculated as

$$1-\beta=\bar{\Phi}(z_{1-\alpha/2}-\Delta\sqrt{nr_1r_2}), \qquad (1)$$

where $\overline{\Phi}(z) = 1 - \Phi(z)$ and $\Phi(z) = P(Z \le z)$ is the cumulative distribution function of the standard normal distribution, $N(0,1)$. By solving (1) with respect to n, we obtain the required total sample size as

$$n = \frac{(z_{1-\alpha/2} + z_{1-\beta})^2}{r_1 r_2 \Delta^2},$$

or $n_k = n \times r_k$ for group k. For one-sided testing, replace $\alpha/2$ with α. This sample size is based on a large sample approximation to a *t*-distribution, so that this formula underestimates the sample size for small sample sizes. If the final sample size by the formula based on normal approximation is smaller than 30, we may consider increasing it by about 10%.

In summary, the sample size calculation for a two-sample t-test is conducted as follows:

- In addition to type I error probability α and power $1-\beta$, specify

  (a) $\Delta = \sigma^{-1} | \mu_1 - \mu_2 |$, standardized effect size

  (b) r_k = the prevalence of group k $(r_1 + r_2 = 1)$

- Calculate the sample size

$$n = \frac{(z_{1-\alpha/2} + z_{1-\beta})^2}{r_1 r_2 \Delta^2}.$$

Example 18.1

Suppose that we want to detect a difference of 0.5σ in the population means with two-sided $\alpha = 0.05$ and power $1-\beta = 0.9$. Then $z_{1-\alpha/2} = 1.96$ and $z_{1-\beta} = 1.282$. Assuming an equal proportion of two groups in the population (that is, $r_1 = r_2 = 0.5$), we obtain the required sample size $n = 171$. PROC POWER in SAS/STAT can directly handle this scenario, as shown in the following code:

Program 18.1 SAS Code for Two-Sample *t*-Test

```
proc power;
     twosamplemeans
     nfractional
     meandiff = 0.5                /* mean difference               */
     stddev   = 1                  /* sigma                         */
     groupweights = (0.5 0.5)      /* r1 r2                         */
     sides = 2                     /* 1: one sided 2: 2: two-sided  */
     power =0.9                    /* power                         */
     alpha =0.05                   /* alpha                         */
     ntotal=.;                     /* Sample Size                   */
run;
```

Output from Program 18.1

```
                    The POWER Procedure
          Two-sample t Test for Mean Difference

                 Fixed Scenario Elements

           Distribution                     Normal
           Method                            Exact
           Number of Sides                       2
           Alpha                              0.05
           Mean Difference                     0.5
           Standard Deviation                    1
           Group 1 Weight                      0.5
           Group 2 Weight                      0.5
           Nominal Power                       0.9
           Null Difference                       0

                 Computed Ceiling N Total

              Fractional      Actual     Ceiling
                N Total        Power     N Total

              170.062568       0.902         171
```

18.2.2 Wilcoxon Rank Sum Test

It is known that t-tests are sensitive to outliers. The Wilcoxon rank sum test (WRST) has been widely used as a robust test. We assume that for group $k(=1,2)$, $X_{k1},\ldots,X_{k,n_k}$ are IID random variables from a distribution with cumulative distribution function $F(x-\theta_k)=P(X_{ki}\le x)$. For $\Delta=\theta_1-\theta_2$, we want to test $H_0:\Delta=0$ vs. $H_a:\Delta\ne 0$. Mann and Whitney (1947) propose to use $W=(n_1n_2)^{-1}\sum_{i=1}^{n_1}\sum_{j=1}^{n_2}I(X_{1i}>X_{2j})$ for testing the hypothesis. The expected value of W is $P(X_{1i}>X_{2j})$, the probability that a randomly chosen measurement from group 1 is greater than a randomly chosen measurement from group 2. Thus, the test statistic will be close to 1/2 if H_0 is true, and closer to 0 or 1 if H_a is true.

For large $n(=n_1+n_2)$, we reject H_0 if the absolute value of

$$T=\frac{W-\nu_0}{\sigma_0}$$

is larger than $z_{1-\alpha/2}$, where $\nu_0=1/2$ and $\sigma_0^2=(n+1)/(12n_1n_2)$ are the mean and variance of W under H_0, respectively.

Let $f(x)=\partial F/\partial x$ denote the probability density function of $F(x)$. The appendix shows that, under H_a, W has mean

$$\nu_a=\int_{-\infty}^{\infty}F(x+\Delta)f(x)dx$$

and variance

$$\sigma_a^2 = \frac{\sigma_1^2}{n_1} + \frac{\sigma_2^2}{n_2},$$

where

$$\sigma_1^2 = \int_{-\infty}^{\infty} F^2(x+\Delta) f(x)dx - \{\int_{-\infty}^{\infty} F(x+\Delta) f(x)dx\}^2,$$

and

$$\sigma_2^2 = \int_{-\infty}^{\infty} F^2(x-\Delta) f(x)dx - \{\int_{-\infty}^{\infty} F(x-\Delta) f(x)dx\}^2.$$

Then,

$$T = Z\frac{\sigma_a}{\sigma_0} + \frac{v_a - v_0}{\sigma_0},$$

where $Z = (W - v_a)/\sigma_a$ is an asymptotically $N(0,1)$ random variable. Given power $1-\beta$,

$$1-\beta = P(|T| > z_{1-\alpha/2} \mid H_a) = P(Z\frac{\sigma_a}{\sigma_0} + \frac{|v_a - v_0|}{\sigma_0} > z_{1-\alpha/2}).$$

$$= \overline{\Phi}(\frac{\sigma_0}{\sigma_a}(z_{1-\alpha/2} - \frac{|v_a - v_0|}{\sigma_0})),$$

where $\overline{\Phi}(z) = P(Z > z)$. By replacing n_k with nr_k in σ_0^2 and σ_a^2, and solving with respect to n, we obtain the required sample size

$$n = \frac{1}{12r_1r_2}\{\frac{z_{1-\alpha/2} + z_{1-\beta}\sqrt{12(r_2\sigma_1^2 + r_1\sigma_2^2)}}{v_a - 1/2}\}^2.$$

Although the testing does not require the specification of the distribution function $F(x)$, a sample size calculation does. The alternative hypothesis is specified by two distributions with a location shift. The assumption of a location shift model is not required in order to carry out the rank sum test, but it is needed if we want to make inferences about medians or means. It is, of course, needed in the sample size calculation as presented here.

While a *t*-test requires a finite variance of the observations, WRST does not. For example, if F has a Cauchy distribution, we can use WRST, but not a *t*-test.

A sample size calculation for WRST assuming normal distributions can be described as follows:

- In addition to type I error probability α and power $1-\beta$, specify

  (a) $\Delta = \sigma^{-1}(\mu_1 - \mu_2)$, standardized effect size

  (b) r_k = the prevalence of group k $(r_1 + r_2 = 1)$

- Calculate

$$v_a = \int_{-\infty}^{\infty} \Phi(x+\Delta)\phi(x)dx$$

$$\sigma_1^2 = \int_{-\infty}^{\infty} \Phi^2(x+\Delta)\phi(x)dx - \{\int_{-\infty}^{\infty} \Phi(x+\Delta)\phi(x)dx\}^2$$

and

$$\sigma_2^2 = \int_{-\infty}^{\infty} \Phi^2(x-\Delta)\phi(x)dx - \{\int_{-\infty}^{\infty} \Phi(x-\Delta)\phi(x)dx\}^2,$$

where $\phi(x)$ and $\Phi(x)$ are the probability density function and the cumulative distribution function of $N(0,1)$, respectively.

- Calculate the sample size

$$n = \frac{1}{12r_1r_2}\{\frac{z_{1-\alpha/2} + z_{1-\beta}\sqrt{12(r_2\sigma_1^2 + r_1\sigma_2^2)}}{v_a - 1/2}\}^2.$$

Example 18.2

Suppose that we want to detect a difference of 0.5σ in the population means with two-sided $\alpha = 0.05$ and power $1-\beta = 0.9$. Then $z_{1-\alpha/2} = 1.96$ and $z_{1-\beta} = 1.282$. Assuming an equal proportion of two groups in the population (that is, $r_1 = r_2 = 0.5$), we obtain the required sample size $n = 177$. Note that the two-sample *t*-test requires a slightly smaller $n = 171$, but, in case there are outliers in the final data, the Wilcoxon rank test may be more powerful.

Program 18.2 SAS Code for Wilcoxon Rank Sum Test

```
%macro  WilcoxonRankSumTest( delta=,      /* Standardized effect size     */
                             r1 =  ,      /* prevalence of group 1        */
                             r2 =  ,      /* prevalence of group 2        */
                             sides=,      /* number of test sides: 1 or 2 */
                             alpha=,      /* alpha                        */
                             power=       /* power                        */
                             );
proc iml;
  start CDFPDFDELTA(t);
      m=t+&delta; c=cdf('normal',m,0,1); p=pdf('normal',t,0,1); v=c*p;
return(v);
  finish;
  start CDF2PDFDELTA(t);
      m=t+&delta; c=cdf('normal',m,0,1)**2; p=pdf('normal',t,0,1); v=c*p;
return(v);
  finish;
```

```
  start CDFPDF_DELTA(t);
      m=t-&delta; c=cdf('normal',m,0,1); p=pdf('normal',t,0,1); v=c*p;
return(v);
  finish;
  start CDF2PDF_DELTA(t);
      m=t-&delta; c=cdf('normal',m,0,1)**2; p=pdf('normal',t,0,1); v=c*p;
return(v);
  finish;
  start s1(t);
      m=t+&delta; c=cdf('normal',m,0,1); p=pdf('normal',t,0,1); v=c*p;
return(v);
  finish;

  interval = .M || .P;
  call quad(nu1,"CDFPDFDELTA",   interval);
  call quad(s1, "CDF2PDFDELTA",  interval);
  call quad(nu2,"CDFPDF_DELTA",  interval);
  call quad(s2, "CDF2PDF_DELTA", interval);

  sigma1 = s1-nu1**2; sigma2 = s2-nu2**2;
  p1=1-&alpha/&sides; z_alpha = probit(p1);
  p2=&power; z_beta  = probit(p2);
  n =
(1/(12*&r1*&r2))*((z_alpha+z_beta*sqrt(12*(&r2*sigma1+&r1*sigma2)))/(nu1-
0.5))**2;
  delta=&delta;r1 =&r1; r2=&r2;sides =&sides;alpha=&alpha;power=&power;
  print  'Sample Size';
  print 'Wilcoxon Rank Sum Test for Mean Difference';
  print delta r1 r2 sides alpha power;
  print n;
quit;
run;
%mend WilcoxonRankSumTest;

/*---------------------- Run the macro for Example 2. -------------------*/

%WilcoxonRankSumTest(delta=0.5, r1 = 0.5, r2 = 0.5, sides=2, alpha=0.05,
power=0.9);
```

Output from Program 18.2

```
                    Sample Size
         Wilcoxon Rank Sum Test for Mean Difference

      delta       r1       r2      sides      alpha      power
        0.5      0.5      0.5          2       0.05        0.9

                          n
                      176.41709
```

18.3 Binary Variables

In this section, we investigate two-sample tests for binary outcome variables with or without stratification. We use a weighted Mantel-Haenszel test for stratified analysis to adjust for covariates that are unbalanced between two groups.

18.3.1 Two-Sample Test on a Binary Outcome

Suppose that, for group $k(=1,2)$, X_k denotes the number of responders from n_k independent subjects. If group k has a response probability p_k, then X_k is a binomial distribution with n_k independent trials and response probability p_k. We want to test $H_0: p_1 = p_2$ vs. $H_a: p_1 \neq p_2$. Let $\hat{p}_k = X_k/n_k$ and $\hat{p} = (X_1 + X_2)/(n_1 + n_2)$ denote the sample proportion for group k and the pooled data, respectively. Then, for large n_1 and n_2 (say, $n_1, n_2 > 30$),

$$T = \frac{\hat{p}_1 - \hat{p}_2}{\sqrt{\hat{p}\hat{q}(n_1^{-1} + n_2^{-1})}}$$

follows the standard normal distribution under H_0, where $\hat{q} = 1 - \hat{p}$. Hence, given type I error probability α, we reject H_0 if $|T| > z_{1-\alpha/2}$. It is easy to show that T^2 is identical to the chi-squared test with 1 degree of freedom for a 2×2 table.

Let p_1, p_2 denote the response probability under a specific alternative hypothesis for sample size calculation, and $\Delta = p_1 - p_2$. Then, for large $n(= n_1 + n_2)$, $\hat{p}$ converges to $\bar{p} = r_1 p_1 + r_2 p_2$, where $r_k = n_k/n$. Under H_a,

$$T \approx \frac{\hat{p}_1 - \hat{p}_2 - \Delta}{\sqrt{\bar{p}\bar{q}(n_1^{-1} + n_2^{-1})}} + \frac{\Delta}{\sqrt{\bar{p}\bar{q}(n_1^{-1} + n_2^{-1})}}$$

$$= Z + \Delta\sqrt{\frac{nr_1r_2}{\bar{p}\bar{q}}},$$

where $Z : N(0,1)$ and $\bar{q} = 1 - \bar{p}$. Hence, given n, the power is calculated as

$$1 - \beta = \overline{\Phi}(z_{1-\alpha/2} - \Delta\sqrt{nr_1r_2}\, 0). \tag{2}$$

By solving (2) with respect to n, we obtain the required total sample size as

$$n = \frac{(z_{1-\alpha/2} + z_{1-\beta})^2\, \bar{p}\bar{q}}{r_1 r_2 (p_1 - p_2)^2}.$$

In summary, the sample size calculation for two-sample binomial proportions is conducted as follows:

- In addition to type I error probability α and power $1-\beta$, specify

  (a) p_1, p_2 = binomial proportions under H_a

  (b) r_k = the prevalence of group k $(r_1 + r_2 = 1)$

- Calculate the sample size

$$n = \frac{(z_{1-\alpha/2} + z_{1-\beta})^2 \overline{p}\overline{q}}{r_1 r_2 (p_1 - p_2)^2},$$

where $\overline{p} = r_1 p_1 + r_2 p_2$ and $\overline{q} = 1 - \overline{p}$.

Example 18.3

Suppose that we want to detect a difference of $p_1 = 0.4$ and $p_2 = 0.5$ with two-sided $\alpha = 0.05$ and power $1 - \beta = 0.9$. Assuming an equal proportion of two groups in the population (that is, $r_1 = r_2 = 0.5$), we obtain the required sample size $n = 1038$.

Program 18.3 SAS Code for Two-Sample Binomial Proportions

```
proc power;
     twosamplefreq  test=pchi
     groupproportions =(0.4 0.5) /* binomial proportions to be detected  */
     groupweights = (1 1)        /* (w1, w2):Weight of two groups,(r1,r2)*/
     sides = 2                   /* 1: one sided 2: 2: two-sided         */
     power =0.9                  /* power                                */
     alpha =0.05                 /* alpha                                */
     ntotal=.;                   /* sample size                          */
    run;
```

Output from Program 18.3

```
The POWER Procedure
Pearson Chi-square Test for Two Proportions

Fixed Scenario Elements

Distribution                         Asymptotic normal
Method                            Normal approximation
Number of Sides                                      2
Alpha                                             0.05
Group 1 Proportion                                 0.4
Group 2 Proportion                                 0.5
Group 1 Weight                                       1
Group 2 Weight                                       1
Nominal Power                                      0.9
Null Proportion Difference                           0

Computed N Total

Actual        N
Power     Total

0.901      1038
```

18.3.2 Weighted Mantel-Haenszel Test

In an observational study, patients are not randomly assigned to treatment groups with equal probability. Instead, the probability of assignment varies from patient to patient, possibly depending on the patient's baseline covariates. This often results in non-comparable treatment groups due to imbalance of the baseline covariates and consequently invalidates the standard methods commonly employed in data analysis. To overcome this problem, Rosenbaum and Rubin (1983, 1984) developed the propensity score method.

Suppose that there are J strata formed by propensity score stratification. Let n denote the total sample size and n_j the sample size in stratum j ($\sum_{j=1}^{J} n_j = n$). The data on each subject comprise the response variable $x = 1$ for response and 0 for no response and j and k for the stratum and treatment group, respectively, to which the subject is assigned ($1 \le j \le J; k = 1,2$). Frequency data in stratum j can be described as follows:

	Group		
Response	1	2	Total
Yes	x_{j11}	x_{j12}	x_{j1}
No	x_{j21}	x_{j22}	x_{j2}
Total	n_{j1}	n_{j2}	n_j

Let $O_j = x_{j11}$, $E_j = n_{j1}x_{j1}/n_j$, and

$$V_j = \frac{n_{j1}n_{j2}x_{j1}x_{j2}}{n_j^2(n_j - 1)}.$$

Then, the weighted Mantel-Haenszel (WMH) test is given by

$$T = \frac{\sum_{j=1}^{J} \hat{w}_j (O_j - E_j)}{\sqrt{\sum_{j=1}^{J} \hat{w}_j^2 V_j}},$$

where the weights $\hat{w}_j$ converge to a constant w_j as $n \to \infty$. The weights are $\hat{w}_j = 1$ for the original Mantel-Haenszel test and $\hat{w}_j = \hat{q}_j = x_{j2}/n_j$ for the statistic proposed by Gart (1985).

Let $a_j = n_j/n$ denote the allocation proportion for stratum j ($\sum_{j=1}^{J} a_j = 1$), and $b_{jk} = n_{jk}/n_j$ denote the allocation proportion for group k within stratum j ($b_{j1} + b_{j2} = 1$). Let p_{jk} denote the response probability for group k in stratum j and $q_{jk} = 1 - p_{jk}$. Under $H_0 : p_{j1} = p_{j2}, 1 \le j \le J$, T is approximately $N(0,1)$. The optimal weights maximizing the power depend on the allocation proportions $\{(a_j, b_{1j}, b_{2j}), j = 1,\ldots,J\}$ and effect sizes $(p_{j1} - p_{j2}, 1,\ldots,J)$ under H_1.

In order to calculate the power of WMH, we have to derive the asymptotic distribution of $\sum_{j=1}^{J} \hat{w}_j (O_j - E_j)$ and the limit of $\sum_{j=1}^{J} \hat{w}_j^2 V_j$ under H_1. We assume that the success probabilities $(p_{jk}, 1 \le j \le J, j = 1,2)$ satisfy $p_{j2}q_{j1}/(p_{j1}q_{j2}) = \phi$ for $\phi \ne 1$ under H_1. Note that a constant odds ratio across strata holds if there exists no interaction between the treatment and the propensity score when the binary response is regressed on the treatment indicator and the propensity score using a logistic regression. The following derivations are based on H_1. It can be verified that

$$O_j - E_j = \frac{n_{j1}n_{j2}}{n_j}(\hat{p}_{j1} - \hat{p}_{j2})$$
$$= \frac{n_{j1}n_{j2}}{n_j}(\hat{p}_{j1} - p_{j1} - \hat{p}_{j2} + p_{j2}) + \frac{n_{j1}n_{j2}}{n_j}(p_{j1} - p_{j2})$$
$$= na_j b_{j1} b_{j2}(\hat{p}_{j1} - p_{j1} - \hat{p}_{j2} + p_{j2}) + na_j b_{j1} b_{j2}(p_{j1} - p_{j2}).$$

Thus, under H_1, $\sum_{j=1}^{J} \hat{w}_j(O_j - E_j)$ is approximately normal with mean $n\Delta$ and variance $n\sigma_1^2$, where

$$\Delta = \sum_{j=1}^{J} w_j a_j b_{j1} b_{j2}(p_{j1} - p_{j2})$$
$$= (1-\phi)\sum_{j=1}^{J} w_j a_j b_{j1} b_{j2} \frac{p_{j1}q_{j1}}{q_{j1} + \phi p_{j1}}$$

and

$$\sigma_1^2 = n^{-1}\sum_{j=1}^{J} w_j^2 \frac{n_{j1}^2 n_{j2}^2}{n_j^2}\left(\frac{p_{j1}q_{j1}}{n_{j1}} + \frac{p_{j2}q_{j2}}{n_{j2}}\right)$$
$$= \sum_{j=1}^{J} w_j^2 a_j b_{j1} b_{j2}(b_{j2}p_{j1}q_{j1} + b_{j1}p_{j2}q_{j2}).$$

Also under H_1, we have

$$\sum_{j=1}^{J} w_j^2 V_j = n\sigma_0^2 + o_p(n),$$

where

$$\sigma_0^2 = \sum_{j=1}^{J} w_j^2 a_j b_{j1} b_{j2}(b_{j1}p_{j1} + b_{j2}p_{j2})(b_{j1}q_{j1} + b_{j2}q_{j2}).$$

Hence, the power of WMH is given as

$$1-\beta = P(|T| > z_{1-\alpha/2} \mid H_1)$$
$$= P\left(\frac{\sigma_1}{\sigma_0}Z + \sqrt{n}\frac{|\Delta|}{\sigma_0} > z_{1-\alpha/2}\right)$$
$$= \overline{\Phi}\left(\frac{\sigma_0}{\sigma_1}z_{1-\alpha/2} - \sqrt{n}\frac{|\Delta|}{\sigma_1}\right),$$

where Z is a standard normal random variable and $\overline{\Phi}(z) = P(Z > z)$. Thus, the sample size required for achieving a desired power of $1-\beta$ can be obtained as

$$n = \frac{(\sigma_0 z_{1-\alpha/2} + \sigma_1 z_{1-\beta})^2}{\Delta^2}. \tag{3}$$

Following Jung, Chow, and Chi (2007), the sample size calculation for the weighted Mantel-Haenszel test can be carried out as follows:

1. Specify the input variables
   - Type I and II error probabilities (α, β).
   - Success probabilities for group 1 $p_{11},\ldots,p_{J1}$, and the odds ratio ϕ under H_1.
     Note that $p_{j2} = \phi p_{j1}/(q_{j1} + \phi p_{j1})$.
   - Incidence rates for the strata, $(a_j, j = 1,\ldots,J)$. (Yue [2007] proposes to use $a_j \approx 1/J$.)
   - Allocation probability for group 1 within each stratum, $(b_{j1}, j = 1,\ldots,J)$.

2. Calculate n by

$$n = \frac{(\sigma_0 z_{1-\alpha/2} + \sigma_1 z_{1-\beta})^2}{\Delta^2},$$

   where

$$\Delta = \sum_{j=1}^{J} a_j b_{j1} b_{j2} (p_{j1} - p_{j2})$$

$$\sigma_1^2 = \sum_{j=1}^{J} a_j b_{j1} b_{j2} (b_{j2} p_{j1} q_{j1} + b_{j1} p_{j2} q_{j2})$$

$$\sigma_0^2 = \sum_{j=1}^{J} a_j b_{j1} b_{j2} (b_{j1} p_{j1} + b_{j2} p_{j2})(b_{j1} q_{j1} + b_{j2} q_{j2}).$$

Example 18.4

Suppose that we want to compare the response probabilities between control ($k = 1$) and experimental ($k = 2$) groups. We consider partitioning the combined data into $J = 5$ strata, and the allocation proportions are projected as $(a_1, a_2, a_3, a_4, a_5) = (.15,.15,.2,.25,.25)$ and $(b_{11}, b_{21}, b_{31}, b_{41}, b_{51}) = (.4,.4,.5,.6,.6)$. Also, suppose that the response probabilities for the control group are given as $(p_{11}, p_{21}, p_{31}, p_{41}, p_{51}) = (.5,.6,.7,.8,.9)$, and we want to calculate the sample size required for a power of $1-\beta = 0.8$ to detect an odds ratio of $\phi = 2$ using two-sided $\alpha = 0.05$. For $\phi = 2$, the success probabilities for the experimental group are given as $(p_{12}, p_{22}, p_{32}, p_{42}, p_{52}) = (.6667,.7500,.8235,.8889,.9474)$. Under these settings, by (3), we need $n = 447$ for Mantel-Haenszel.

Program 18.4 SAS Code for Weighted Mantel-Haenszel Test with Strata

```
%macro WMHTestwithStrata (  J = ,   /* number of strata                       */
                            inA= ,  /* incidence rates for the strata         */
                            inB= ,  /* allocation probability for control group */
                            inP1=,  /* success probability for control group  */
                            phi =,  /* odds ratio under H1                    */
                            power=, /* power                                  */
                            alpha=, /* alpha                                  */
                            sides=   /* 1: one-sided test  2: Two-sided test */
                          );

 proc iml;
   %let K = 2; /* two groups */
   A=&inA; B =&inB;P1=&inP1;
   P2 =J(&J,1,0);Q1 =J(&J,1,0); Q2 =J(&J,1,0);
   do j=1 to &J;
      Q1[j]=1-P1[j];
      P2[j]=&phi*P1[j]/(Q1[j]+&phi*P1[j]);
      Q2[j]=1-P2[j];
   end;
   z_p1=1-&alpha/&sides; z_alpha = probit(z_p1);
   z_p2=&power;  z_beta  = probit(z_p2);
   delta = 0; s0_sq= 0; s1_sq= 0;

   do j=1 to &J;
    delta = delta+A[j]*B[j]*(1-B[j])*(P1[j]-P2[j]);
    s1_sq= s1_sq+A[j]*B[j]*(1-B[j])*((1-
B[j])*P1[j]*Q1[j]+B[j]*P2[j]*Q2[j]);
    s0_sq= s0_sq+A[j]*B[j]*(1-B[j])*(B[j]*P1[j]+(1-
B[j])*P2[j])*(B[j]*Q1[j]+(1-B[j])*Q2[j]);
   end;
   n = (1/(delta**2))*((sqrt(s0_sq)*z_alpha+sqrt(s1_sq)*z_beta)**2);

   print 'Sample Size Calculation';
   print 'Weighted Mantel-Haenszel Test with Strata';
   alpha = &alpha; power = &power; phi= &phi; sides = &Sides;
   print   alpha power phi sides ;
   print A B P1 P2;
   print delta s0_sq s1_sq;
   print n;
 quit;
 run;
%mend WMHTestwithStrata;

/*----------------  Run the macro for Example 18.4. ---------------------*/

%WMHTestwithStrata(
   J = 5 ,                                       /* number of strata         */
   inA= %str({0.15, 0.15, 0.2, 0.25, 0.25}), /*Incidence Rates for Strata*/
   inB= %str({0.4 , 0.4,  0.5, 0.6,  0.6}),  /* Allocation Probability   */
   inP1=%str({0.5 , 0.6,  0.7, 0.8,  0.9}),  /* Success Probability      */
   phi = 2,                                      /* odds Ratio Under H1      */
   power =0.8,                                   /* Power                    */
   alpha = 0.05,                                 /* Alpha                    */
   sides = 2                                     /* Two-sided test           */
  );
```

Output from Program 18.4

```
                  Sample Size Calculation
         Weighted Mantel-Haenszel Test with Strata

              alpha       power        phi      sides
              0.05         0.8           2          2

                 A           B          P1         P2
              0.15         0.4         0.5 0.6666667
              0.15         0.4         0.6       0.75
               0.2         0.5         0.7 0.8235294
              0.25         0.6         0.8 0.8888889
              0.25         0.6         0.9 0.9473684

                   delta      s0_sq      s1_sq
              -0.025752 0.0381275 0.0367178

                               n
                           446.21501
```

18.4 Two-Sample Log-Rank Test for Survival Data

Suppose that n_k subjects are accrued to a study from group $k(=1,2)$. For subject $i(=1,...,n_k)$ in group $k(=1,2)$, let T_{ki} denote the survival variable (that is, time to an event of interest), with marginal cumulative hazard function $\Lambda_k(t)$. We want to test the null hypothesis,

$$H_0 : \Lambda_1(t) = \Lambda_2(t) \textit{ for all } t \geq 0$$

against the alternative hypothesis,

$$H_a : \Lambda_1(t) \neq \Lambda_2(t) \textit{ for some } t \geq 0.$$

Because a cumulative hazard function uniquely determines the distribution, H_0 implies that $(T_{1i}, i=1,...,n_1)$ and $(T_{2i}, i=1,...,n_2)$ have the same distributions.

Due to loss to follow up or termination of study before all subjects experience events, survival times are censored for some subjects. Let C_{ki} denote the censoring time for the subject i in group k. Then, we observe $\{(X_{ki}, \delta_{ki}), 1 \leq i \leq n_k, k=1,2\}$, where $X_{ki} = \min(T_{ki}, C_{ki})$ and $\delta_{ki} = I(T_{ki} \leq C_{ki})$. We assume that C_{ki} and T_{1i} are independent within each group.

The log-rank test (Peto and Peto, 1972) is given by

$$W = \int_0^\infty \frac{Y_1(t)Y_2(t)}{Y_1(t)+Y_2(t)} \{d\hat{\Lambda}_1(t) - d\hat{\Lambda}_2(t)\},$$

where $\hat{\Lambda}_k(t) = \int_0^t Y_k(s)^{-1} dN_k(s)$ is the Nelson-Aalen estimator (Nelson, 1969; Aalen, 1978) of $\Lambda_k(t)$, $N_k(t) = \sum_{i=1}^{n_k} N_{ki}(t)$, $N_{ki}(t) = \delta_{ki} I(X_{ki} \le t)$, $Y_k(t) = \sum_{i=1}^{n_k} Y_{ki}(t)$, and $Y_{ki}(t) = I(X_{ki} \ge t)$. For large n with $n_k/n = r_k$ and $0 < r_k < 1$, $W/\hat{\sigma}$ is approximately normal with mean 0 and variance 1 under H_0, where

$$\hat{\sigma}^2 = \int_0^\infty \frac{Y_1(t)Y_2(t)}{\{Y_1(t)+Y_2(t)\}} \{dN_1(t) + dN_2(t)\},$$

Refer to Fleming and Harrington (1991), for example. We reject H_0 if the absolute value of $W/\hat{\sigma}$ is larger than $z_{1-\alpha/2}$.

For sample size and power calculation, we assume a proportional hazards model $\Delta = \Lambda_2(t)/\Lambda_1(t)$. The power of the log-rank test depends on the number of events, rather than the number of patients. By Rubinstein and colleagues (1981), the number of events D_1 and D_2 in the two groups, required for a two-sided α test to detect a hazard ratio of $\Delta(<1)$ with power $1-\beta$, is given as

$$\left(\frac{\log \Delta}{z_{1-\alpha/2} + z_{1-\beta}}\right)^2 = D_1^{-1} + D_2^{-1}. \tag{4}$$

In order to calculate D_k, we need to specify the survival distributions under H_a and the common censoring distribution. Suppose that the subjects are accrued at a constant rate for a period of A and followed for an additional period of B after the completion of accrual. The total study period is $A+B$. Then, assuming no loss to follow up, the censoring distribution is uniform between B and $A+B$, as in the following:

$$G(t) = P(C_{ki} \ge t) = \begin{cases} 1 & \text{if } t < B \\ 1+(B-t)/A & \text{if } B \le t \le A+B \\ 0 & \text{otherwise.} \end{cases}$$

One of the most popular survival models in sample size calculation is the exponential distribution,

$$S_k(t) = P(T_{ki} \ge t) = \exp(-\lambda_k t)$$

for group k. Then, the probability that a subject in arm k experiences an event is given as

$$d_k = P(T_{ki} \le C_i) = \int_0^\infty S_k(t) dG(t) = 1 - \frac{\exp(-\lambda_k B)\{1-\exp(-\lambda_k A)\}}{A\lambda_k},$$

so that we have $D_k = n_k d_k = n r_k d_k$. By plugging this in (4) and solving with respect to n, we obtain

$$n = (\frac{1}{r_1 d_1} + \frac{1}{r_2 d_2})(\frac{z_{1-\alpha/2} + z_{1-\beta}}{\log \Delta})^2.$$

We assumed no loss to follow up in calculating d_k, but this assumption can be easily loosened by assuming a distribution for the time to loss to follow up.

In summary, a sample size is calculated as follows:

- In addition to type I error probability α and power $1-\beta$, specify

  (a) $\lambda_1, \lambda_2 =$ hazard rates under H_a $(\Delta = \lambda_2/\lambda_1)$

  (b) $r_k =$ the prevalence of group k $(r_1 + r_2 = 1)$

  (c) $A =$ accrual period, $B =$ additional follow-up period

- Calculate the probability of an event for a subject in group $k(=1,2)$

$$d_k = 1 - \frac{\exp(-\lambda_k B)\{1-\exp(-\lambda_k A)\}}{A\lambda_k},$$

- Calculate the sample size

$$n = (\frac{1}{r_1 d_1} + \frac{1}{r_2 d_2})(\frac{z_{1-\alpha/2} + z_{1-\beta}}{\log \Delta})^2.$$

Example 18.5

Suppose that the control group $(k=1)$ has a median survival time of $\mu_1 = 3$ years, and the experimental group will be considered acceptable if it extends the median survival by 50% (that is, $\mu_2 = 4.5$ years). Under the exponential survival model, the annual hazard rates are $\lambda_1 = 0.231$ and $\lambda_2 = 0.154$ $(\Delta = 0.667)$. Also, suppose that $(r_1, r_2) = (0.3, 0.7)$, and patients were uniformly accrued for $A = 3$ years and the final analysis is conducted $B = 2$ years after the completion of accrual. Then, we have $(d_1, d_2) = (0.5455, 0.4115)$, $n = 613$ ($n_1 = 184, n_2 = 429$), and $(D_1, D_2) = (100, 177)$. PROC POWER in SAS/STAT(Program 18.5.2) also provides sample sizes for the log-rank test based on Lakatos (1988), which, unlike our formula, calculates the limit of the variance estimator of the log-rank test under the null hypothesis. As demonstrated here, it gives a slightly smaller sample size, $n = 593$, under the design setting.

Program 18.5.1 SAS Code for Two-Sample Log-Rank Tests for Survival Data

```
%macro SS_TwoSmpleLogRank(
            Accrual  =,    /* accrual period                          */
            Follow   =,    /* additional follow-up period              */
            inR      =,    /* group allocation proportion(a1, a2)      */
            inLambda =,    /* hazard rates under the alternative       */
            alpha    =,    /* alpha                                    */
            power    =,    /* power                                    */
            sides    =     /* 1: One-sided test  2: Two-sided test     */
                          );
 proc iml;
  %let K = 2;   r = &inR; Group = J(&K,1,0); lambda = &inLambda;
  delta = lambda[2]/lambda[1]; d_prob = J(&K, 1,0);
  n = J(&K, 1,0); D = J(&K, 1,0);
  do i=1 to &K;
    group[i] = i;
    d_prob[i]=1-(exp(-lambda[i]*&Follow))*(1-exp(-lambda[i]*&Accrual))
              /(&Accrual*lambda[i]);
  end;
  z_p1=1-&alpha/&sides; z_alpha = probit(z_p1);
  z_p2=&power; z_beta  = probit(z_p2);
  Total =
int((1/(r[1]*d_prob[1])+1/(r[2]*d_prob[2]))*((z_alpha+z_beta)/log(delta))**
2)+1;
  do i=1 to &K; n[i]= r[i]*Total; D[i]= d_prob[i]*n[i]; end;
  print ' Sample Size Calculation';
  print 'for Two-Sample Log-Rank Test for Survival Data';
  Accrual=&Accrual; Follow_Up= &Follow;
  print 'Accrual Period : ' &Accrual;
  print ' Follow Up period : ' &Follow;
  print Group lambda delta r d_prob;
  print Group n D;
  print Total;
  quit;
 run;
%mend SS_TwoSmpleLogRank;

/*-------------- Run the macro for Example 18.5.1 ------------------------
---*/

%SS_TwoSmpleLogRank(
    Accrual  =3,                     /* accrual period                      */
    Follow   =2,                     /* additional follow-up period         */
    inR      =%str({0.3, 0.7}),      /* group allocation proportion(r1, r2)*/
    inLambda =%str({0.231, 0.154}),/* hazard rates under the alternative */
    alpha    =0.05,                  /* alpha                               */
    power    =0.9,                   /* power                               */
    sides    =2                      /* two-sided test                      */
        );
```

Output from Program 18.5.1

```
                    Sample Size Calculation
          for Two-Sample Log-Rank Test for Survival Data

                 Accrual Period :          3
               Follow Up period :          2

          GROUP     LAMBDA      DELTA          R    D_PROB
              1      0.231 0.6666667         0.3  0.5455053
              2      0.154                   0.7  0.411467

                    GROUP          N          D
                        1      183.9  100.31843
                        2      429.1  176.56049

                             TOTAL
                              613
```

Program 18.5.2 SAS Code (PROC POWER) for Example 18.5

```
proc power;
    twosamplesurvival test=logrank
    nfractional
    groupmedsurvtimes = 3 | 4.5
    accrualtime = 3
    followuptime = 2
    groupweights = (0.3,0.7)
    alpha = 0.05
    sides=2
    power = 0.9
    ntotal = .
   ;
run;
```

Output from Program 18.5.2

```
                        The POWER Procedure
                 Log-Rank Test for Two Survival Curves

                       Fixed Scenario Elements

  Method                                Lakatos normal approximation
  Form of Survival Curve 1                               Exponential
  Form of Survival Curve 2                               Exponential
  Number of Sides                                                  2
  Accrual Time                                                     3
  Follow-up Time                                                   2
  Alpha                                                         0.05
  Group 1 Median Survival Time                                     3
  Group 2 Median Survival Time                                   4.5
  Group 1 Weight                                                 0.3
  Group 2 Weight                                                 0.7
  Nominal Power                                                  0.9
  Number of Time Sub-Intervals                                    12
  Group 1 Loss Exponential Hazard                                  0
  Group 2 Loss Exponential Hazard                                  0


                     Computed Ceiling N Total

                 Fractional     Actual     Ceiling
                    N Total      Power     N Total
                 592.792138      0.900         593
```

18.5 Two-Sample Longitudinal Data

In a longitudinal study, we measure the outcome of research interest repeatedly from each subject over a time period. When there are two groups of subjects, one popular primary objective is the between-group comparison of change rate in the expected value of a response variable over time. Typically, the repeated measurements within each subject are correlated. Because of the robustness to possible misspecification of the correlation structure among the repeated measurements, the generalized estimating equation (GEE) method has been one of the most popular methods to fit the regression models and to test on the change rates (Liang and Zeger, 1986). In this section, we discuss sample size estimation methods for such testing. We consider cases where the response variable is continuous or dichotomous.

18.5.1 Generalized Estimating Equations

Suppose that there are n_k subjects in treatment group $k(=1,2)$, $n_1+n_2=n$. Let, for group k, $N_k=\sum_{i=1}^{n_k} m_{ki}$ denote the total number of observations and $r_k=n_k/n$ the allocation proportion $(r_1+r_2=1)$. For subject i $(i=1,...,n_k)$ in group k, let y_{kij} denote the outcome variable at measurement time t_{kij} $(j=1,...,m_{ki})$ with $\mu_{kij}=E(y_{kij})$ that is expressed as

$$g(\mu_{kij})=a_k+b_k t_{kij},$$

where $g(\cdot)$ is a known link function. In other words, we assume that there exists a link function $g(\cdot)$ linearizing the trajectory in response over time. To simplify the discussions, we use the identity link $g(\mu)=\mu$ for continuous outcome variables and the logit link $g(\mu)=\log\{\mu/(1-\mu)\}$ for binary outcome variables, but the generalization to the use of other links is simple.

The coefficient b_k represents the change rate per unit time in mean response if y is continuous and the change rate in log-odds if y is binary. The measurement times may vary subject by subject due to missing measurements, patients' visits for measurements at unscheduled times, loss to follow up, or other causes. In this chapter, we assume that any missing data is missing completely at random (Rubin, 1976).

The repeated measurements $(y_{kij}, 1\le j\le m_{ki})$ within each subject tend to be correlated. However, the true correlation structure is usually unknown or of secondary interest. Liang and Zeger (1986) proposed a consistent estimator, called the *GEE estimator*, based on a working correlation structure. Using either the identity or logit link, the GEE estimator $(\hat{a}_k,\hat{b}_k)$ based on the working independence structure solves $U_k(a,b)=0$, where

$$U_k(a,b)=\frac{1}{\sqrt{n_k}}\sum_{i=1}^{n_k}\sum_{j=1}^{m_{ki}}\{y_{kij}-\mu_{kij}(a,b)\}\begin{pmatrix}1\\ t_{kij}\end{pmatrix}$$

and $\mu_{kij}(a,b)=g^{-1}(a+bt_{kij})$.

18.5.1.1 Continuous Outcome Variable Case

In the continuous outcome variable case, we have a closed form solution to $U_k(a,b)=0$

$$\hat{b}_k = \frac{\sum_{i=1}^{n_k}\sum_{j=1}^{m_{ki}}(t_{kij}-\bar{t}_k)y_{kij}}{\sum_{i=1}^{n_k}\sum_{j=1}^{m_{ki}}(t_{kij}-\bar{t}_k)^2}$$

and $\hat{a}_k = \bar{y}_k - \hat{b}_k\bar{t}_k$, where $\bar{t}_k = N_k^{-1}\sum_{i=1}^{n_k}\sum_{j=1}^{m_{ki}} t_{kij}$ and $\bar{y}_k = N_k^{-1}\sum_{i=1}^{n_k}\sum_{j=1}^{m_{ki}} y_{kij}$.

By Liang and Zeger (1986), as $n\to\infty$, $\sqrt{n_k}(\hat{b}_k - b_k)\to N(0,v_k)$ in distribution. Here v_k is consistently estimated by

$$\hat{v}_k = \frac{\sum_{i=1}^{n_k}\{\sum_{j=1}^{m_{ki}}(t_{kij}-\bar{t}_k)\hat{\varepsilon}_{kij}\}^2}{\{\sum_{i=1}^{n_k}\sum_{j=1}^{m_{ki}}(t_{kij}-\bar{t}_k)^2\}^2}$$

where $\hat{\varepsilon}_{kij} = y_{kij} - \hat{a}_k - \hat{b}_k t_{kij}$.

18.5.1.2 Binary Outcome Variable Case

Let $p_{kij}=\mu_{kij}$ in the binary outcome variable case. We have to solve the equation using a numerical method, such as the Newton-Raphson algorithm: at the l-th iteration,

$$\begin{pmatrix}\hat{a}_k^{(l)}\\ \hat{b}_k^{(l)}\end{pmatrix} = \begin{pmatrix}\hat{a}_k^{(l-1)}\\ \hat{b}_k^{(l-1)}\end{pmatrix} + n_k^{-1/2}A_k^{-1}(\hat{a}_k^{(l-1)},\hat{b}_k^{(l-1)})U_k(\hat{a}_k^{(l-1)},\hat{b}_k^{(l-1)}),$$

where

$$A_k(a,b) = -n_k^{-1/2}\frac{\partial U_k(a,b)}{\partial(a,b)} = \frac{1}{n_k}\sum_{i=1}^{n_k}\sum_{j=1}^{m_{ki}} p_{kij}(a,b)q_{kij}(a,b)\begin{pmatrix}1 & t_{kij}\\ t_{kij} & t_{kij}^2\end{pmatrix}$$

$$p_{kij}(a,b) = g^{-1}(a+bt_{kij}) = \frac{e^{a+bt_{kij}}}{1+e^{a+bt_{kij}}} \qquad (5)$$

and $q_{kij}(a,b) = 1 - p_{kij}(a,b)$.

By Liang and Zeger (1986), for large n, $\sqrt{n_k}(\hat{a}_k - a_k, \hat{b}_k - b_k)^T$ is asymptotically normal with mean 0 and variance V_k that can be consistently estimated by

$$\hat{V}_k = A_k^{-1}(\hat{a}_k, \hat{b}_k)\hat{\Sigma}_k A_k^{-1}(\hat{a}_k, \hat{b}_k)$$

where

$$\hat{\Sigma}_k = \frac{1}{n_k}\sum_{i=1}^{n_k}\{\sum_{j=1}^{m_{ki}}\hat{\varepsilon}_{kij}\begin{pmatrix}1\\ t_{kij}\end{pmatrix}\}^{\otimes 2},$$

$\hat{\varepsilon}_{kij} = y_{kij} - p_{kij}(\hat{a}_k, \hat{b}_k)$ and $c^{\otimes 2} = cc^T$ for a vector c. Let $\hat{v}_k$ be the (2,2)-component of $\hat{V}_k$.

18.5.2 Sample Size Calculation

Suppose that we want to test the rate of change between two groups (that is, $H_0 : b_1 = b_2$). Based on the asymptotic results from the previous section, we can reject $H_0 : b_1 = b_2$ in favor of $H_1 : b_1 \neq b_2$ when

$$\left| \frac{\hat{b}_1 - \hat{b}_2}{\sqrt{\hat{v}_1/n_1 + \hat{v}_2/n_2}} \right| > z_{1-\alpha/2}, \qquad (6)$$

where $z_{1-\alpha/2}$ is the $100(1-\alpha/2)$ percentile of a standard normal distribution.

In this section, we derive a sample size formula for the two-sided α test (6) to detect $H_1 :| b_2 - b_1 |= \Delta(> 0)$ with power $1-\beta$. When designing a study, we usually schedule fixed visit times $t_1 < \cdots < t_m$ for m repeated measurements from each subject. We often set $t_1 = 0$ for the baseline measurement time. When the study is conducted, however, the subjects may skip some visit times due to various reasons, which results in missing values, or they may not follow the visit schedule correctly so that the observed visit times may be variable. Jung and Ahn (2003) show through simulations in a continuous outcome variable case that the sample size formula based on fixed measurement times is very accurate even when the observed measurement times are widely distributed around the scheduled times.

By simple algebra, we can derive a sample size formula to detect the specified difference $| b_2 - b_1 |= \Delta$ with power $1-\beta$,

$$n = \frac{(z_{1-\alpha/2} + z_{1-\beta})^2 (v_1/r_1 + v_2/r_2)}{\Delta^2}, \qquad (7)$$

where $v_k = \lim_{n\to\infty} \hat{v}_k$. The expression of v_k is slightly different between continuous and binary outcome variable cases, as shown in the following subsections.

In order to allow for missing values, let δ_j denote the proportion of patients with observations at t_j and $\delta_{jj'}$ the proportion of patients with observations at both t_j and $t_{j'}$. Also, let $\rho_{jj'} = corr(y_{kij}, y_{kij'})$. We assume that the missing pattern and correlation structure are common in two treatment groups. We discuss specific models for missing pattern and correlation structure in Section 18.5.3.

18.5.2.1 Continuous Variable Case

We assume that the continuous outcome variable has a constant variance $var(y_{kij}) = \sigma^2$ over time, which is common between two treatment groups. Jung and Ahn (2003) show that $v_1 = v_2 = v$ is expressed as

$$v = \frac{\sigma^2(s^2 + c)}{s^4},$$

where

$$s^2 = \sum_{j=1}^{m} \delta_j (t_j - \tau)^2$$

$$c = \sum\sum_{j \neq j'} \delta_{jj'} \rho_{jj'} (t_j - \tau)(t_{j'} - \tau)$$

and

$$\tau = \frac{\sum_{j=1}^{m} \delta_j t_j}{\sum_{j=1}^{m} \delta_j}.$$

Hence, (7) is simplified to

$$n = \frac{v(z_{1-\alpha/2} + z_{1-\beta})^2}{\Delta^2 r_1 r_2}. \tag{8}$$

Note that we do not have to specify the true values for $\{(a_k, b_k), k = 1,2\}$ but only the difference $|b_2 - b_1| = \Delta$ in sample size calculation. The sample size is proportional to the variance of measurement error σ^2 and decreases as r_1 approaches $1/2$.

18.5.2.2 Binary Variable Case

Let $p_{kj} = a_k + b_k t_k$ denote the success probabilities under H_1. Jung and Ahn (2005) show that

$$v_k = \frac{s_k^2 + c_k}{s_k^4},$$

where

$$s_k^2 = \sum_{j=1}^{m} \delta_j p_{kj} q_{kj} (t_j - \tau_k)^2$$

$$c_k = \sum\sum_{j \neq j'} \delta_{jj'} \rho_{jj'} \sqrt{p_{kj} q_{kj} p_{kj'} q_{kj'}} (t_j - \tau_k)(t_{j'} - \tau_k),$$

and

$$\tau_k = \frac{\sum_{j=1}^{m} \delta_j p_{kj} q_{kj} t_j}{\sum_{j=1}^{m} \delta_j p_{kj} q_{kj}}.$$

As shown here, the sample size formula under the binary outcome variable case depends on the probabilities $(p_{kj}, j = 1,...,m)$ under H_1, so that we need to specify all regression parameters $\{(a_k, b_k), k = 1,2\}$. Let $\Delta = b_2 - b_1$ denote the difference in slope between two groups under H_1. If pilot data exist for the control group (group 1), then we may use the estimates as the parameter values, a_1 and b_1. If $t_1 = 0$ is the baseline, the intercepts in the two groups are set the same (that is, $a_1 = a_2$). By setting $b_2 = b_1 + \Delta$, we can specify all regression coefficients under H_1.

If no pilot data are available, we may specify the binary probabilities at the baseline, p_{11}, and at the end of follow up, p_{1m}, for the control group. Then we obtain (a_1, b_1) by

$$b_1 = \frac{g(p_{1m}) - g(p_{11})}{t_m - t_1}, \tag{9}$$

$$a_1 = g(p_{11}) - b_1 t_1 = g(p_{11}).$$

And we set $a_2 = a_1$ (since $p_{11} = p_{21}$ at the baseline) and $b_2 = b_1 + \Delta$.

18.5.3 Modelling Missing Pattern and Correlation Structure

Calculation of n (or v_k) requires projection of the missing probabilities and the true correlation structure.

18.5.3.1 Missing Pattern

In order to specify $\delta_{jj'}$, we need to estimate the missing pattern. If missing at time t_j is independent of missing at time $t_{j'}$ for each patient, then we have $\delta_{jj'} = \delta_j \delta_{j'}$ and we call this type *independent missing*.

In some studies, subjects missing at a measurement time may be missing at all following measurement times, as in the labor pain study discussed in Example 18.6. This type of missing is called *monotone missing*. In this case, we have $\delta_{jj'} = \delta_{j'}$ for $j < j'$ ($\delta_1 \geq \cdots \geq \delta_m$). In monotone missing cases, one may want to specify the proportion of patients who will contribute exactly the first j observations, say η_j. Then, noting that $\eta_j = \delta_j - \delta_{j+1}$ for $j = 1,...,m-1$ and $\eta_m = \delta_m$, we can obtain δ_j recursively starting from δ_m. Note also that $\sum_j \eta_j = \delta_1$, which equals 1 if all patients have measurements at the first measurement time t_1.

In summary, we consider two missing patterns as candidates to the true one: (a) independent missing, where $\delta_{jj'} = \delta_j \delta_{j'}$, and (b) monotone missing, where $\delta_{jj'} = \delta_{j'}$ for $j < j'$ ($\delta_1 \geq \cdots \geq \delta_m$).

18.5.3.2 Correlation Structure

Now, we specify the true correlation structure $\rho_{jj'}$. A reasonable model for $\varepsilon_{ij} = y_{ij} - g^{-1}(a + bt_{ij})$ may be

$$\varepsilon_{ij} = u_i + e_{ij},$$

where u_i is a subject-specific error term with variance σ_u^2 and e_{ij} is a serially correlated within-subject error term with variance σ_e^2 and correlation coefficients $\tilde{\rho}_{jj'}$. Assuming that u_i and e_{ij} are independent, we have

$$cov(\varepsilon_{ij}, \varepsilon_{ij'}) = \sigma_a^2 + \sigma_e^2 \tilde{\rho}_{jj'}.$$

Often, the variation between subjects (σ_u^2) is much larger than that within subjects (σ_e^2). In this case, we have

$$cov(\varepsilon_{ij}, \varepsilon_{ij'}) \approx \sigma_u^2$$

and an exchangeable correlation structure, $\rho_{jj'} = \rho$ for $j \neq j'$, may be a reasonable approximation to the true one.

On the other hand, if the variation within the subject (σ_e^2) dominates over the variation between subjects (σ_u^2), then we will have

$$cov(\varepsilon_{ij}, \varepsilon_{ij'}) \approx \sigma_e^2 \tilde{\rho}_{jj'},$$

so that a serial correlation structure may be a reasonable approximation to the true one. One of the most popular serial correlation structures, especially when measurement times are not equidistant, is a continuous autocorrelation model with order 1, AR(1), for which $\rho_{jj'} = \rho^{|t_j - t_{j'}|}$.

We consider two correlation structures as candidate approximations to the true one: (i) exchangeable, where $\rho_{jj'} = \rho$, and (ii) AR(1), where $\rho_{jj'} = \rho^{|t_j - t_{j'}|}$.

18.5.3.3 Examples

For sample size calculation, the following parameters need to be specified commonly in both continuous and discrete outcome variable cases:

- Type I and II errors α and β, respectively.
- The size of difference to detect, $|b_2 - b_1| = \Delta$.

- Allocation proportion for group k, r_k.
- Correlation structure and the associated correlation parameter ρ, (that is, (i) $\rho_{jj'} = \rho$ for exchangeable or (ii) $\rho_{jj'} = \rho^{|t_j - t_{j'}|}$ for AR(1)).
- Proportion of patients with an observation at t_j, δ_j.
- Missing pattern: (a) independent missing ($\delta_{jj'} = \delta_j \delta_{j'}$) or (b) monotone missing ($\delta_{jj'} = \delta_{j'}$ for $j < j'$).

In addition, we need to specify $\sigma^2 = var(\varepsilon_{ij})$ in the continuous outcome variable case and the regression coefficients $\{(a_k, b_k), k = 1,2\}$ under H_1 in the binary outcome variable case.

We demonstrate our sample size formula with real longitudinal studies.

Example 18.6 Continuous Outcome Case
In a study on labor pain (Davis, 1991), 83 women in labor were assigned to either a pain medication group (43 women) or a placebo group (40 women). At 30-minute intervals, the self-reported amount of pain was marked on a 100mm line, where 0 = no pain and 100 = extreme pain. The maximum number of measurements for each woman was $m = 6$, but there were numerous missing values at later measurement times with monotone missing pattern. A simple approach to such a study objective might be to estimate and compare the slopes of pain scores over time in the two treatment groups. In this study, the outcome variable is continuous. Suppose that we want to design a new study on labor pain based on the data reported by Davis (1991). As in the original study, we assume monotone missing. In this study, the measurement times were equispaced, so that we set $t_j = j - 1$ ($j = 1,...,6$) for convenience. From the data, we obtained $\sigma^2 = 815.84$. Suppose we want to detect a difference of σ in mean pain score between two groups at t_6. So, we project $\Delta = \sigma/(t_6 - t_1) = 5.71$ in a new study. We consider a balanced design (that is, $r_1 = r_2 = 1/2$). Also, from the data, the proportion of observed measurements are

$$(\delta_1, \delta_2, \delta_3, \delta_4, \delta_5, \delta_6) = (1,.90,.78,.67,.54,.41).$$

From these results, we obtain $\tau = 2.02$ and $s^2 = 11.42$.

Suppose that we want to detect a difference of $\Delta = 5.71$ with 80% of power ($z_{1-\beta} = 0.84$) using a two-sided $\alpha = .05$ ($z_{1-\alpha/2} = 1.96$) test. Under an exchangeable correlation structure, we obtain $\rho = .64$ and $c = -3.13$ from the data, so that we have $v = 815.84 \times (11.42 - 3.13)/11.42^2 = 51.84$. Hence, from (8), the required sample size is calculated as

$$n = [\frac{51.84 \times (1.96 + 0.84)^2}{5.71^2}] + 1 = 50.$$

where $[x]$ is the largest integer not exceeding x.

Under AR(1), we obtain from the data $\rho = .80$ and $c = 2.31$, so that the required sample size for detecting $\Delta = 5.71$ with 80% of power using a two-sided $\alpha = .05$ test is given as $n = 83$. The sample size under AR(1) is larger than that under an exchangeable correlation, by about 66%, in this example.

Program 18.6 SAS Code for Two-Group Comparision of Repeated Continuous Measurement

```
%macro SS_RepeatedContinuousMeasurement(
               missingPattern = , /* 1: independent missing 2: monotone missing     */
               corrStructure  = , /* 1: compound symetric , 2: AR(1)                */
               rho            = , /* associated correlation parameter               */
               m              = , /* number of measurement time points              */
               sigma_sq       = , /* variance                                       */
               inR            = , /* group allocation proportion(r1, r2)            */
               inDelta        = , /* proportion of observed measurements            */
               alpha          = , /* alpha                                          */
               power          = , /* power                                          */
               sides          = , /* 1: one-sided test  2: two-sided test           */
               print    = 0       /* 0:default 1: detail                            */
                                 );
proc iml;
  %let K = 2; r = &inR; delta = &inDelta; t = J(&m,1,0);
  do j=1 to &m; t[j] = j-1; end;
  %if &inDelta eq %then %do; delta=J(&m,1,0);do j=1 to &m; delta[j]=1-(j-1)/20; end;
%end;
  d = sqrt(&sigma_sq)/(t[&m]-t[1]);
  start g(p); gp = log(p/(1-p)); return (gp); finish g;
  start prob(a,b,t); p = 1/(1+exp(-a-b*t)); return (p); finish prob;
  start rho(i,j,r,c);
    if c=1 then do; /* CS */ if i=j then rho_ij =1;else rho_ij = r; end;
    else do; /* AR(1) */ dist = abs(i-j); rho_ij = r**dist; end;
    return (rho_ij);
  finish rho;
  tau_num =0;  tau_denum = 0;
  do j=1 to &m; tau_num = tau_num+delta[j]*t[j]; tau_denum = tau_denum+delta[j]; end;
  tau= tau_num/tau_denum; s_sq=0;
  do j=1 to &m; s_sq = s_sq+delta[j]*((t[j]-tau)**2); end;
  c=0;
  do i=1 to &m;
     do j=1 to &m;
          if i ^= j then do;
             if &missingPattern = 1 then do; delta_ij = delta[i]*delta[j]; end;
         else do; if j > i then max_ij=j; else max_ij=i; delta_ij=delta[max_ij]; end;
         c = c+delta_ij*rho(i,j,&rho,&corrStructure)*(t[i]-tau)*(t[j]-tau);
               end;
      end;
   end;
   v = &sigma_sq*(s_sq+c)/(s_sq**2);
   z_p1=1-&alpha/&sides; z_alpha = probit(z_p1); z_p2=&power;  z_beta   = probit(z_p2);
   n = int((v*(z_alpha+z_beta)**2)/(d**2*r[1]*r[2]))+1;
   print 'Sample Size Calculation for a Two-Group Comparision';
   print ' of Repeated Continous Measurements';
   alpha  =&alpha; power=&power; rho=&rho; sides=&sides;
   sigma_sq=&sigma_sq;
   print alpha power rho sides;
   if &missingPattern = 1 then do;print ' Missing Pattern: Independent '; end;
   else if &missingPattern = 2 then do; print ' Missing Pattern: Monotone '; end;
   if &corrStructure=1 then do; print ' Correlation Structure : Compound Symetric
';end;
   else if &corrStructure = 2 then do; print ' Correlation Structure : AR(1) '; end;
   %if &print = 1 %then %do; print delta; print tau s_sq c v ; %end;
   print d sigma_sq;
   print n;
   quit;
run;
%mend SS_RepeatedContinuousMeasurement;
```

```
/*--Run the macro for Example 18.6 when Correlation Structure = Compound Symetric --*/

%SS_RepeatedContinuousMeasurement(
      missingPattern = 2,            /* monotone missing                          */
      corrStructure  = 1,            /* compound symetric                         */
      rho            = 0.64,         /* associated correlation parameter          */
      m              = 6,            /* number of measurement time points         */
      sigma_sq       = 815.84,       /* variance                                  */
      inR          = %str({0.5, 0.5}), /* group allocation proportion(r1, r2)     */
      inDelta      = %str({1, 0.9, 0.78, 0.67, 0.54, 0.41}),
                                     /* proportion of observed measurements       */
      alpha        = 0.05,           /* alpha                                     */
      power        = 0.8,            /* power                                     */
      sides         = 2,             /* two-sided test                            */
      print         = 1
       );

/*--- Run the macro for Example 18.6 when Correlation Structure = AR(1) ---------*/

%SS_RepeatedContinuousMeasurement(
    missingPattern  = 2,             /*  monotone missing                         */
    corrStructure  = 2,              /* AR(1)                                     */
    rho              = 0.8,          /*  associated correlation parameter         */
    m              = 6,              /* number of measurement time points         */
    sigma_sq         = 815.84,       /* variance                                  */
    inR            = %str({0.5, 0.5}),/* group allocation proportion(r1, r2)      */
    inDelta        = %str({1, 0.9, 0.78, 0.67, 0.54, 0.41}),
                                     /* proportion of observed measurements       */
    alpha          = 0.05,           /* alpha                                     */
    power          = 0.8,            /* power                                     */
    sides            = 2,            /* two-sided test                            */
    print = 1
       );
```

Output from Program 18.6

```
/*----------------- When Correlation Structure = Compound Symetric --------*/


                    Sample Size Calculation for a Two-Group Comparision
                             of Repeated Continous Measurements

                              ALPHA      POWER        RHO     SIDES
                              0.05        0.8       0.64         2

                                  Missing Pattern: Monotone
                          Correlation Structure : Compound Symetric

                               TAU       S_SQ          C          V
                         2.0186047 11.418512 -3.133345 51.842656

                                              D  SIGMA_SQ
                                     5.7125826    815.84

                                              N
                                             50
```

(continued)

Output from Program 18.6 *(continued)*

```
/*-------------------- When Correlation Structure = AR(1) ----------------*/

                  Sample Size Calculation for a Two-Group Comparision
                          of Repeated Continous Measurements

                            ALPHA       POWER         RHO       SIDES
                             0.05         0.8         0.8           2

                             Missing Pattern: Monotone
                           Correlation Structure : AR(1)

                            TAU       S_SQ           C           V
                      2.0186047  11.418512  2.3055968   85.87567

                                          D   SIGMA_SQ
                                  5.7125826     815.84

                                          N
                                         83
```

Example 18.7 Binary Outcome Case

The Genetics vs. Environment In Scleroderma Outcome Study (GENISOS) is an observational study designed as a collaboration of the University of Texas-Houston Health Science Center with the University of Texas Medical Branch at Galveston and the University of Texas-San Antonio Health Science Center (Reveille et al., 2001). *Scleroderma*, or *systemic sclerosis*, is a multisystem disease of unknown etiology characterized by cutaneous and visceral fibrosis, small blood vessel damage, and autoimmune features (Medsger, 1997). The study subjects are regularly followed to check for the occurrence of pulmonary fibrosis. In this case, the outcome is a binary variable.

Suppose that we want to develop a study to examine the effect of a new drug in preventing the occurrence of pulmonary fibrosis in subjects with scleroderma compared to no intervention. The parameter values specified here for sample size calculation are approximated by the estimates from the current data set of GENISOS.

We want to estimate the sample size for the new study using $\alpha = .05$ and $1-\beta = .8$. As in GENISOS, presence or absence of pulmonary fibrosis is assessed at baseline and at months 6, 12, 18, 24, and 30. Because the measurement times are equidistant, we set $t_j = j-1$ ($j = 1,...,6$) for the $m = 6$ time points. The within-group correlation structure of the repeated measurements conforms to AR(1) with the adjacent correlation equal to $\rho = .8$ (that is, $\rho_{jj'} = .8^{|j-j'|}$). We consider assigning an equal number of scleroderma patients in each of two groups (that is, $r_1 = r_2 = 1/2$).

Approximately 75% of scleroderma patients do not have pulmonary fibrosis at the baseline in the ongoing GENISOS. We project that the proportion of subjects without pulmonary fibrosis is 75% at baseline (that is, $p_{1,1} = .75$) and 50% at 30 months (that is, $p_{1,6} = .50$) in a placebo group. We assume that a new therapy will prevent or delay further occurrence of pulmonary fibrosis. That is, the proportion of subjects without pulmonary fibrosis will remain 75% during the 30-month study in a new therapy group (in other words, $p_{2,1} = p_{2,6} = .75$). From these values and (9), we obtain

$$b_1 = \frac{g(.5) - g(.75)}{5 - 0} = -0.220,$$

and $a_1 = g(.75) = 1.099$. Similarly, we obtain (a_2, b_2)=(1.099, 0), so that $\Delta = 0-(-0.220) = 0.220$. By (5), the probabilities of no pulmonary fibrosis at the 6 time points are obtained as $(.750,.707,.659,.608,.555,.500)$ for the placebo group and $(.750,.750,.750,.750,.750,.750)$ for the treatment group.

The proportions of observed measurements are expected to be

$$(\delta_1, \delta_2, \delta_3, \delta_4, \delta_5, \delta_6) = (1,.95,.90,.85,.80,.75).$$

Suppose that we expect independent missing. Then, we obtain $\delta_{jj'}$ from the specified δ_j values using $\delta_{jj'} = \delta_j \delta_{j'}$. Now we have all the parameter values required, and we obtain $v_1 = 0.305$ and $v_2 = 0.353$. Finally, from (7), we obtain

$$n = [\frac{(1.96+0.84)^2(0.305/0.5+0.353/0.5)}{0.220^2}]+1 = 215.$$

If we assume monotone missing ($\delta_{jj'} = \delta_{j\vee j'}$), we obtain $v_1 = 0.324$, , $v_2 = 0.308$ and $n = 229$.

Program 18.7 SAS Code for Two-Group Comparision of Repeated Binary Measurement

```
%macro SS_RepeatedBinaryMeasurement(
      missingPattern =    , /* 1: independent missing 2: monotone missing       */
      corrStructure =     , /* 1: compound symetric , 2: AR(1)                  */
      rho           =     , /*  associated correlation parameter                */
      m             =     , /* number of measurement time points                */
      inP1          =     , /* proportion of subjects for control group         */
      inP2          =     , /* proportion of subjects                           */
      inR           =     , /* group allocation proportion(r1, r2)              */
      inDelta  =          , /* proportion of observed measurements              */
      alpha    =          , /* alpha                                            */
      power    =          , /* power                                            */
      sides    =            /* 1: one-sided test   2: two-sided test            */
   );
  proc iml;
   start g(p); gp = log(p/(1-p)); return (gp); finish g;
   start prob(a,b,t); p = 1/(1+exp(-a-b*t)); return (p); finish prob;
   start rho(i,j,r,c);
    if c=1 then do; /* CS */ if i=j then rho_ij =1; else rho_ij = r; end;
    else if c = 2 then do; /* AR(1) */ dist = abs(i-j); rho_ij = r**dist; end;
    return (rho_ij);
   finish rho;
   %let K = 2;
   P1=&inP1;  P2=&inP2; r =&inR; a=J(&K,1,0);  b=J(&K,1,0); t=J(&m,1,0);
   tau = J(&K,1,0);  s_sq = J(&K,1,0); v = J(&K,1,0); c_sq = J(&K,1,0);
   do j=1 to &m;  t[j] = j-1; end;
   %if &inDelta eq %then %do;
       delta = J(&m,1,0);
       do j=1 to &m; delta[j] = 1-(j-1)/20; end;
   %end;
   b[1] = (g(P1[&m])-g(P1[1]))/(t[&m]-t[1]); a[1] = g(P1[1])-B[1]*t[1];
   b[2] = (g(P2[&m])-g(P2[1]))/(t[&m]-t[1]); a[2] = g(P2[1])-B[1]*t[1];
   d = b[2]-b[1];
   do j=1 to &m;
      T[j] = j-1; P1[j]= prob(a[1], b[1], t[j]); P2[j]= prob(a[2], b[2], t[j]);
   end;
   tau1_num =0; tau1_denum = 0; tau2_num =0; tau2_denum = 0;
   do j=1 to &m;
     tau1_num = tau1_num+delta[j]*P1[j]*(1-P1[j])*t[j];
     tau1_denum = tau1_denum+delta[j]*P1[j]*(1-P1[j]);
```

```
      tau2_num = tau2_num+delta[j]*P2[j]*(1-P2[j])*t[j];
      tau2_denum = tau2_denum+delta[j]*P2[j]*(1-P2[j]);
   end;
   tau[1]= tau1_num/tau1_denum; tau[2]= tau2_num/tau2_denum;
   s1=0;s2=0;
   do j=1 to &m;
      s1 = s1+delta[j]*P1[j]*(1-P1[j])*((t[j]-tau[1])**2);
      s2 = s2+delta[j]*P2[j]*(1-P2[j])*((t[j]-tau[2])**2);
   end;
   s_sq[1]=s1; s_sq[2]=s2; c1=0; c2=0; c12=0;
   do i=1 to &m;
      do j=1 to &m;
            if i ^= j then do;
               if &missingPattern = 1 then do;
              delta_ij = delta[i]*delta[j];
               end;else do;
                  if j > i then max_ij = j; else max_ij = i; delta_ij = delta[max_ij];
           end;
           c1=c1+delta_ij*rho(i,j,&rho,&corrStructure)*
              sqrt(P1[i]*(1-P1[i])*P1[j]*(1-P1[j]))*((t[i]-tau[1])*(t[j]-tau[1]));
           c2=c2+delta_ij*rho(i,j,&rho,&corrStructure)*
              sqrt(P2[i]*(1-P2[i])*P2[j]*(1-P2[j]))*((t[i]-tau[2])*(t[j]-tau[2]));
          end;
      end;
   end;
   c_sq[1]=c1; c_sq[2]=c2;
   do k =1 to &K; v[k] = (s_sq[k]+c_sq[k])/(s_sq[k]**2); end;
   z_p1=1-&alpha/&sides; z_alpha = probit(z_p1);
   z_p2=&power; z_beta  = probit(z_p2);
   n = int((z_alpha+z_beta)**2*(v[1]/r[1]+v[2]/r[2])/d**2)+1;

   print 'Sample Size Calculation for a Two-Group Comparision';
   print ' of Repeated Binary Measurements';
   alpha  =&alpha; power=&power; rho=&rho; sides=&sides;
   print alpha power rho sides;
   if &missingPattern = 1 then do; print ' Missing Pattern: Independent '; end;
   else if &missingPattern = 2 then do;print ' Missing Pattern: Monotone '; end;
   if &corrStructure = 1 then do; print ' Correlation Structure : Compound Symetric ';
   end; else if &corrStructure = 2 then do; print ' Correlation Structure : AR(1) ';
   end;
   print P1 P2 delta v ; print d; print n;
   quit;
run;
%mend  SS_RepeatedBinaryMeasurement;

/*--------------- Run the macro for Example 18.7 ------------------------------*/

%SS_RepeatedBinaryMeasurement(
     missingPattern = 1,          /* 1: independent missing 2: monotone missing    */
     corrStructure  = 2,          /* 1: compound symetric , 2: AR(1)               */
     rho      = 0.8,              /*  associated correlation parameter             */
     m        = 6,                /* number of measurement time points             */
    inP1    = %str({0.75, 0, 0, 0, 0, 0.5}),
                                  /* proportion of subjects for control group      */
    inP2    = %str({0.75, 0.75, 0.75, 0.75, 0.75, 0.75}),
                                  /* proportion of subjects                        */
     inR      = %str({0.5, 0.5}), /* group allocation proportion(r1, r2)           */
     inDelta = ,        /* delta[j] = 1-(j-1)/20, proportion of observed measurements */
     alpha    = 0.05,             /* alpha                                         */
     power    = 0.8,              /* power                                         */
     sides    = 2                 /* 1: one-sided test  2: two-sided test          */
     );


%SS_RepeatedBinaryMeasurement(
    missingPattern = 2,          /*  monotone missing                              */
    corrStructure = 2,           /* AR(1)                                          */
     rho      = 0.8,                /* associated correlation parameter            */
     m        = 6,                  /* number of measurement time points           */
    inP1    = %str({0.75, 0, 0, 0, 0, 0.5}),
```

```
                              /* proportion of subjects for control group     */
inP2     = %str({0.75, 0.75, 0.75, 0.75, 0.75, 0.75}),
                           /* proportion of subjects                          */
 inR      = %str({0.5, 0.5}),     /* group allocation proportion(r1, r2)       */
 inDelta = ,        /* delta[j] = 1-(j-1)/20, proportion of observed measurements */
 alpha    = 0.05,              /* alpha                                        */
 power    = 0.8,               /* power                                        */
 sides    = 2                  /* 1: one-sided test  2: two-sided test         */
 );
```

Output from Program 18.7

```
/*--------------When Missing Pattern Is Independent Missing ----------------*/

                    Sample Size Calculation for a Two-Group Comparision
                              of Repeated Binary Measurements

                              ALPHA      POWER        RHO      SIDES
                               0.05        0.8        0.8          2

                               Missing Pattern: Independent
                               Correlation Structure : AR(1)

                                 P1         P2      DELTA          V
                               0.75       0.75          1  0.3048798
                          0.7065921       0.75       0.95  0.3534175
                          0.6590733       0.75        0.9
                          0.6081268       0.75       0.85
                          0.5547107       0.75        0.8
                                0.5       0.75       0.75

                                             D
                                     0.2197225

                                             N
                                           215

/*-------------- When Missing Pattern Is Monotone Missing ------------------*/

                    Sample Size Calculation for a Two-Group Comparision
                              of Repeated Binary Measurements

                              ALPHA      POWER        RHO      SIDES
                               0.05        0.8        0.8          2

                                 Missing Pattern: Monotone
                               Correlation Structure : AR(1)

                                 P1         P2      DELTA          V
                               0.75       0.75          1  0.3236844
                          0.7065921       0.75       0.95  0.3804059
                          0.6590733       0.75        0.9
                          0.6081268       0.75       0.85
                          0.5547107       0.75        0.8
                                0.5       0.75       0.75

                                             D
                                     0.2197225

                                             N
                                           229
```

18.6 Discussion

In designing an observational study, we should choose a statistical testing method that will be used when analyzing the final data. For an accurate sample size calculation, the sample size formula should be directly derived from the power function of the chosen testing method.

There are two types of parameters included in sample size formulas: primary and nuisance parameters. The primary parameters are those shown in the statistical hypotheses (for example, means, binomial proportions, and hazard rates), and the nuisance parameters (for example, prevalence rates, accrual period in survival data, correlation coefficients, and missing type and probabilities in longitudinal data) are those of no or secondary interest. Because both types of parameters determine the final sample size, it is important to specify the parameter values as accurately as possible. If a database exists, we usually estimate the values of nuisance parameters and the primary parameter value of the control group from the database. Although r_k may be chosen by the prevalence of a disease, we may decide to use different allocation proportions from the prevalence rates in the natural population depending on the relative cost to accrue subjects in two groups. The primary parameter value for the case group is usually chosen based on the clinical significance of the associated intervention on the outcome variable, which is measured in terms of the difference or ratio of the primary parameter values between the two groups. When there is uncertainty in some of these parameters, we may conduct a sensitivity analysis on the power to demonstrate that the power would be adequate under a range of scenarios.

Appendix: Asymptotic Distribution of Wilcoxon Rank Sum Test under H_a

Let $\widetilde{X}_{ki} = X_{ki} - \theta_k$. Then $\widetilde{X}_{11},\ldots,\widetilde{X}_{1n_1},\widetilde{X}_{21},\ldots,\widetilde{X}_{2n_2}$ are IID with cumulative density function (CDF) $F(x)$. Noting that

$$W = \frac{1}{n_1 n_2}\sum_{i=1}^{n_1}\sum_{j=1}^{n_2} I(\widetilde{X}_{1i} > \widetilde{X}_{2j} - \Delta),$$

we have $W = \int_{-\infty}^{\infty}\hat{F}_2(x+\Delta)d\hat{F}_1(x)$, where $\hat{F}_k(x) = n_k^{-1}\sum_{i=1}^{n_k} I(\widetilde{X}_{ki} \le x)$ is the empirical CDF of $\widetilde{X}_{k1},\ldots,\widetilde{X}_{kn_k}$ that uniformly converges to $F(x)$ as $n_k \to \infty$. Let $v_a = P(\widetilde{X}_{1i} > \widetilde{X}_{2j} - \Delta) = \int_{-\infty}^{\infty} F(x+\Delta)dF(x)$. For a large n, $W - v_a$ is expressed as

$$\int_{-\infty}^{\infty}\hat{F}_2(x+\Delta)d\hat{F}_1(x) - \int_{-\infty}^{\infty}F(x+\Delta)dF(x)$$

$$= \int_{-\infty}^{\infty}F(x+\Delta)d\{\hat{F}_1(x)-F(x)\} + \int_{-\infty}^{\infty}\{\hat{F}_2(x+\Delta)-F(x+\Delta)\}dF(x) + o_p(n^{-1}),$$

where $o_p(n^{-1}) = \int_{-\infty}^{\infty}\{\hat{F}_2(x+\Delta)-F(x+\Delta)\}d\{\hat{F}_1(x)-F(x)\}$ is negligible for a large n.

Because

$$\int_{-\infty}^{\infty} F(x+\Delta)\hat{F}_1(x) = \frac{1}{n_1}\sum_{i=1}^{n_1} F(\widetilde{X}_{1i}+\Delta)$$

and

$$\int_{-\infty}^{\infty} \hat{F}_2(x+\Delta)dF(x) = \frac{1}{n_2}\sum_{i=1}^{n_2} \overline{F}(\widetilde{X}_{2i}-\Delta),$$

we have $var(W) = \sigma_1^2/n_1 + \sigma_2^2/n_2$, where

$$\sigma_1^2 = var\{F(\widetilde{X}_{1i}+\Delta)\}$$

$$\sigma_2^2 = var\{\overline{F}(\widetilde{X}_{2i}-\Delta)\} = var\{F(\widetilde{X}_{2i}-\Delta)\}.$$

References

Aalen, O. 1978. "Nonparametric inference for a family of counting processes." *Annals of Statistics* 6: 701–726.

Carroll, R. J., and D. Ruppert. 1988. *Transformation and Weighting in Regression*. New York: Chapman and Hall/CRC.

Davis, C. S. 1991. "Semi-parametric and non-parametric methods for the analysis of repeated measurements with applications to clinical trials." *Statistics in Medicine* 10: 1959–1980.

Fleming, T. R., and D. P. Harrington. 1991. *Counting Processes and Survival Analysis*. New York: John Wiley & Sons, Inc.

Gart, J. J. 1985. "Approximate tests and interval estimation of the common relative risk in the combination of 2×2 tables." *Biometrika* 72: 673–677.

Jung, S. H., and C. Ahn. 2003. "Sample size estimation for GEE method for comparing slopes in repeated measurements data." *Statistics in Medicine* 22: 1305–1315.

Jung, S. H., and C. W. Ahn. 2005. "Sample size for a two-group comparison of repeated binary measurements using GEE." *Statistics in Medicine* 24(17): 2583–2596.

Jung, S. H., S. C. Chow, and E. Chi. 2007. "A note on sample size calculation based on propensity analysis in non-randomized trials." *Journal of Biopharmaceutical Statistics* 17: 35–41.

Lakatos, E. 1988. "Sample sizes based on the log-rank statistic in complex clinical trials." *Biometrics* 44: 229–241.

Liang, K. Y., and S. L. Zeger. 1986. "Longitudinal data analysis using generalized linear models." *Biometrika* 73: 13–22.

Mann, H. B., and D. R. Whitney. 1947. "On a test of whether one of two random variables is stochastically larger than the other." *The Annals of Mathematical Statistics* 18: 50–60.

Medsger, Jr., T. A. 1997. "Systemic sclerosis (scleroderma): clinical aspects. In *Arthritis and allied conditions: a textbook of rheumatology*. 13th ed. Edited by W. J. Koopman. Baltimore, MD: Williams & Wilkins, pp 1433–1464.

Nelson, W. 1969. "Hazard plotting for incomplete failure data." *Journal of Quality Technology* 1(1): 27–52.

Peto, R., and J. Peto. 1972. "Asymptotically efficient rank invariant test procedures (with discussion)." *Journal of the Royal Statistical Society, Series A: General* 135: 185–206.

Reveille, J. D., M. Fischbach, T. McNearney, et al. 2001. "Systemic sclerosis in 3 US ethnic groups: a comparison of clinical, sociodemographic, serologic, and immunogenetic determinants." *Seminars in Arthritis and Rheumatism* 30(5): 332–346.

Rosenbaum, P. R., and D. B. Rubin. 1983. "The central role of the propensity score in observational studies for causal effects." *Biometrika* 70: 41–55.

Rosenbaum, P. R., and D. B. Rubin. 1984. "Reducing bias in observational studies using subclassification on the propensity score." *Journal of the American Statistical Association* 79: 516–524.

Rubin, D. B. 1976. "Inference and missing data." *Biometrika* 63: 581–590.

Rubinstein, L. V., M. H. Gail, and T. J. Santner. 1981. "Planning the duration of a comparative clinical trial with loss to follow-up and a period of continued observation." *Journal of Chronic Diseases* 34(9/10): 469–479.

SAS Institute Inc. 2009. *SAS/STAT 9.2 User's Guide, Second Edition*. Cary, NC: SAS Institute Inc.

Yue, L. Q. 2007. "Statistical and regulatory issues with the application of propensity score analysis to non-randomized medical device clinical studies." *Journal of Biopharmaceutical Statistics* 17: 1–13.

Index

D

E

M

S

Z

Made in the USA
Lexington, KY
27 July 2014